NOBEL PRIZES
THAT CHANGED
MEDICINE

NOBEL PRIZES
THAT CHANGED
MEDICINE

editor

Gilbert Thompson
Imperial College, UK

Imperial College Press

ICP

Published by

Imperial College Press
57 Shelton Street
Covent Garden
London WC2H 9HE

Distributed by

World Scientific Publishing Co. Pte. Ltd.
5 Toh Tuck Link, Singapore 596224
USA office: 27 Warren Street, Suite 401-402, Hackensack, NJ 07601
UK office: 57 Shelton Street, Covent Garden, London WC2H 9HE

British Library Cataloguing-in-Publication Data
A catalogue record for this book is available from the British Library.

NOBEL PRIZES THAT CHANGED MEDICINE

ISBN-13 978-1-84816-825-1
ISBN-10 1-84816-825-X
ISBN-13 978-1-84816-826-8 (pbk)
ISBN-10 1-84816-826-8 (pbk)

Typeset by Stallion Press
Email: enquiries@stallionpress.com

Printed by FuIsland Offset Printing (S) Pte Ltd Singapore

CONTENTS

v

FOREWORD

This admirable book, a compilation of crisp essays on Nobel Prizes and Nobel Prize winners of the better part of the last century, demonstrates the way our lives have been enriched by these scientists. When I became a medical student in the mid-1950s I was aware of the momentous impact of the discoveries of penicillin and insulin, I soon learned about vitamin B12 and pernicious anaemia and marvelled that catheters could safely be placed in the heart via veins in the forearm. I confess I had no appreciation of the revolution in genetics that had been ignited a few years earlier in Cambridge, nor later in the 1960s as a young doctor did I have any inkling that the shadowy discipline of radiology would soon be transformed by the invention of the CT scanner — itself a product of the revolution in computational science started several decades earlier. Technology is a driver of advances in medicine, and the CT scanner developed in parallel with the capacity to measure, through the invention of radioimmunoassay, minute quantities of biologically active substances in blood samples; as a result research and medical practice in endocrinology and many other branches of medicine was transformed. In Cambridge in the 1980s I had the privilege of knowing César Milstein and by that time his monoclonal antibody technology had greatly enhanced the power of radioimmunoassay, but the idea that monoclonal antibodies would be of major therapeutic benefit was met with widespread scepticism. Now it is estimated that about a third of drugs in late development are monoclonal antibodies and the lives of patients with chronic disabling diseases such as rheumatoid arthritis and cancer have been transformed — all because of Milstein's determination to elucidate the mechanisms underlying the immune system's extraordinary repertoire of antibody responses. In the 1980s the molecular biology revolution had started to permeate most areas of medicine, and molecular medicine had become widely used to describe these activities: the 'DNA makes RNA makes protein' construct underpinned molecular medicine and was at the heart of the case for the Genome Project. But lying in wait was another surprise — RNA interference — which has transformed our understanding of gene regulation: it has already become a routine tool in biological research and has great promise as a therapy to control pathological gene expression. 'Translational' has become a pervasive term in medical research: government bodies and research charities urge their grant-giving bodies to prioritise funding according to the translational potential of the research they fund. They would do well to read Gilbert Thompson's book.

Keith Peters

PREFACE

Discovery! To give birth to an idea, to discover a great thought — an intellectual nugget, right under the dust of a field that many a brain-plough had gone over before. To be the first — that is the idea.

Mark Twain, 1869

Alfred Nobel was born in Stockholm in 1833 but moved to St Petersburg with his family when he was nine. Subsequently he trained as a chemical engineer and became interested in the explosive properties of nitro glycerine. To overcome the latter's inherent instability he combined it with *kieselguhr* (diatomaceous earth) and patented this invention as Dynamite. His inventive and entrepreneurial skills allied to a rapidly expanding market for explosives meant he was a rich man when he died in 1896. His will stipulated that his fortune should be used to set up a fund, the interest from which would be spent on prizes to be awarded annually for the most important discoveries made in the fields of Chemistry, Physics, Physiology or Medicine, Literature and Peace. There was speculation at the time that Alfred's generosity was triggered by the publication several years previously of an obituary in a French newspaper titled 'The merchant of death is dead', which mistakenly confused his brother's death with his own. Whatever the motive, his legacy has ensured that the name Nobel will forever be synonymous with excellence.

The winner of the Nobel Prize in Physiology or Medicine is chosen by the Nobel Assembly at the Karolinska Institute and success is regarded as the ultimate accolade for any scientist undertaking biomedical research. Inaugurated in 1901 it has been awarded one hundred times up to 2009, gap years when no awards were made reflecting the disruption caused by two World Wars. After 1946 it became increasingly common for the prize to be shared between two or three individuals (but not more), which has resulted in 195 Nobel Laureates in Physiology or Medicine to date. Of these, 47% have been American, 13% British and 8% German. Each of the other 18 nationalities represented has had up to 5% of the prize winners but only 4% of the latter were women. The average age of recipients at the time of the award was 57, the youngest being 32 and the oldest 89. The prize cannot be awarded posthumously.

The scientific advances honoured by these one hundred awards encompass a wide range of topics, as shown in the Table in the Appendix. At the risk of oversimplification they can be grouped arbitrarily as follows:

1. **The role of infectious agents in disease.** Many of the earlier awards fall into this category, notably for research into the causes of malaria, tuberculosis and yellow fever, and for the development of a vaccine against poliomyelitis. More recent discoveries include the role of human immunodeficiency virus (HIV) in AIDS, human papillomavirus (HPV) in cervical cancer, prions in Creutzfeldt–Jacob disease and *Helicobacter pylori* in peptic ulceration.

2. **Advances in human physiology and metabolism.** This section includes the discovery of cyclic AMP as the second messenger of hormone action; the discovery of the LDL receptor and its role in cholesterol homeostasis; the role of nitric oxide in the vascular system; and the discovery of neuropeptides and prostaglandins.

3. **Immunological mechanisms and immunity.** Discoveries in this field include the identification of blood groups, which paved the way for blood transfusion; immunological tolerance, which has been crucial to organ transplantation; HLA antigens and their role in transplantation and disease; and the production of monoclonal antibodies, which has had major therapeutic consequences.

4. **Genetic research.** This rapidly expanding field has increasingly dominated the prize list during the past decade but dates back to 1933 when the role of chromosomes in heredity was discovered. Subsequent advances include the famed demonstration of the double helical structure of DNA; the deciphering of the genetic code; and recently, the discovery of RNA interference and gene targeting.

5. **Technological advances in the diagnosis of disease.** This small but select category consists of discoveries that have revolutionised clinical diagnosis, namely the invention of the electrocardiograph (ECG); the introduction of cardiac catheterisation; and the invention of computer-assisted tomography (CAT) and magnetic resonance imaging (MRI).

6. **Therapeutic discoveries.** One of the earliest and most dramatic achievements was the isolation and use of insulin to treat diabetes in 1923. This was followed by the discoveries that pernicious anaemia could be cured by vitamin B12 and adrenal insufficiency remedied with cortisone, which paved the way for the development of steroids as immunosuppressive and anti-inflammatory agents. Other pharmacological discoveries that have won the Prize include the sulphonamides, penicillin, streptomycin, β blockers and H2 antagonists.

Detailed information on the particulars of a specific award or Laureate is available on the Nobel Foundation's website. In contrast, this book aims to provide a less formal and more personal view of the science and scientists involved by inviting prominent academics to each write a chapter about a Nobel Prize-winning discovery in their own area of expertise and to evaluate its impact on medical science. The choice of chapters was not easy (and will probably be questioned), with examples from each of the categories listed above being included. Chapter 12 is anomalous in that it describes research that earned the Chemistry Prize whereas all the remainder deal with prizes awarded for Physiology or Medicine. However, this only serves to emphasise the impact that basic science can have on medical practice.

The overall objective of this book is to inform, entertain and stimulate the reader, including those who are pursuing or are considering a career in biomedical research. To paraphrase Napoleon, every young scientist carries a Nobel Prize in his rucksack!

Perhaps the final word on this topic should come from a Laureate, in this instance Michael Brown who shared the Prize in Physiology or Medicine with Joe Goldstein in 1985 (see Chapter 11). During the Nobel banquet he told the following story concerning a Nobel Prize winner who stopped his car at a roadside garage in a small town in the US to fill up. His wife recognised the pump attendant and, jumping out, she rushed up to the man and embraced him passionately. On returning to the car she was confronted by her furious husband: 'What on earth do you think you're doing, kissing that jerk?' 'I'm sorry, darling, but he was my first sweetheart and my feelings for him came rushing back when I recognised him. We were very much in love in those days, so much so that we nearly got married. I do apologise for getting so carried away.' Mollified, her husband said, 'Just as well you didn't marry him or you would never have done all the things we've done together since I became a Nobel Laureate.' 'If I'd married him,' replied his wife, 'he'd have got the Nobel Prize, not you!'

Gilbert Thompson

ACKNOWLEDGEMENTS

I am extremely grateful to Sir Keith Peters for writing the Foreword and to each and every author of a chapter for unselfishly devoting the time and effort that this task involved. I am grateful also to Elizabeth Manson for assisting with the indexing and to Jacqueline Downs and her colleagues at Imperial College Press for help and guidance during the publication process.

Gilbert Thompson

CONTRIBUTORS

Timothy J. Aitman, FRCP, DPhil, FMed Sci.
Professor of Clinical and Molecular Genetics
MRC Clinical Sciences Centre and Imperial College, Hammersmith
Hospital, London.

Stephen Bloom, MD, DSc, FSB, FRCP, FRCPath, FMed Sci.
Professor of Medicine
Division of Diabetes, Endocrinology and Metabolism, Imperial
College, Hammersmith Hospital, London.

Jaimini Cegla, MSc, MRCP.
Specialty Registrar in Chemical Pathology (Metabolic Medicine)
Division of Diabetes, Endocrinology and Metabolism, Imperial
College, Hammersmith Hospital, London.

Keith M. Channon, MD, FRCP, FMed Sci.
Professor of Cardiovascular Medicine
Department of Cardiovascular Medicine,
University of Oxford, Oxford.

Rod Flower, PhD, DSc, FMed Sci, FRS.
Professor of Biochemical Pharmacology
William Harvey Research Institute, St Barts & The London School of
Medicine & Dentistry, Queen Mary University of London, London.

Chris Hawkey, FMed Sci.
Professor of Gastroenterology
Nottingham Digestive Diseases Centre, Nottingham University
Hospital, Nottingham.

A. Victor Hoffbrand, DM, FRCP, FRCPath, FRCP (Edin),
DSc, FMed Sci.
Emeritus Professor of Haematology
University College London.
Honorary Consultant Haematologist
Royal Free Hospital, London.

Richard P. Hull, MB BChir, MRCP (UK).
Wellcome Trust Clinical PhD Fellow
MRC Clinical Sciences Centre, & Imperial College, Hammersmith
Hospital, London.

Ellis Kempner, PhD
Scientist Emeritus
National Institutes of Health, Bethesda, Maryland.

John MacDermot, MD, PhD, FRCP, FMed Sci.
Emeritus Professor of Clinical Pharmacology
Imperial College, London.

Celia P. Milstein, MSc, ScD.
Retired scientist
Newnham College, Cambridge.

Sir Keith Peters, FRS, FMed Sci.
Emeritus Regius Professor of Physic
University of Cambridge, Cambridge.

James Scott, FRS, FMed Sci.
Professor of Cardiovascular Medicine
National Heart & Lung Institute, Imperial College, London.

Tony Seed, BM, PhD, FRCP.
Emeritus Professor of Medicine
Imperial College Faculty of Medicine, Imperial College, Charing
Cross Hospital, London.

Eric Sidebottom, BM, DPhil.
Retired Lecturer in Experimental Pathology
Sir William Dunn School of Pathology, Oxford.

Anne K. Soutar, PhD.
Professor of Molecular Genetics
MRC Clinical Sciences Centre, Imperial College, Hammersmith
Hospital, London.

Robert Tattersall, MD, FRCP.
Retired Professor of Clinical Diabetes
University of Nottingham, Nottingham.

Adrian M. K. Thomas, FRCP, FRCR, FBIR.
Honorary Librarian, The British Institute of Radiology
Clinical Director for Radiology, South London Healthcare, NHS
Trust, London.

Gilbert R. Thompson, MD, FRCP.
Emeritus Professor of Clinical Lipidology
Metabolic Medicine, Imperial College, Hammersmith Hospital,
London.

Herman Waldmann, FRS, ScD (Hon).
Professor of Pathology
Sir William Dunn School of Pathology, Oxford.

Chapter 1

THE DISCOVERY OF INSULIN

Robert Tattersall

1.1 Introduction

In 1923 the Nobel Prize for Physiology or Medicine was awarded to
Frederick Grant Banting (1891–1941) and John James Rickard
Macleod (1876–1935) for the discovery of insulin and has been a
source of controversy ever since. What is controversial is not the
importance of the discovery but the identity of the Laureates and particularly whether Macleod had done enough to be included. These
issues will be explored in this chapter but first it should be explained
why people thought that the pancreas might produce an anti-diabetic
substance or hormone.

1.2 The Pancreas and Diabetes

In his 1866 book, *Diabetes: Its Various Forms and Different
Treatments,* the English physician George Harley (1829–1896) suggested that there were different types of diabetes.[1] In one the sufferer
was 'fat and ruddy' which Harley attributed to excessive formation of
sugar by the liver. The other was due to 'defective assimilation' with
emaciation one of the earliest and most prominent symptoms. These
corresponded to what the French physician Etienne Lancereaux
(1829–1910) later called *diabète gras* and *diabète maigre* and what we
call Types 2 and 1. Their prognoses were succinctly summed up by
the Toronto physician Walter Campbell (1891–1981) who wrote,
'Before the First World War there were only two kinds of diabetics,
those who died quickly and those who stuck around slowly deterio-
rating for a long time. For the first group there was little or nothing

one could do; the second type had certain inconveniences to put up with.'[2]

The first clue that the two types might have different causes came in 1889 when Oskar Minkowski (1858–1931), working in Strasbourg, discovered serendipitously that pancreatectomy in the dog caused a severe wasting type of diabetes.[3,4] One possible explanation was that the pancreas destroyed a toxin which interfered with glucose metabolism but Minkowski and others believed that it produced an internal secretion. In 1894, Gustave Laguesse (1861–1927) suggested that this was produced by the 'small irregularly polygonal cells, with brilliant cytoplasm, diffusely scattered in the pancreatic parenchyma', which had been discovered in 1861 by a medical student Paul Langerhans (1847–1888). In 1905 Ernest Starling (1866–1927) coined the word hormone from the Greek ορμαω = to stir up. In 1909, a Belgian physiologist Jean de Meyer (1878–1934) named the hypothetical anti-diabetic hormone insulin.

One powerful piece of evidence for the existence and importance of internal secretions was the dramatic effects of (sheep) thyroid extract, which in 1891 had been shown, either subcutaneously or by mouth, to cure myxoedema in humans.[5] It seemed likely that pancreatic extracts would have a similar effect on diabetes, and the decade after Minkowski's pancreatectomy experiment was marked by attempts to cure diabetes by pancreas feeding and injecting. Most were done by physicians on an *ad hoc* basis without any clear end points except whether the patient felt better and had less glycosuria. All were failures, but between 1900 and 1921 at least five investigators came close to discovering insulin.[6]

In bony fish, such as the cod and haddock, the islets are separate from the exocrine pancreas and in 1903 in Aberdeen a zoologist, John Rennie (1865–1928), and a physician, Thomas Fraser (1872–1951), took advantage of this to prepare extracts of the islets. They treated several patients by mouth and one with hypodermic injections but gave up after the latter produced what seemed to be a toxic reaction. In 1922, the *Lancet* suggested that they might have discovered insulin if they had a simple method of measuring blood sugar — the one they used needed 50 ml of blood and took about 3 hours!

In 1906, a Berlin physician Georg Zuelzer (1870–1949) produced a pancreatic extract which in eight patients eliminated glycosuria and ketonuria without any change in diet. This, patented in America as Acomatol, was tested in Minkowski's department in Breslau (now Wroclaw in Poland) on three dogs and three patients, but, although confirming that it suppressed glycosuria, the side effects, especially fever, were so severe that it was concluded it would never be safe for therapeutic use. In 1928, Minkowski said, 'In retrospect I blame myself that — considering the indubitable action of these extracts on the glycosuria — we did not make an effort to explore the causes of side effects, and that we resigned ourselves with the statement of the uselessness of the extract for the treatment of human diabetes.'[4]

Another who nearly discovered insulin was Ernest Scott (1877–1966) at the University of Chicago. His extract produced a significant drop in glycosuria and in his thesis in 1911 he concluded that:

(i) There is an internal secretion from the pancreas controlling the sugar metabolism.
(ii) By proper methods this secretion may be extracted and still retain its activity.
(iii) This secretion is easily destroyed by oxidation or by the action of the digestive enzymes of the pancreas.
(iv) The secretion is insoluble, or nearly so, in strong alcohol but is readily soluble in acidulated water.
(v) The failure of previous workers to procure satisfactory results was due to their not preventing oxidation or the action of the digestive enzymes.

Unfortunately by the time his paper was published, a sentence had been inserted (by his professor AJ Carson who believed in the detoxification theory of pancreatic action) warning that, '*It does not follow that these effects are due to the internal secretion of the pancreas in the extract*' [my italics].[7] After moving to Kansas, Scott maintained his interest in the internal secretion of the pancreas and in 1912 visited JJR Macleod, then Professor of Physiology in Cleveland, Ohio but, according to Scott, Macleod was 'not interested, he just shrugged it off'.

In New York in 1912 John Raymond Murlin (1874–1960) put his idea of trying to find an active extract to his boss, Graham Lusk, whose response was, 'Oh, but Minkowski tried that and failed.' Neverthess, Murlin went ahead with his idea of combining duodenal mucosa and pancreas in the hope that secretin might be an adjuvant. When the extract was given subcutaneously to a diabetic patient it did diminish the excretion of sugar. In March 1913, he made a new extract which completely eliminated glycosuria in a depancreatised dog but Lusk convinced him that this was because its kidneys had been damaged by too much alkali. Murlin later discovered and named glucagon.

In 1919, Israel Kleiner (1885–1966) at the Rockefeller Institute in New York published the results of intravenous injection of a pancreatic extract in 16 depancreatised dogs. In most there was a substantial reduction of blood sugar between 60 and 90 minutes after the injection. Kleiner thought the temporary effect of his extract in dogs might be duplicated in man and might be useful in emergencies. He also noted that it was simple to make and did not have any toxic effects. Kleiner never tried it in humans and his contract at the Rockefeller Institute was terminated by Frederick Allen in 1919 on the grounds that this sort of research was futile. Allen may be said to have had a conflict of interest since he was the inventor of the under-nutrition treatment which kept those who had the fortitude to follow it half alive.[8]

In 1920 there were still many who did not believe that there was an internal secretion of the pancreas and even believers were depressed about the possibility of isolating it, fearing that it might not be stored in the pancreas or that it might be species specific. It was also abundantly clear to clinicians and physiologists that attempts to cure severe diabetes by feeding or injecting pancreatic extracts had been an abject failure.

Given this background (of which he was ignorant) the chutzpah of Banting in approaching Macleod was amazing.

1.3 Banting and Macleod[9]

Fred Banting was born on a farm in Ontario and began his medical studies in 1912 at the University of Toronto. In 1917 he was sent with the Canadian Army Medical Corps to Europe where he was wounded at the battle of Cambrai and awarded the Military Cross. He hoped to become a surgeon at the Toronto Hospital for Sick Children but, after missing out on this prestigious position, set up practice in London, Ontario. This was not a success and to earn extra money he got a part-time job as a demonstrator at the University of Western Ontario. At the end of October 1920, he had to lecture to the students on carbo-hydrate metabolism of which he knew little. While preparing, he read an article, 'The Relation of the Islets of Langerhans to Diabetes with Special Reference to Cases of Pancreatic Lithiasis' by Moses Barron (1884–1975), Professor of Pathology at the University of Minnesota. Barron reported a case in which a stone had blocked the pancreatic duct leading to atrophy of the acinar tissue but leaving the islets intact. This was not new since it was well known, at least to physiologists, that this was what happened when the duct was ligated in experimental ani-mals. In his notebook, Banting wrote:

> Diabetus [sic].
> Ligate pancreatic ducts of dog. Keeping dogs alive until acini degenerate leaving Islets.
> Try to isolate the internal secretion of these to relieve glycosurea [sic].

Banting mentioned his idea to a university colleague, who suggested he should consult JJR Macleod, the Professor of Physiology in Toronto (Fig. 1.1). Macleod, Jack to his friends, qualified in medicine at Aberdeen in 1889 and then spent a year studying physiological chem-istry in Leipzig. He became a demonstrator in physiology at the London Hospital in 1900 and in 1903, when still only 27, was invited to apply for the Chair at Western Reserve University, Cleveland, US.[10] In 1906 he contributed three chapters to a book *Recent Advances in Physiology and Biochemistry* edited by Leonard Hill, his former boss at the London Hospital. One chapter was 74 pages on carbohydrate metabolism, a sub-ject on which he had not done any research. He soon rectified this with a series of papers entitled 'Studies in experimental glycosuria I-XII' pub-lished in the *American Journal of Physiology* between 1907 and 1917. His magnum opus was a textbook *Physiology and Biochemistry in Modern Medicine*, first published in 1918, in which he wrote all but 8 of the 101 chapters. In 1918 he moved to Toronto where his research was mainly

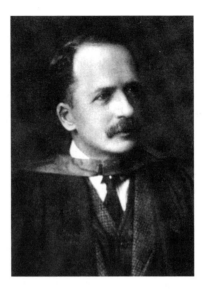

Fig. 1.1. JJR Macleod in academic robes, 1923 (Thomas Fisher Rare Book Library, University of Toronto).

concerned with acid base balance. In 1922, after the event, Macleod claimed that he had 'devoted practically all my spare time during the past 18 years to the investigation of the problem of diabetes, and like every other worker in this field I have constantly had in mind the discovery of some "internal secretion" whose absence might be the cause of diabetes'. This was not true. He had gradually wound down his carbohydrate research although he did study the blood sugar of turtles with his research students Charles Best (1899–1978) and Clark Noble (1900–1978). Furthermore, like many other physiologists he shared the general pessimism about finding the internal secretion of the pancreas, even if it existed. As late as 1921, he wrote:

> The removal of some hormone necessary for proper sugar metabolism is, however, by no means the only way in which the results [of pancreatectomy] can be explained, for we can assume that the pancreas owes its influence over sugar metabolism to some change occurring in the composition of the blood as this circulates through the gland — a change which is dependent on the integrity of the gland and not on any one enzyme or hormone which it produces.[11]

The meeting between Macleod and Banting took place on 7 November 1920. As when Scott had asked his advice in 1912, Macleod did not seem particularly interested, writing afterwards, 'I found that Dr Banting had only a superficial textbook knowledge of the work that had been done on the effects of pancreatic extracts in diabetes and that he had very little practical familiarity with the methods by which such a problem could be investigated in the laboratory'.[12,13] For his part, Banting wrote that Macleod 'put me off by saying that many men had worked for years in well-equipped laboratories and had not even proved that there was an internal secretion of the pancreas'. Finally, Macleod said that negative results would be of great physiological value. According to Banting, he repeated this three times, and when introducing the project to Best, Macleod opined that 'It would likely all go up in smoke'. Nevertheless, he offered to help Banting who procrastinated about whether to leave his practice in London, Ontario but contacted Macleod again in April 1921 and was told that the offer still stood. He was given a small disused and dirty room in the physiology department. Macleod's students Charles Best and Clark Noble were given the chance to make money by helping Banting and tossed a coin to decide who should do the first month. It was originally agreed that they should do a month each but, in Noble's words, 'When (Best's) month was up, we agreed mutually that there was no reason to change horses in mid stream'.

Banting needed an assistant because he did not know how to measure blood sugar and Macleod had wisely insisted on this as the end point of the experiment. One crucial factor in their ultimate success was that, during his research with Macleod, Best learned the recently introduced Lewis–Benedict method which needed as little as 0.2 ml blood whereas Paulesco (*vide infra*) used Pflüger's method, which needed 25 ml. Another stumbling block was that Banting had never done a pancreatectomy, an operation used only in animal research. On 14 May Macleod showed Banting how to do Hédon's two-stage pancreatectomy and during the rest of the month Banting and Best did several more operations. In the middle of June Macleod went on holiday to Scotland although he could be (and was) contacted by letter, which took a month. How much advice Banting obtained in this way was later disputed. Banting said that if he needed advice he went to the Professor of Pharmacology, Velyien Henderson (1877–1945), and never got any from Macleod. When Macleod returned from holiday at the end of September, Banting and Best already had some evidence that their pancreatic extracts lowered the blood sugar of dogs and Banting presented a list of demands including a salary and improved facilities. At first Macleod refused saying that Banting's research was no more important than any other in the department. Eventually he did produce better facilities and Banting was given a salaried job in the department of pharmacology.

At a journal club on 14 November 1921 Banting and Best (Fig. 1.2) gave a preliminary presentation of their work to colleagues and students (Fig. 1.3). This caused further resentment because, according to Banting, Macleod in his introduction said everything Banting was going to say as well as using the pronoun 'we' throughout. One important suggestion at this meeting was that the best way of showing that the extract worked would be if regular administration could prolong the life of diabetic dogs. This was difficult because the duct-ligation method of obtaining dog insulin was slow, cumbersome and expensive. It involved delicate operations, many dogs and a four- to seven-week wait while the acinar tissue degenerated. Banting's solution was to use foetal calf pancreas which Best got from the local abattoir. The rationale was that calf pancreas contained a high proportion of islets in relation to acinar tissue. An important breakthrough came on 6 December 1921 when Banting decided to use alcohol instead of saline in making their extract (an idea Macleod had suggested some months before). It worked well and led them to wonder whether fresh adult beef pancreas might be equally good. That it was must have been a surprise because the original rationale for duct ligation was that the internal secretion would be destroyed by proteolytic enzymes from the exocrine pancreas. In fact, although Macleod and many others believed this, the German physiologist Rudolf Heidenhain (1834–1897) had shown in 1875 that fresh pancreas did not have any proteolytic qualities. The intact gland contains an inactive

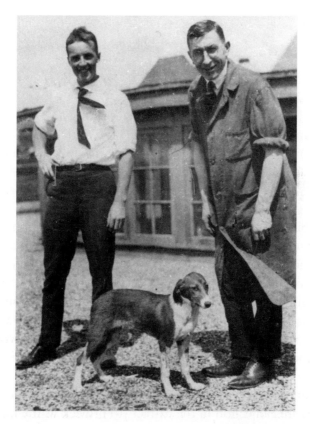

Fig. 1.2.   FG Banting and CH Best with a dog on the roof of the Medical Building, University of Toronto, August 1921.

precursor, trypsinogen, which is only converted into trypsin by contact with duodenal juice.

At the same time Banting and Best were joined by the biochemist Bert Collip — it might be more accurate to say that he was foisted on them by Macleod who regarded him as a proper scientist in contrast to the volatile surgeon Banting. James Bertram Collip (1892–1965) had originally trained at the University of Toronto and by 1920 was Associate Professor of Biochemistry in Edmonton, Alberta. In 1921 he was working with Macleod on a Rockefeller travelling fellowship. Sometime in December 1921 Collip began making extracts from whole pancreas and found that they reduced the blood sugar of

UNIVERSITY OF TORONTO

PHYSIOLOGICAL JOURNAL CLUB

Nov 14th — 4 o'clock — room 17

Speakers — Dr Banting

Mr Best

Subject — Pancreatic Diabetes

Fig. 1.3. Announcement of the journal club. The notice of the meeting where the original paper on insulin was presented (Best CH. *Canad Med Assoc J* 1962; 87: 1046–1051).

normal rabbits, which was important in providing a cheap way of testing the potency of a batch. He also used his extract on a diabetic dog and showed that it restored liver glycogen. Banting presented his and Best's results at the American Association of Biological Sciences on 30 December 1921. This was not a success, partly because of his extreme nervousness but also because he could not answer the critical questions of the assembled experts. Macleod was chairman of the meeting and intervened to help, again, according to Banting, talking about 'we'. Later Banting commented that Macleod had not contributed one idea of value except to suggest measuring haemoglobin before and after injection of the extract (to prove that the fall in blood sugar was not due to dilution).

1.4 The First Clinical Test

The first use of insulin (a pancreatic extract made by Charles Best) in a human being was on 11 January 1922 when a house physician at Toronto General Hospital injected what he described as 15 cc of 'thick brown muck' (known to the clinical staff as Macleod's serum) into the buttocks of the 14-year-old Leonard Thompson who had been on the Allen starvation regime since 1919 and weighed only 65 lbs. After the injection his blood sugar fell from 24.4 to18.3 mmol/L (440 to 320 mg/dl) but no clinical benefit was seen and he developed a sterile abscess at one injection site. It was accepted that this test had been a failure but the experiment was resumed on 23 January when he was given 5 cc of a pancreatic extract made by Collip and then 10 cc more over the next 24 hours. This time the results were spectacular. Thompson's blood sugar fell from 29 mmol/L (520 mg/dl) on the morning of 29 January to 6.7 mmol/l (120 mg/dl) the next morning. He continued on Collip's extract for the next ten days with marked clinical improvement and complete elimination of his glycosuria and ketonuria. Subsequently he lived a relatively normal life, working intermittently and even playing baseball. He died in 1935 of bronchopneumonia and at autopsy had marked atheroma of the aorta and coronary arteries.[14]

This test caused resentment in that Banting was excluded because he did not have treatment rights at Toronto General Hospital. Therefore it was supervised by Walter Campbell who chose Leonard Thompson because, 'We thought it should be tried on the most severe cases we could find, for two reasons. If nothing happened their number was up anyway, and, more important, if effective in such patients, the results could not be gainsaid'.[2]

Banting asked Collip for details of how he had made the effective extract and Collip refused to tell him. This led to a confrontation in which Banting grabbed Collip by the collar. Clark Noble drew a cartoon which showed Banting sitting on and trying to choke Collip which he entitled 'The discovery of insulin'. After peace had been restored the first clinical results were published in the March 1922 *Canadian Medical Association Journal* where the authors reported that up to 22 February they had treated seven cases, Leonard Thompson being the only one described in detail. Dramatically the paper concluded:

(i) Blood sugar can be markedly reduced, even to normal values.
(ii) Glycosuria can be abolished.
(iii) The acetone bodies can be made to disappear from the urine.
(iv) The respiratory quotient shows evidence of increased utilisation of carbohydrates.
(v) A definite improvement is observed in the general condition of these patients and, in addition, the patients themselves report a subjective sense of wellbeing and increased vigour for a period following the administration of these preparations.[15]

Given the 30-year history of false dawns since 1889, it is not surprising that the reports from Toronto were greeted with scepticism, especially in Europe. However the imprimateur of the North American scientific community was given at a meeting of the Association of American Physicians on 3 May 1922 when Macleod presented the clinical results. Nobody present seems to have doubted them and a standing vote of appreciation was given to Macleod and his associates, something which had never happened before in the history of the Association.

In Toronto, production was handed over to the Connaught Laboratories, a small industrial plant set up in 1914 to make vaccines and antitoxins, but its efforts were dogged by problems. Therefore, in May 1922 it was decided to call in Eli Lilly and Co. of Indianapolis, an ethical pharmaceutical company with experience in production and standardisation of glandular extracts.

The Dean of the University of Toronto set up an 'insulin committee' to manage the problems of the patent, finances and monitoring the quality of insulin. At the end of May the university gave Lilly exclusive rights to produce and sell insulin for one year. Lilly's part of the bargain was to provide it free to selected clinicians (who Lilly's research director later described as 'the insulin aristocrats'), to have all batches tested in Toronto and to assign the patent for any improvements to the university. Insulin was first supplied to the aristocrats in August 1922 and their experiences were published in a special edition of Allen's *Journal of Metabolic Research* which, although dated Nov–Dec 1922, did not come out until 1923 — the last contribution was received on 9 May 1923! The journal contained 10 papers and was 438 pages long. In his 1962 reminiscences Walter Campbell wrote that by the end of 1922,

> We had studied 50 patients for many months, including patients with coma, acidosis, gangrene and various infections. There is little doubt that we ourselves were over-impressed by the dramatic repair of patients in such dire extremity as we will never encounter again, and we even had visions of islet cell repair taking place, far beyond anything that has yet been seen. We saw such remarkable repair of malignantly progressing tuberculosis in a young diabetic, under adequate treatment with diet and insulin, as would still astonish the chest physician of today. Other infections, too, responded, far beyond our expectations. Acidosis was now no great problem.[2]

Before and after photographs of children who had been resurrected offered dramatic evidence of the power of insulin. The most famous are those of Kansas Professor of Medicine Ralph Major's patient Billy Leroy in his June 1923 paper in the *Journal of the American Medical Association*. This 3-year-old boy had diabetes for 2 years and weighed only 6.8 kg. After 3 months on a regimen of 55 g carbohydrate and 25 units of insulin daily his weight had doubled and his urine was sugar free.[16]

Even in a world without fax or e-mail, news of the discovery spread rapidly. One reason for this was the more international outlook of medical journals in those days; American, English, French and German journals all reported medical meetings in other countries and printed abstracts of papers from other journals. In *Index Medicus* in 1922 there were only 19 references to 'insulin' or an equivalent term (such as pancreatic extract): 7 each in the *Lancet* and *British Medical Journal* and 5 in the *Journal of the American Medical Association*. In 1923 there were 320: 108 in Britain, 88 in the *Journal of the American Medical Association*, 86 in the 3 main German journals and 41 in the French *Presse Medicale*. In just the first half of 1924 the number of references reached 317.[17]

In October 1922 the Danish Nobel Prize winner August Krogh (1874–1949) was lecturing in the US and contacted Macleod wondering 'if it might be consistent with the plans of your collaborators and yourself to have experiments carried out also in Denmark'. Krogh's wife Marie had been diagnosed with diabetes a year earlier so that he had a personal as well as professional interest. He suggested that his friend Dr Hagedorn would 'be able to do very good work with the insulin' and that pancreata and money would be easy to get. Production in Denmark began in December 1922 in Hagedorn's home. Krogh played an important part in the award of the Nobel Prize.

1.5 The Nobel Prize

It is very unusual for Nobel Prizes to be awarded within two years of a discovery and to people being nominated for the first time. Banting and Macleod were nominated for the first time in 1923: Banting by George

W. Crile (Cleveland), Francis G. Benedict (Boston) and Krogh; and Macleod by George N. Stuart (Cleveland) and Krogh. Krogh considered nominating Collip as well but thought he had not done enough. Charles Best was never nominated and was thus ruled out because only nominated candidates can be considered.

Krogh's reasons for proposing Banting and Macleod were that Banting ('a young and apparently very talented man') had the idea but that it could not have been progressed without the assistance of Macleod. Written evaluations of Banting's and Macleod's scientific contributions were provided by two members of the Nobel Committee, John Sjöqvist (Professor of Chemistry and Pharmacy) and Hans Christian Jacobaeus (Professor of Internal Medicine). Sjöqvist arrived at the same conclusion as Krogh, but Jacobaeus found the decision more difficult because Macleod's contribution was 'not apparent from the literature'.

There seems no doubt that the decision was made more hastily than usual and what must have swayed the committee is that by the time of their final decision in October 1923, there was already abundant evidence of the value of insulin, especially in the previously fatal diabetes of children and young people and the treatment of diabetic coma. Banting was furious at having to share the prize with Macleod and his first instinct was to refuse it. The Chairman of the Insulin Committee persuaded him that he must accept as this was the first Nobel ever awarded to a Canadian whereupon Banting decided to share his money with Best. Later Macleod did the same with Collip.

One controversy which will never be resolved is whether the Romanian, Nicholas Paulesco (1869–1931) should have shared the prize with Banting and Macleod.[18] In contrast to the 'amateurs' Banting and Best, Paulesco was a professional physiologist of international renown. His interest in diabetes began in 1891 when he worked in Paris with Etiènne Lancereaux. Paulesco left Paris in 1900 to take up the Chair of Physiology in Bucharest and never went back to France. In 1908 he invented a way of approaching the pituitary gland by the temporal route without causing cerebral injury and was thereby able to show that the pituitary was essential to life. His monograph *The Hypophysis of the Brain* was acknowledged by Harvey

Cushing as being a seminal work and one which stimulated and maintained Cushing's interest in the pituitary.

As early as 1899 Paulesco wrote that, 'Among others, together with Professor Dastre, I undertook a work whose scope was the isolation and study of the active product of the internal secretion of the pancreas. This work will be published soon.' In fact no publication resulted and he probably did not return to his pancreatic research until 1916. In his *Textbook of Medical Physiology*, written in French and published in Bucharest in 1920, he included a 15 page chapter entitled 'Personal Research' in which he described an aqueous pancreatic extract, called pancreine, which resulted in 'disappearance of the symptoms of diabetes' in depancreatised dogs.

In the autumn and winter of 1920 he did a new set of experiments which were published in French journals in July and August 1921.[19,20] One cannot but agree with Paulesco's supporters[21] that these papers report a beautifully conceived and executed series of experiments and in April 1922 he obtained a patent for 'Pancréine and the Process of its Production'. His application included the sentence 'In order that Pancréine be used in the treatment of human diabetes, it must be prepared in large quantities — which requires a lot of capital'.

When Paulesco heard of Banting and Macleod's award he wrote to the President of the Nobel Foundation citing his paper in the *Archives Internationales de Physiologie* and saying, 'I seek the opportunity to protest against the fact that this distinction was accorded to some people who did not deserve it. Indeed, the discovery of these physiologic and therapeutic effects belongs to me in their entirety.' After summarising the results of his experiments, he continued, 'Thus, the treatment of diabetes was already discovered and nothing remained but its application in man'. Unfortunately for Paulesco there is no appeal against Nobel Prize assignments and there the matter rested.

1.6 The Long-term Impact of the Discovery

Populist accounts of the discovery of insulin often imply that it revolutionised the treatment of diabetes overnight. In fact it was such a radically different treatment from any in the medical armamentarium of the time that many doctors were frightened to use it. In 1923, Hugh Maclean, Professor of Medicine at St Thomas' was hardly reassuring when he stated, 'Every medical man employing insulin should be thoroughly impressed with the fact that he is using a powerful and dangerous, though easily controlled, remedy, and that any neglect on his part may end in disaster'.[22] The editor of *The Medical Journal of Australia*, attacked insulin as a dangerous and unproven remedy claiming that, 'No doubt hundreds of diabetics will be hastened to their graves (and that) it is too potent for safe use in advanced conditions.'[23]

The most dramatic effects were seen in the previously universally fatal diabetic coma (ketoacidosis). The famous American diabetes specialist Elliott Joslin (1869–1962) and colleagues reviewed their first 33 cases treated with insulin between 1 January 1923 and 1 April 1925. The most important statistic was that 31 survived and these results were attributed to 'promptly applied medical care. Rest in bed, special nursing attendance, warmth, evacuation of the bowels by enema, the introduction of liquids into the body, lavage of the stomach (and) cardiac stimulants'.[24] They were at pains to play down the idea that since insulin had been available, coma no longer needed to be taken seriously, writing that, 'Coma patients recover as the result of hard work by day and night of doctors, usually young, who apply the most modern methods of medical practice'.

At first insulin was very expensive and English physicians used it as a last resort. Newly diagnosed diabetics were admitted to hospital or a nursing home and put on a severely restricted diet. Only if they still had glycosuria on 40–50 g of carbohydrate per day was insulin started. How far patients were encouraged to be active participants in their own treatment probably depended on the views of their physician and many not only prescribed an excessively rigid routine but were also authoritarian. For example Jack Eastwood, a retired headmaster writing in 1986, remembered that when he developed diabetes in 1925 at the age of 13:

I was taken to a Harley Street specialist and spent three weeks in a nursing home, during which time my diet and insulin requirements were settled. I returned home to be looked after by my parents in accordance with the

detailed instructions given to them. My diet was strictly controlled, especially on the carbohydrate side: for two years all my food was weighed and
no excesses at all were allowed.

In 1931 Eastwood won a scholarship to Oxford where he imple-
mented a 'not less intelligent method of treatment that had become
normal in my case by the time I left university'. He ate lunch in an
ordinary restaurant, played golf nearly every afternoon (such was university life in the 1930s!) and then had a normal four course dinner
in hall, eating whatever was necessary to give himself carbohydrate 65
g, protein 35 g and fat 30 g. His basic regimen was two injections a
day but he tested himself before every meal and often gave extra
insulin after lunch. Eventually he decided to eat normal meals and
have an injection before each of 'the amount of insulin that I knew
from experience would be needed to cope with the food about to be
eaten, due allowance being made for what I expected to be doing during the next few hours'. In 1935 he visited a specialist for the last time
and was told there was no need to go again since he knew more about
controlling his own diabetes than the specialist.[25]

Most authorities believed that the aim of treatment should be
physiological normality and patients were told that their urine should
not contain sugar at any time. Inevitably this led to hypoglycaemic
attacks and in self defence many patients decided it was safer and more
comfortable to run with 'a little sugar in the urine'. In the mid-1930s
some physicians realised that rigid treatment was acting as a psychological strait jacket, especially in the young, and advocated a free diet
and no attempt to maintain sugar-free urine. This coincided with the
introduction of long acting insulins — protamine insulinate in 1936
and protamine zinc insulin (PZI) in 1937 — and led to two decades
in which many patients lived with permanently high blood sugars.
Between 1935 and 1950 diabetes specialists were disturbed to find
that so called juvenile diabetics whose lives had been saved by insulin
were developing complications such as blindness and renal failure,
which, before insulin, had only been seen in middle aged and elderly
diabetics. As the Canadian physician, Israel Rabinowitch (1890–1983)
put it in 1944, 'There is nothing more disturbing than the diabetic

who acquires the disease in childhood, who apparently is a picture of robust health — who looks and feels perfectly well — but whose blood vessels have been degenerating insidiously for years; who, in the early 20s or 30s and probably married and with a family, is beginning to feel the effect of the degenerative changes, either because of a progressive hypertension, kidney failure, disturbance of sight due to retinitis or a sudden attack of coronary thrombosis'.[26] Ruth Reuting followed up 50 patients of Elliott Joslin who had originally been identified in 1929 when the only criteria were that they should be under 40 and have had diabetes for more than 5 years. By 1949 a third had died at an average age of 24.9 years with an average diabetes duration of 17.6 years. Of the 19 deaths, 8 were due to cardiovascular-renal disease, 4 to pulmonary TB and 4 to other infections. Among the survivors she reported that, 'ominous signs of hypertension, azotemia and proteinuria are evident in significant numbers and 27 of the 29 living patients had X-ray evidence of vascular calcification'.[27] These tragedies led to a long running debate about whether complications were due to poor glucose control or were an inevitable, possibly inherited, consequence of the disease. The issue was not resolved until 1993 when the results of the American Diabetes Control and Complications Trial (DCCT) clearly showed that near normoglycaemia prevented or delayed the onset of complications.[28]

References

1. Harley G. *Diabetes: Its Various Forms and Different Treatments.* London: Walton and Maberly; 1866.
2. Campbell WR. Anabasis. *Canad Med Assoc J* 1962; 87: 1055–1061.
3. Nothmann MM. The history of the discovery of pancreatic diabetes. *Bull Hist Med* 1954; 28: 272–274.
4. Minkowski O. Historical development of the theory of pancreatic diabetes. *Diabetes* 1989; 38: 1–6.
5. Murray GR. Note on the treatment of myxoedema by hypodermic injections of an extract of the thyroid gland of a sheep. *Br Med J* 1891; 2: 796–797.

6. Tattersall RB. Pancreatic organotherapy for diabetes 1889–1921. *Medical History* 1995; 39: 288–316.

7. Richards DW. The effect of pancreas extract on depancreatised dogs: Ernest L Scott's thesis of 1911. *Persp Biol Med* 1966; 10: 84–95.

8. Cox C. *The Fight to Survive: A Young Girl, Diabetes and the Discovery of Insulin*. New York: Kaplan Publishing; 2009.

9. Bliss M. *The Discovery of Insulin*. Chicago: University of Chicago Press; 1982.

10. Williams MJ. J.J.R. Macleod: the co-discoverer of insulin. *Proc Royal Coll Phys Edinburgh* 1993; 23 (supplement 1): 1–125.

11. Macleod JJR. *Physiology and Biochemistry in Modern Medicine*. 3rd ed. London: Henry Kimpton; 1921.

12. Stevenson L. J.J.R. Macleod: history of the researches leading to the discovery of insulin. *Bull Hist Med* 1978; 52: 295–312.

13. Bliss M. Texts and documents: Banting's, best's, and collip's accounts of the discovery of insulin. *Bull Hist Med* 1982; 56: 554–568.

14. Burrow GN, Hazlett BE, Phillips MJ. A case of diabetes mellitus. *N Engl J Med* 1982; 306: 340–343.

15. Banting FG, Best CH, Collip JB *et al.* Pancreatic extracts in the treatment of diabetes mellitus: preliminary report. *Canad Med Assoc J* 1922; 12: 141–146.

16. Major RH. The treatment of diabetes mellitus with insulin. *J Am Med Assoc* 1923; 80: 1597–1600.

17. Hetenyi G. The day after: how insulin was received by the medical profession. *Persp Biol Med* 1995; 38: 396–405.

18. Murray I. Paulesco and the isolation of insulin. *J Hist Med* 1971; 26: 150–157.

19. Paulesco NC. Action de l'extrait pancréatique injecté dans le sang chez un animal diabetique. *Comptes Rendus des Séances de la Société de Biologie* 1921; 85: 555–559.

20. Paulesco NC. Recherche sur le rôle du pancréas dans l'assimilation nutritive. *Archives Internationales de Physiologie* 1921; 17: 85–103.

21. Ionescu-Tirgoviste C. *The Rediscovery of Insulin*. Bucharest: Editura Geneze; 1996.

22. Maclean H. The use of insulin in general practice. *Lancet* 1923; 2: 829–833.

23. Martin FIR. *A History of Diabetes in Australia*. Victoria, Australia: Miranova Publishers; 1998.
24. Joslin EP, Root HF, White P. Diabetic coma and its treatment. *Med Clin N Amer* 1925; 8: 1873–1919.
25. Eastwood JD. Insulin and independence. *Br Med J* 1986; 293: 1659–1661.
26. Rabinowitch IM. Prevention of premature arteriosclerosis in diabetes mellitus. *Can Med Assoc J* 1944; 51: 300–306.
27. Reuting RE. Progress notes on fifty diabetic patients followed 25 or more years.
28. The diabetes control and complications trial research group. The effect of intensive treatment of diabetes on the development and progression of long-term complications in insulin-dependent diabetes mellitus. *N Engl J Med* 1993; 329: 977–986.

Chapter 2

THE DISCOVERY OF THE CURE FOR PERNICIOUS ANAEMIA, VITAMIN B12

A. Victor Hoffbrand

2.1 Introduction

The Nobel Prize in Physiology or Medicine was awarded in 1934 to George Whipple, George Minot and William Murphy (Fig. 2.1) for their discovery of a cure for pernicious anaemia (PA). Minot and Murphy fed 45 patients with PA half a pound of raw or lightly cooked beef liver daily. They observed an increase in the reticulocyte count within a week, a rapid improvement in tongue and digestive symptoms and a feeling of well-being; blood counts normalised within 60 days. The choice of liver was based on Whipple's experiments on dogs, which had been repeatedly bled and kept on a standard diet. He found that the addition of liver to the diet gave the best results of any food in stimulating blood regeneration and correcting the experimentally-induced anaemia.

The discovery of a dietary deficiency as the cause of the anaemia in PA led to the isolation of vitamin B12 in 1948. It also stimulated the nutritional research of Lucy Wills, which resulted in the isolation of folic acid in 1941. Research on these two vitamins, still active today, has revealed important biochemical pathways and has had enormous clinical implications, not only in haematology and gastroenterology but also in the fields of congenital defects, cardiovascular disease, cancer and neurology. An excellent review, 'The Conquest of Pernicious Anemia', was published in 1940 by William Bosworth Castle.[1] More recently, Israel Chanarin[2] and Victor Hoffbrand and David Weir[3] have reviewed the history of pernicious

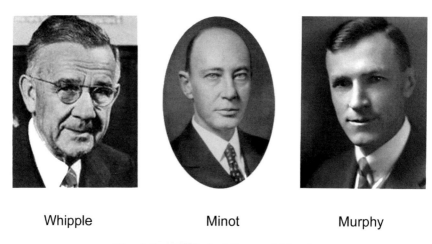

| Whipple | Minot | Murphy |

Fig. 2.1.   Whipple, Minot and Murphy.

anaemia and of folic acid respectively. Biographies of the three Nobel Prize winners and other major researchers in the field are included in Wintrobe's book, *Hematology: the Blossoming of a Science*.[4]

2.2 Brief Biographies

2.2.1 *George Whipple*

George Hoyt Whipple (1878–1976) was born on 28 August in Ashland, New Hampshire. He was the son and grandson of general practitioners. He attended Yale and then Johns Hopkins, working in biochemistry and acting as a senior student instructor, qualifying in medicine in 1905. He met many distinguished men at that time, including William Osler. He worked in the pathology department and performed research on liver injury and regeneration between 1907 and 1914. He then moved to San Francisco and for the next seven years was Director of the Hooper Foundation for Medical Research and Professor of Research Medicine. In 1921 he moved to Rochester, New York, as Dean, helping to found a new Medical and Dental School.

His research on the liver got him interested in bile pigments and jaundice. This led to the research, much of it with CW Hooper, on haemoglobin formation, using dogs with a bile fistula. The laboratory was run by Mrs Robscheit-Robbins who took special care of the dogs. Whipple was a self-disciplined, conscientious and determined research worker who believed in the steady accumulation of data and their objective analysis. He took infinite pains in his medical research and in his hobby, fly-fishing.

2.2.2 George Minot

George Richards Minot (1885–1950) was born on 2 December in Boston. His ancestors included many distinguished scientists and doctors. In his youth he studied butterflies and moths. He qualified with a Bachelor's degree in 1908 and in medicine in 1912. He received his clinical training at the Massachusetts General Hospital, which one of his ancestors had helped found.

Minot's interest in haematology arose from contact with Assistant Professor J. Homer Wright, who developed the blood stain eosin and methylene blue (Wright's stain) still in use today. He worked in Johns Hopkins Hospital where he became interested in PA, although mainly working on blood coagulation with William Howell, whose student Jay McLean discovered heparin.

He returned to Boston in 1915 when his research into dietary treatment of PA began. In 1922 he became Physician-in-Chief at the Collis P. Huntington Memorial Hospital and later was on the staff of the Peter Bent Brigham Hospital. In 1928 he succeeded William Peabody as Head of the Thorndike Laboratories and was appointed Professor of Medicine at Harvard University.

Minot had a wide interest in blood transfusion, coagulation, platelets, leukaemia and lymphomas. He developed diabetes mellitus in 1921 and was one of the first to be treated with insulin, his disease emphasising to him the necessity for strict dietary control. He was painstaking in eliciting the exact diets of his patients and in recording the details.

2.2.3 William Murphy

William Parry Murphy (1892–1987) was born on 6 February in Wisconsin, the son of a congregational minister. He gained a Bachelor's degree from Oregon University in 1914 and then taught physics and mathematics for two years before entering Harvard Medical School and graduating in 1922. He worked at the Peter Bent Brigham Hospital from 1923 until he retired in 1958. He was chosen by Minot to join him in a rigorous trial of a special diet to treat PA. Murphy was already performing clinical research in diabetes and he learned to perform reticulocyte counts and to accurately document clinical and haematological responses. He continued with trials of liver fractions by mouth or by intramuscular injections after the initial success with raw liver.

2.3 The Medical Problem

The diagnosis of the disease we now call Addisonian pernicious anaemia at the time when Minot and Murphy began their studies depended on characterising the blood changes and distinguishing them from those in other forms of anaemia. The associated clinical features of PA included jaundice, glossitis, neurological symptoms, and gastric atrophy and achlorhydria.

Thomas Addison of Guy's Hospital is considered to have first described pernicious anaemia in 1855 in his monograph, 'On the Constitutional and Local Effects of Disease of the Suprarenal Capsules'.[5] Addison described a 'very remarkable form of general anaemia, occurring without any discoverable cause whatsoever, during life or at post-mortem'. He did not describe jaundice, sore mouth or tongue or neurological signs, nor did he give its microscopic appearances. These were later described by Anton Biermer in 1872[6] who reported 15 cases, 14 fatal, of a 'progressiver perniciöser anemia', mainly occurring among poor people, especially multiparous women in their 30s. It is most likely that these were cases of megaloblastic anaemia due to folate deficiency.

In 1874, the fact that the red cell count was low in relation to the haemoglobin level was reported in PA[7], and in 1877 Hayem documented for the first time the macrocytic red cells.[8] Paul Ehrlich,[9] using his new methods of blood cell staining, described 'megloblastic' nucleated red cells in the blood of PA patients. From then on workers could more clearly separate PA from other chronic refractory anaemias. Ehrlich also discovered reticulocytes by supra-vital staining, later recognised to be young red cells by Theobald Smith in 1901.[10] These cells were found to be low in relation to the degree of anaemia in PA and were to be crucial in the studies of Minot and Murphy in assessing the response to different potential treatments in PA. Indeed Minot, as early as 1916, reported a rise in reticulocytes in PA patients who had undergone splenectomy.[11]

While these advances in the microscopic description of PA were being made, the clinical features of the disease were also becoming apparent. There were descriptions of sore mouth and glossitis being associated with PA during the last quarter of the 19th century. Neurological associations were also reported sporadically and in 1883 Leichtenstern[12] described the characteristic demyelination of posterior nerve tracts in the spinal cord in two cases at autopsy. Lichtheim (1887) first made the correct association of spinal cord lesions with PA.[13] The neurological abnormalities were more fully illustrated in 1900 by Russell, Batten and Collier at the National Hospital, Queen Square, in London but they did not regard these as specific in view of the absence of anaemia in some of the patients.[14] Cabot in 1908[15] gave an incidence of 40% for glossitis and 10% for spinal cord damage, with abnormalities of sensation in the feet and hands more frequent. He also described jaundice in the more anaemic patients. The triad of macrocytic anaemia, glossitis and neuropathy became well recognised but it was clear that they were not necessarily present in every patient, and did not relate to each other in severity. The association of gastric achlorhydria with PA had been previously described but was fully documented by Hurst and Bell in 1922[16] who also insisted on the association of sub-acute degeneration of the cord specifically with PA. Others reported the association with vitiligo and early greying of the hair. It was, however, the anaemia and monitoring of its response that was to prove crucial in finding the cure for this fatal disease.

2.4 Possible Mechanisms

Before the proof by Minot and Murphy of a nutritional basis for PA, there had been considerable debate about the nature of the disease.

This was partly because in the last quarter of the 19th century there was not a clear distinction between PA and other forms of progressive anaemia. The intense cellularity of the bone marrow (at post-mortem) and primitive nature of the cells and low reticulocyte count suggested to some it was a form of leukaemia or a primary disorder of blood formation or due to some toxin damaging the marrow. Ehrlich[17] considered such a toxin might also cause peripheral blood destruction. Jaundice was ascribed to red cell breakdown due to a toxin. The correction of some cases of PA by expulsion of a tapeworm was thought to be due to removal of a source of such a toxin. The low reticulocyte count often combined with low white cell and platelet counts, were in keeping with marrow failure and, although some thought the response to liver therapy indicated removal of a toxin, Minot and Murphy correctly concluded that it worked by replacing a missing dietary factor. In 1927, Peabody,[18] examining bone marrow aspirates before and after feeding of liver, wrote that there was some factor in liver 'that promotes the development and differentiation of mature red cells'. It was in 1956 that Clement Finch (who died in 2010 aged 95) elegantly showed, using radioactive iron studies, the massive ineffective erythropoiesis with death in the marrow of the majority of red cell precursors in severe untreated PA, fully explaining why such a hypercellular marrow could be associated with such a low cell output.[19] As early as 1922 Whipple had described the large amounts of haemoglobin breakdown products in PA in relation to the small numbers of circulating red cells.[20]

2.4.1 *The nutritional deficiency concept*

At about the beginning of the 20th century, the deficiency diseases beri-beri, pellagra and scurvy were clearly delineated.[21] Whipple's experiments on dogs had shown the beneficial effects of dietary supplements and particularly of liver on blood regeneration. However, it is now clear that this response to liver was probably due to the ready availability of its iron rather than to its high vitamin B12 and folate content.

There had been sporadic reports of improvement in the disease in small numbers of PA patients treated with various dietary supplements. It was, however, George Minot who focused on the dietary treatment of the disease. He had experienced the lack of response to iron and arsenic, two standard treatments at the time for anaemia. As early as 1912 while at Johns Hopkins he had become interested in the diets of PA patients and he took detailed dietary histories of his patients when he returned to Boston, advising them to add liver and meat to their diets. He then embarked on the trial with William Murphy of a diet 'rich in complete proteins and low in fat'. The 45 patients were fed 120–240 g of liver daily and 120 g of muscle meat, leafy vegetables, fruit, eggs and milk (Fig. 2.2). It was difficult for the patients to get all this down, so much encouragement from the investigators and their assistants was needed. This was reinforced when the patients began to feel better and showed increased reticulocyte counts within a week or so. Minot was himself on a

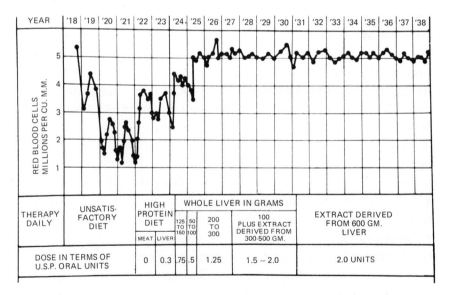

Fig. 2.2.   Haematological response of one of the first patients with PA treated with oral liver. (Reproduced from Castle WB. The conquest of pernicious anemia. In: *Blood, Pure and Eloquent*, 1980: McGraw-Hill Book Company, with the permission of The McGraw-Hill Companies).

strict diet for his diabetes and showed a compulsive attention to those of his patients. Nevertheless it took 2 years to complete studies on 45 patients.

On 4 May 1926 Minot and Murphy reported to the Association of American Physicians correction of the anaemia in a nearly consecutive series of 45 patients.[22] The full details were published later that year.[23]

2.4.2 *Why liver therapy worked*

Although based on a faulty deduction from Whipple's work (it is now clear that the response of the venesected dogs to liver was due to the ready availability of its iron rather than to its high vitamin B12 and folate content), beef liver was effective in PA because of the large amounts of vitamin B12 it provided. This is about a microgram per gram so 240 g liver provided approximately 240 μg daily. The normal daily requirement is now known to be about 1 μg. A haematological response in PA can be obtained with this very low dose. A normal diet contains roughly 15 μg of which 1 μg is absorbed by the active intrinsic factor mechanism. This amount does not provide sufficient vitamin B12 in the absence of intrinsic factor, as occurs in PA. The much larger amount of vitamin B12 Minot and Murphy fed their patients, however, allowed sufficient vitamin B12 to be absorbed, in the absence of intrinsic factor, by passive diffusion through the buccal, gastric and upper small intestinal mucosae. Between 0.1% and 1.0% of an oral dose of vitamin B12 can be absorbed by this mechanism, and it was this passively absorbed vitamin B12 from the large amounts present in liver that elicited a haematological response in their patients.

Beef liver also contains folate, about 300 μg/100 g. It is now known that folate in large doses can elicit a haematological response in untreated vitamin B12 deficiency. The amount of folate absorbed from 240 g of liver would, however, be less than is needed to elicit a reticulocyte response in untreated PA.[24] Folate may, however, have augmented the response to the vitamin B12 present in the liver.

2.5 Subsequent Research

Minot and Murphy's Nobel Prize-winning work led to a number of important lines of further research which are discussed next. These include:

(i) Trials of increasingly purified, effective fractions of liver in untreated PA which resulted in the isolation of vitamin B12, also called cobalamin, by two groups in 1948. The Nobel Prize in Chemistry was subsequently awarded to Dorothy Hodgkin for the elucidation of its three-dimensional molecular structure.

(ii) The demonstration of the physiological mechanism by which vitamin B12 absorption occurs through the ileum after combining with intrinsic factor made by the stomach.

(iii) The demonstration by Lucy Wills of the cure of other forms of macrocytic anaemia with a separate nutritional factor. This turned out to be folic acid which had been isolated before vitamin B12 in 1941.

(iv) Elucidation of those megaloblastic anaemias caused by vitamin B12 deficiency and those by folate deficiency and the development of tests to distinguish between them. The demonstration that PA itself is an acquired autoimmune disease of the stomach.

(v) Research into the biochemical functions of the two vitamins, their inter-relations and how their deficiencies cause megaloblastic anaemia and its associated clinical manifestations.

(vi) The development of anti-folate drugs for treating leukaemia and other forms of malignant disease.

(vii) Studies of how vitamin B12 deficiency causes neurological disease and whether vitamin B12 or folate therapy might prevent other neurological diseases, particularly in the elderly.

(viii) The recognition that vitamin B12 and folate deficiencies or abnormalities of their metabolism may be relevant in a wide range of cardiovascular diseases, and also to cancer.

2.5.1 *Isolation of vitamin B12*

George Minot approached Edwin J. Cohn, Professor of Physical Chemistry at Harvard, suggesting that he prepared fractions of liver that could be tested by mouth or parenterally on patients, with observation of the reticulocyte response as a quick method of purifying the active compound and making the treatment more palatable to the patients. He and Murphy thought the active substance would be found in the protein fraction. To their surprise, bulky liver proteins turned out to be inactive.[25] On the other hand, a water soluble liver fraction, G, was extremely active. This fraction became commercially available after collaboration with Eli Lilly and Co. and was widely used. To everyone's surprise, Ganssler then reported from Germany[26] that an active, protein-free preparation could be made from as little as 5 g of liver.

The subsequent purification of the active compound from liver in the Merck Laboratories in the US and by workers at Glaxo Laboratories in England was accelerated by microbiological assays using *Lactobacillus* organisms.[27] One of these, *Lactobacillus Leichmannii*, was subsequently to be used clinically until the 1970s to measure vitamin B12 in human tissues and serum.

As the active factor was purified, it became apparent that it was coloured red. It was isolated in 1948 by both commercial teams as cyanocobalamin and called vitamin B12.[28, 29] It was rapidly shown that only a few micrograms were required daily by injection to correct the anaemia in PA[30] (Table 2.1). The two main physiological forms of the vitamin were then found to be methyl-cobalamin and deoxyadenosyl-cobalamin (initially called coenzyme B12). In 1956 Dorothy Hodgkin and colleagues described the structure of cyano- and deoxyadenosyl-cobalamin based on three-dimensional crystallography[31] (Fig. 2.3). For this work and her work on the structure of insulin, Hodgkin received the Nobel Prize in Chemistry in 1964.

2.5.2 *Extrinsic and intrinsic factors*

Early major research into the mechanism of PA was performed in the same Thorndike Laboratories in Boston where Minot was working and

Table 2.1.   Progress in concentrating the anti-PA constituent of liver. (Reproduced from Castle WB. The conquest of pernicious anemia. In: *Blood, Pure and Eloquent*; 1980: McGraw-Hill Book Company, with the permission of The McGraw-Hill Companies).

Year	Substance	Dry Weight (G)*
Clinical era		
1926	Whole beef liver (240 g)	60.0
1928	Liver fraction G (oral)	12.75
1930	Crude liver extract	0.35
1936	Refined liver extract	0.015
Microbiological era		
1945	Folic acid	0.001
1948	Vitamin B12	0.000001

* Comparably effective therapeutic daily dosage when given by injection, unless otherwise indicated.

where he became Director in 1928. William Bosworth Castle had been assistant to Francis Peabody, the first Director since 1922. After Minot and Murphy's reports, he asked the question, why did patients with PA have to eat large amounts of liver every day while the rest of the population could eat normal quantities of meat or liver without developing anaemia? In the light of the well-known observation of gastric atrophy and achlorhydria in PA, he began a series of experiments into the nature of the stomach factor lacking in patients with PA.[32,33] He ate 300 g of rare hamburger steak daily and, an hour after this meal, aspirated his own stomach contents and allowed the digestion of the steak to continue in 'the test tube' for a few hours until it was liquid. He then fed this digest through a flexible gastric tube to PA patients daily over a ten day period. He mistakenly, on the basis of reports from other laboratories, considered steak equivalent to liver for treating PA. The patients showed a reticulocyte response at six days rising to a maximum at ten days with a subsequent rise in red cell count and improvement in well-being. Steak alone (200 g fed daily as the only source of animal protein), for the previous ten days, did not produce such a response in the patients. The reduced amount (200 g rather than 300 g) was chosen because 100 g of the beef was lost in the normal subject before aspiration.

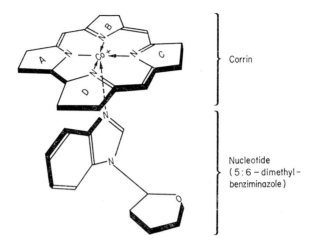

Fig. 2.3. The basic structure of vitamin B12 (cobalamin). Cyano-, hydroxo-, methyl- and deoxyadenosyl-cobalamin have the appropriate side group attached to the cobalt atom.

Castle called the factor in the steak 'extrinsic factor' (now known to be vitamin B12) and the factor in gastric juice 'intrinsic factor'. Castle became the third Director of the Thorndike Laboratories in 1948 when Minot retired. He was a most impressive man of great physical as well as intellectual stature. I had the pleasure of meeting him briefly in 1967 when I was undertaking research on folate in Maurice Friedkin's laboratory in Boston.

Subsequent experiments by Castle and others led to the isolation of intrinsic factor by Ralph Gräsbeck in 1966, aided by the availability of radioactive vitamin B12.[34] It was shown to be a glycoprotein. Forty litres of gastric juice yielded 8 mg of intrinsic factor which could bind 240 μg of vitamin B12. Booth and Mollin[35] later showed that the role of intrinsic factor was to promote vitamin B12 absorption through the distal ileum in humans.

2.5.3 *Discovery of folic acid*

Lucy Wills, a graduate with first class honours from Cambridge University, was working in the Department of Chemical Pathology at the Royal Free Hospital in London when, in 1928, she was invited to go to Bombay to investigate the macrocytic anaemia ('pernicious anaemia') of pregnancy. She observed that the anaemia was more common in those living on a diet lacking protein, fruit and vegetables. On the basis of a similar anaemia she could produce in rats fed a similarly poor diet, which she could correct by adding yeast or a yeast extract, she tried feeding yeast to the anaemic pregnant women. She gave them 30 g of yeast or yeast extract, Marmite, every day and observed excellent haematological responses.[36] Like Minot and Murphy, she used reticulocyte counts for early detection of improvement. She also showed responses to crude liver extract but when she subsequently tried purified liver preparations that were effective in PA, these were inactive in her anaemic pregnant women.[37] This implied that a different compound was involved in the macrocytic anaemia of pregnancy from that needed to treat PA (with gastric achlorhydria) in older subjects.

Several lines of research converged before the isolation of folic acid in 1941. The vitamin received many names: vitamin M (for monkeys), vitamin Bc (for chickens), Norit eluate factor and Factor S before it became clear that there were a large number of natural folate compounds. Again microbiological assays for folate using *Lactobacillus casei* and *Streptococcus lactis R* (*Streptococcus faecalis*) were valuable in the purification process. The name 'folic' was introduced because green leaves were a rich source (it was isolated from large amounts of spinach)[38] and it was also isolated from liver.[39] The term 'folic acid' is now used for the parent compound that is given therapeutically and 'folate' to describe the whole group of compounds which make up the vitamin. These compounds are usually reduced to di- or tetra-hydro forms, have single carbon unit additions e.g. methyl, methylene or formyl and, inside cells, are polyglutamated to form the active coenzymes and to ensure cell retention.

Lucy Wills on her return to London fed Marmite to patients with a variety of macrocytic anaemias. Her handwritten notebooks, which were in my office when I was appointed to the Chair of Haematology at the Royal Free Hospital in 1973,[3] are now kept in the hospital's archives. She and others rapidly showed which macrocytic anaemias responded to Marmite e.g. in pregnancy or sprue[40] and which others responded to the purified liver fractions (vitamin B12). In the author's opinion, Lucy Wills should have received the Nobel Prize for her discovery of folate. She was a remarkably active and cheerful lady, a socialist who came to work on a bicycle when many of her colleagues arrived in Rolls Royce cars. She died in 1964. Her life story has been recorded in detail by Daphne Roe.[41]

After 1941, before vitamin B12 was isolated, pure synthetic folic acid was used to treat patients with all kinds of macrocytic or megaloblastic anaemias.[42] Responses were found in all types, but it became apparent that in PA the response was often suboptimal and poorly sustained, and that the neurological defect was not corrected or could become worse or even appear for the first time, even though the anaemia might be in remission. Folic acid in large doses could by-pass (at least temporarily) the block in folate metabolism affecting DNA synthesis caused by vitamin B12 deficiency (see below). Presumably some folic acid was converted to the folate coenzyme 5,10 methylenetetrahydrofolate. It could not, however, correct all the biochemical abnormalities caused by vitamin B12 deficiency, including the defect causing neurological damage.

2.5.4 Two vitamins

After the isolation of the two vitamins and the identification of their natural derivatives, the biochemical pathways in which they are involved — particularly their roles in 1-carbon metabolism and their interactions — were discovered. It became clear which diseases, such as PA, ileal resection, intestinal blind loops and fish tapeworm, were associated with vitamin B12 (cobalamin) deficiency and which, such as coeliac disease, tropical sprue, pregnancy and haemolytic anaemias were associated with folate deficiency. The types of diet causing the deficiencies also became clear. Avoidance of animal products (veganism) caused vitamin B12 deficiency, a poor quality diet ('tea and toast') caused deficiency of folate. It was also recognised that all vitamin B12 in nature came from micro-organisms; animals acquired the vitamin by absorbing it from the rumen or, as in the case of humans, eating animal produce. In the 1960s, PA was found to be an autoimmune disease of the stomach, with intrinsic factor and parietal cell antibodies in the serum and lack of gastric intrinsic factor accompanying the characteristic gastric atrophy and achlorhydria.

Microbiological assays were used in the isolation of the two vitamins and additional microbiological assays were adapted to measure their concentrations in body fluids and tissues. These assays of serum and, for folate, red cells were employed for many years to test for deficiencies of the two vitamins in clinical practice until they were replaced by immunoassays, more suitable for automation. All these aspects are reviewed in detail in Chanarin's monograph.[43]

2.5.5 *Vitamin B12/folate interactions*

Much research has been devoted to elucidating how the deficiencies cause anaemia and why the appearances of the blood and bone marrow are identical, whichever the deficiency. The most plausible explanation is that folate deficiency causes anaemia by impairing DNA synthesis because of the need for the folate coenzyme 5,10-methylenetetrahydrofolate polyglutamate in the synthesis of thymidine monophosphate from deoxyuridine monophosphate (Fig. 2.4). This is a rate limiting step in DNA synthesis. The deficiency impairs DNA synthesis by reducing the amount of thymidine triphosphate, one of the four immediate DNA precursors, available at the DNA replication fork.

Vitamin B12 deficiency indirectly lowers the level of this folate coenzyme and so impairs DNA synthesis. Vitamin B12 as methylcobalamin is needed in the conversion of methyltetrahydrofolate (methylTHF) to tetrahydrofolate (THF) from which all folate polyglutamate coenzymes are then synthesised inside cells (Fig 2.4). MethylTHF is the form in which all cells, including those of the bone marrow, receive folate from plasma. This is because the small intestine converts all dietary folates to methylTHF which is therefore the dominant form of the vitamin in portal and systemic plasma. MethylTHF enters cells but is not itself a substrate from which folate polyglutamates can be synthesised.[44] In vitamin B12 deficiency,

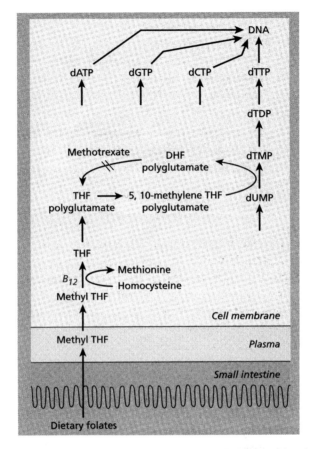

Fig. 2.4.   The role of methyl-cobalamin in folate metabolism and biochemical basis of megaloblastic anaemia (see text). A, adenine; C, cytosine; G, guanine; T, thymine; U, uracil; MP, DP, TP, mono-, di-, tri- phosphate; DHF, dihydrofolate; THF, tetrahydrofolate.

methylTHF accumulates in plasma because of the intracellular block in its conversion to THF whereas the intracellular levels of all folates are reduced.

The nature of the defect in DNA synthesis in vitamin B12 or folate deficiency has also been established. It was initially suggested that DNA lacking the base thymine might explain the chromosome breaks and cell death but the base composition of megaloblastic DNA is normal. Hoffbrand and colleagues[45] suggested instead that because of starvation of dTTP, the dividing cell was unable to elongate DNA from the multiple replicon origins opened up during mitosis. The evidence for excess initiation of DNA synthesis over DNA chain elongation came from experiments showing reduced replicating fork movement and impaired formation of bulk DNA in untreated megaloblastic cells, as well as in cells treated with the antimetabolites hydoxyurea or methotrexate, which also inhibit DNA synthesis. Failure of completion of DNA synthesis at multiple points along the chromosome was proposed to lead to failure of condensation of chromosomes, their fragility and susceptiblity to DNAases. It has also been suggested that mis-incorporation of uracil may be important in causing abnormality of DNA synthesis in vitamin B12 and folate deficiencies, but this could not explain the megaloblastic anaemias due to genetic defects or drugs acting at points in synthesis of DNA other than at thymidylate synthesis.

2.5.6 *Neurological damage*

The explanation for the peripheral nerve and spinal cord damage caused by vitamin B12 deficiency but not by folate deficiency has been more elusive.[46] Failure of methylation of myelin has been proposed but not fully confirmed. Accumulation of methylmalonic acid was also proposed to damage myelin but levels in patients were not found to correlate with whether nerve damage was present or not. Also, nitrous oxide could produce nerve damage by inactivating vitamin B12 without affecting the methylmalonic pathway. Studies are currently taking place into whether supplemental vitamin B12 and folate in the elderly can improve cognitive function, delay the onset and progression of Alzheimer's disease or of senile dementia.

2.5.7 *Systemic effects of vitamin and folate deficiencies*

After the discovery of vitamin B12 and folate, the dominant research into their clinical aspects was carried out by haematologists. However, over the last two or three decades, much of the research has been into cardiovascular, obstetric and malignant disease.

The reaction, methionine synthase, in which methylTHF is converted to THF, and which requires methylcobalamin, results in the methylation of homocysteine to methionine (Fig. 2.4). Homocysteine levels have been found to be raised in the plasma of patients with folate or vitamin B12 deficiency. Very high levels of homocysteine in plasma occur in various inherited enzyme deficiencies affecting its metabolism, including of methionine synthase. These very high levels are associated with severe arterial disease occurring at an early age e.g. children or teenagers. More modestly raised levels, as occur in plasma in vitamin B12 or folate deficiency, have been associated, on the basis of large population studies, with arterial disease in older subjects. Much current research is focused, therefore, on the possible reduction of the incidence of strokes and coronary heart disease with combinations of vitamins (folic acid, vitamin B12 and pyridoxine) given prophylactically in long-term, multi-centre trials.[47] The evidence so far shows a modest reduction in stroke incidence but little effect on the incidence of coronary heart disease or infarcts.

Much has been published on whether vitamin B12 or folate deficiency predisposes to cancer, particularly of the colon or breast, and whether it is safe to fortify the diet with folic acid (as is already carried out in North America and many other countries) or whether this will lead to an increased incidence of cancer. Detailed discussion of this topic is outside the scope of this chapter, but meta-analysis of the numerous large-scale, long-term trials of folic acid (and in some vitamin B12) supplements aimed at determining whether cardiovascular disease can be prevented have shown no evidence for an increased incidence of any form of tumour in those receiving the vitamins compared to controls receiving placebo. Two other important consequences of the discovery of vitamin B12 and folic acid have been the development of antimetabolite drugs, initiated by Farber's treatment of childhood leukaemia with the anti-folate drug aminopterin,[48] and the prevention of neural tube defects with prophylactic folic acid.[49]

2.6 Impact of the Discovery of Vitamin B12 on Medical Practice

Before Minot and Murphy's research, virtually all patients with PA died. It is now one of the easiest and most rewarding diseases to treat, with an essentially 100% survival rate. After the isolation of vitamin B12 as cyanocobalamin in 1948, this became the form of the vitamin used in therapy and still is given monthly in the US. In most other countries it has been replaced for therapy by hydroxocobalmin, which is much better retained in the body, rather than being predominantly excreted, as cyanocobalamin is, in the urine. Standard practice is to 'load' the patient initially with six intramuscular injections each of 1 mg hydroxocobalamin and then to maintain body stores with similar injections every three months. This is for life except in those cases of vitamin B12 deficiency, such as fish tapeworm, where the cause can be permanently corrected. Much vitamin B12 is given as a 'tonic' to patients with all kinds of medical disorders since the injection is cheap, painless and a nice pink colour. The neuropathy due to vitamin B12 deficiency improves but in those cases of spinal cord damage with symptoms present for more than three months, recovery is usually incomplete. There is no evidence that larger or more frequent doses lead to greater neurological improvement than standard doses.

Vitamin B12 can also be given orally as cyanocobalamin. Daily doses of 1000 µg are sufficient to maintain body stores in most patients with PA, a few micrograms being absorbed each day by passive diffusion, as in the liver feeding experiments of Minot and Murphy. Even if patients choose to be treated this way, initial loading should be with parenteral hydroxocobalamin and they should be monitored to be sure they are getting sufficient vitamin B12 by the oral route and are complying with the daily dose regimen. For lesser degrees of vitamin B12 deficiency e.g. malabsorption in the elderly or dietary deficiency of vitamin B12, as in vegans, there is no single established therapeutic regimen. Injections once or twice a year or daily oral cyanocobalamin in doses lower than 1 mg may be used with monitoring of the haematological and vitamin B12 status. Treatment as for PA may also be used and this is also given for life to those who have had a total gastrectomy or an ileal resection or bypass. Unfortunately, radioactive vitamin B12 is no longer available for the diagnosis of vitamin B12 malabsorption and the distinguishing of gastric from intestinal causes. Serum tests for parietal and intrinsic factor antibodies and for gastrin levels help in the diagnosis of PA. Upper gastrointestinal endoscopy is used to confirm gastric atrophy and to exclude gastric polyps or cancer.

The life expectancy of patients with PA has shown a remarkable improvement because of Minot and Murphy's discovery. It is now essentially normal for women[43] and probably, with the decline in the overall incidence of cancer of the stomach, also for men.

References

1. Castle WB. The conquest of pernicious anemia. In: *Blood, Pure and Eloquent*, Wintrobe MM (ed.). New York: McGraw-Hill Book Company; 1980: 283–317.

2. Chanarin I. A history of pernicious anaemia. *Brit J Haemat* 2000; 111: 407–415.

3. Hoffbrand AV, Weir DG. The history of folic acid. *Brit J Haemat* 2001; 113: 579–589.

4. Wintrobe MM. *Hematology, The Blossoming Science*. Philadelphia: Lea & Febiger; 1985.

5. Addison T. *On the Constitutional and Local Effects of Disease of the Suprarenal Capsules*. London: Samuel Highley; 1855.

6. Biermer A. Uber eine form von progressiver perniciöser anämie. *Schweiz. Arzte* 1872; 2: 15.

7. Sörenson ST. Taellinger af blodlegemer i 3 Tilfalde af excessiv oligocythaemi. *Hospitals Tidende* 1874; 1: 513–521.

8. Hayem G. Des alterations anatomique du sang dans l'anémie. In: *Congres Periodiques Internat Sciences Med*, 5'me Session. Geneve: MM Prevost *et al.*; 1877; 895: 211–217.

9. Ehrlich P. Uber regeneration und degeneration rother blutsceibenbei anämien. *Berl Klin Wochenschr* 1880; 17: 405.

10. Smith T. On changes in the red blood corpuscles in the pernicious anemia of Texas cattle fever. *Trans Assoc Am Physicians* 1891; 6: 263–278.

11. Lee RI, Minot GR, Vincent B. Splenectomy in pernicious anemia: studies on bone marrow stimulation. *JAMA* 1926; 67: 719–723.

12. Leichtenstern O. Uber 'progressive perniciöse anämie bei tabeskranken'. *Dtsch Med Wochenschr* 1884; 10: 849–850.

13. Lichtheim L. Zur kenntniss der perniciösen anämie. *Munch Med Wochenschr* 1887; 34: 300–306.

14. Russell JSR, Batten FE, Collier J. Subacute combined degeneration of the spinal cord. *Brain* 1900; 23: 39–110.

15. Hurst AF, Bell JR. The pathogenesis of subacute combined degeneration of the spinal cord, with special reference to its connection with Addisonian's (pernicious) anaemia, achlorhydria and intestinal infection. *Brain* 1922; 45: 266–281.

16. Cabot RC. Pernicious and secondary anaemia, chlorosis, and leukaemia. In: *A System of Medicine*, Osler W, McGrae T (eds). Oxford: Frowde; 1908: 612.

17. Ehrlich P. Uber einigebeobachtungen am anämishenblut. Berl *Klin Wochenschr* 1881; 18: 43.

18. Peabody FW. The pathology of the bone marrow in pernicious anemia. *Am J Pathol* 1927; 3: 179–202.

19. Finch CA, Coleman DH, Motulsky AG *et al.* Erythrokinetics in pernicious anemia. *Blood* 1956; 11: 807–820.

20. Whipple GH. Pigment metabolism and regeneration of hemoglobin in the body. *Arch Intern Med* 1922; 29: 711–731.

21. Funk C. The etiology of deficiency diseases. *J State Med* 1912; 20: 341–368.

22. Minot GR, Murphy WP. Observations on patients with pernicious anemia partaking of a special diet. *Trans Assoc Am Physicians* 1926; 41: 72–75.

23. Minot GR, Murphy WP. Treatment of pernicious anemia by a special diet. *JAMA* 1926; 87: 470–476.

24. Savage DG, Lindenbaum J. Neurological complications of acquired cobalamin deficiency. *Clin Haemat* 1995; 8: 657–678.

25. Minot GR, Cohn EJ, Murphy WP *et al.* Treatment of pernicious anemia with liver extract: effects upon the production of immature and mature red cells. *Am J Med Sci* 1928; 175: 599–606.

26. Gänsslen M. Ein hochwirksamer injizierbarer leberextrakt. *Klin Wochenschr* 1930; 9: 2099–2103.

27. Shorb MS. Unidentified growth factors for *Lactobacillus lactis* in refined liver extracts. *J Biol Chem* 1947; 169: 455–456.

28. Rickes EL, Brink NG, Koniuszy FR *et al.* Crystaline vitamin B12. *Science* 1948; 107: 396–397.

29. Smith EL, Parker LFJ. Purification of antipernicious anaemia factor. *Biochem J* 1948; 43: viii.

30. West R. Activity of vitamin B12 in Addisonian pernicious anemia. *Science* 1948; 107: 398.

31. Hodgkin DC, Kamper J, Mackay M *et al.* Structure of vitamin B12. *Nature* 1956; 178: 64–66.

32. Castle WB. 1. The effect of the administration to patients with pernicious anemia of the contents of the normal human stomach after ingestion of beef muscle. *Am J Med Sci* 1929; 178: 748–763.

33. Castle WB, Townsend WC, Heath CW: 111. The nature of the reaction between normal human gastric juice and beef muscle leading to clinical improvement and increased blood formation similar to the effect of liver feeding. *Am J Med Sci* 1930; 180: 305–335.

34. Grasbeck R, Simons K, Sinkkonnen I. Isolation of intrinsic factor and its probable degradation product as their vitamin B12 complexes from human gastric juice. *Biochem Biophys Acta* 1966; 127: 47–58.

35. Booth CC, Mollin DL. The site of absorption of vitamin B12 in man. *Lancet* 1959; 1: 18–21.

36. Wills L. Treatment of 'pernicious anaemia of pregnancy' and 'tropical anaemia' — with special reference to yeast extract as curative agent. *Brit Med J* 1931; 1: 1059–1064.

37. Wills L, Evans BDF. Tropical macrocytic anaemia: its relation to pernicious anaemia. *Lancet* 1938; 2: 416–421.

38. Mitchell HK, Snell EE, Williams RJ. The concentration of 'folic acid'. *J Am Chem. Soc* 1941; 63: 2284.

39. Pfiffner JJ, Binkley SB, Bloom ES *et al.* Isolation of the antianemia factor (vitaminBc) in crystalline form from liver. *Science* 1943; 97: 404–405.

40. Vaughan J. Tropical macrocytic anaemia. In: *Proceedings of the Royal Society for Medicine* (Discussion of Paper by L Wills) 1932; 25, 122.

41. Roe DA. Lucy Wills (1888–1964): a biographical sketch. *J Nutr* 1978; 107: 1379–1383.

42. Spies TD, Vilter CF, Koch MB. Observations of the anti-anemic properties of synthetic folic acid. *South Med J* 1945; 38: 707–709.

43. Chanarin I. *The Megaloblastic Anemias.* Oxford: Blackwell Scientific Publications; 1969.

44. Lavoie A, Tripp E, Hoffbrand AV. The effect of vitamin B12 on methylfolate metabolism and pteroylpolyglutamate synthesis in human cells. *Clin Sci Mol Med* 1975; 48: 617–630.

45. Hoffbrand AV, Ganeshaguru K, Hooton JWL, Tripp E. Megaloblastic anaemia: initiation of DNA synthesis in excess of DNA chain elongation as the underlying mechanism. *Clinics in Haematology* 1976; 5: 727–745.

46. Weir DG, Scott JM. The biochemical basis of the neuropathy in cobalamin deficiency. *Clinical Haematology* 1995; 8: 479–497.

47. Clarke R, Halsey J, Lewington S *et al.* Effects of lowering homocysteine levels with B vitamins on cardiovascular disease, cancer, and cause-specific mortality: meta-analysis of 8 randomized trials involving 37,485 individuals. *Arch Intern Med* 2010; 170: 1622–1631.

48. Farber S, Diamond LK, Mercer RD *et al.* Temporary remissions in acute leukemia in children produced by folic acid antagonist, 4-aminopteroylglutamic acid (Aminopterin). *N Engl J Med* 1948; 238: 787–793.

49. MRC Vitamin Research Group. Prevention of neural tube defects: results of the Medical Research Council Vitamin Study Group. *Lancet* 1991; 338: 131–137.

Chapter 3

THE DISCOVERY OF PENICILLIN

Eric Sidebottom

3.1 Introduction

The Nobel Prize in Physiology or Medicine in 1945 was awarded to Alexander Fleming, Ernst Chain, and Howard Florey, 'for the discovery of penicillin and its curative effect in various infectious diseases'.[1] The introduction of penicillin as the world's first antibiotic was arguably the most important medical advance of the 20th century. This chapter will address the extraordinary circumstances surrounding that discovery, the relative contributions of the three very different scientists who shared the prize (Fig. 3.1), and the ultimate impact of their discoveries on mankind.

The *discovery* of penicillin is usually attributed to the Scottish scientist Alexander Fleming in 1928. He showed that if *Penicillium notatum* is grown in an appropriate substrate it exudes a substance with antibiotic properties, which he dubbed penicillin. This serendipitous observation began the modern era of antibiotic discovery.[2] However, several other scientists had reported the bacteriostatic effects of *Penicillium* earlier than Fleming.[3] John Burdon Sanderson observed in 1870 that culture fluid covered with mould would produce fewer germs.[4] Joseph Lister, an English surgeon and the father of modern antisepsis, was prompted by Sanderson's discovery to investigate this mould. He described the antibacterial action on human tissue of what he called *Penicillium glaucum*. A nurse at King's College Hospital, whose wounds did not respond to any antiseptic, was given another substance that cured her, and Lister's registrar informed her that it was called Penicillium.[5]

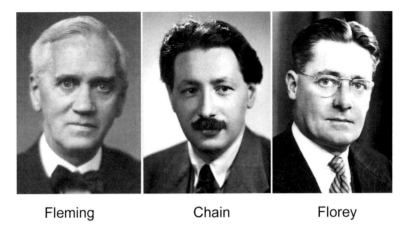

Fleming   Chain   Florey

Fig. 3.1. Winners of the Nobel Prize in Physiology or Medicine 1945 (Dunn School archives).

The role of Merlin Pryce in the discovery creates another uncertainty in the penicillin story.[6] Pryce was a young trainee pathologist who worked in Fleming's laboratory until early 1928 when he was transferred to another laboratory in Almroth Wright's department. On the fateful day in September 1928, Pryce called in to see Fleming on his return from holiday. One version of the story is that Pryce casually picked up Petri dishes from the discard bucket to glance at them and noticed the unusual appearance of the soon-to-be-famous contaminated plate. He passed it to Fleming for his opinion. The more conventional version is that it was Fleming who first picked up the plate and passed it to Pryce to show him the interesting phenomenon it displayed. Apparently twice in his later life Pryce claimed that he was the first to see the plate.

The *development* of penicillin for use as a medicine is attributed to the Australian Howard Walter Florey, together with the German Ernst Chain and the English biochemist Norman Heatley.[7,8] It has often been said that Norman Heatley (Fig. 3.2) only failed to share the Nobel Prize because no more than three people can share one prize. But until 1968, in principle, more than three persons **could** have shared a Nobel Prize, although this had never occurred in practice. The previous wording of the regulations was: 'A prize may be

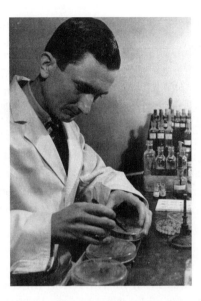

Fig. 3.2. Norman Heatley, 1940 (Dunn School archives).

equally divided between two works, each of which may be considered to merit a prize. If a work which is to be rewarded has been produced by two or more persons together, the prize shall be awarded to them jointly.' In 1968 this section was changed to read that, 'In no case may a prize be divided between more than three persons.'[9]

The statistics of the nomination process (which can only be accessed after 50 years) are themselves interesting. In 1944 there was one nomination for Fleming alone and one for Fleming, Florey, and Chain, and in 1945 there were six for Fleming alone, eight for Fleming and Florey, three for Fleming, Florey, and Richards (the leader of the American team), and only one for Fleming, Florey, and Chain. There were no nominations for Heatley.

There is no doubt that Fleming is by far the most 'famous' of this group. He was the only 20th-century scientist to reach the top 20 in a poll of top Britons of the past thousand years. He was in *Time* magazine's top 100 people of the 20th century. He appeared on the cover of *Time* magazine on 15 May 1944, and was *Picture Post*'s Man of the Year. He consistently appears in lists of 'the world's top 100 best scientists', even in the Top 100 Heroes of Western Culture. I am unaware of Florey ever appearing in such lists, which I find bizarre and will discuss later why this is so and how it came about.

3.2 Biographical Sketches[10]

These sketches are based on the Oxford DNB entries, Fleming by Michael Worboys, Florey by Gwyn Macfarlane, revised by Edward Abraham, and Chain by Edward Abraham (by permission of *Oxford Dictionary of National Biography*, Oxford University Press, 2004, General editors: Colin Matthew & Brian Harrison).

3.2.1 *Alexander Fleming*

Alexander Fleming was born in 1881, the third of four children of Hugh Fleming farmer, of Lochfield, near Darvel, in Ayrshire, who also had four surviving children from a previous marriage. He died when Alexander (known as Alec) was seven.

3.2.1.1 *Education and career*

Fleming's early education was in a small country school at Loudoun Moor, then Darvel School and Kilmarnock Academy. At 14 he went to live with a doctor stepbrother in London, where he spent two years at the Polytechnic Institute in Regent Street. The next four years were spent as a clerk in a shipping office but, on the advice of his stepbrother, in 1901 Alec entered St Mary's Hospital medical school, London, with a senior entrance scholarship. He qualified with an MB, BS of London University in 1908, winning the university gold medal. A year later he graduated FRCS but never practised as a surgeon. Fleming had a natural combativeness and urge to win, which were very apparent in the games he played. This determination to succeed was also evident in his medical and laboratory work, where he took delight in using his technical skill and inventiveness to overcome difficulties.

Immediately after qualification Fleming became an Assistant Bacteriologist at St Mary's. He joined the inoculation department and began the association with its head, Almroth Wright, which shaped his whole career. He worked with Wright in London and then in France during the First World War, and in 1920 he became Lecturer in Bacteriology at St Mary's medical school. In 1928 he was made Professor of Bacteriology at the University of London. He remained in the inoculation department, which eventually became the Wright–Fleming Institute of Microbiology, until he retired in 1948. He was Principal of the institute from 1946 to 1948, and an emeritus professor until 1954.

Until 1942 Fleming was an accomplished but undistinguished metropolitan laboratory scientist whose career had been in the shadow of Wright. Then suddenly, through no actions of his own, at the age of 61, he became an international celebrity because of his association with penicillin. Over the next decade he was fêted across the world and received numerous honours, medals, decorations, and prizes, including sharing the Nobel Prize in Physiology or Medicine with Chain and Florey in 1945. Fleming's name became synonymous with penicillin and the antibiotic revolution of the late 1940s and early 1950s. There is a fascination with what Fleming himself called 'the Fleming myth'; that is, why and how a single scientist was ever made responsible for the discovery of penicillin, and how a reserved hospital bacteriologist became an international celebrity.

3.2.1.2 *The antibiotic revolution and the Fleming myth*

The high profile given to penicillin changed Fleming's standing in science and medicine, starting with his election as a fellow of the Royal Society in 1943. Publicly, Fleming and Florey shared the credit for the revolutionary antibiotic drug, appearing on the same platform at scientific meetings. However, tensions remained and were not eased when Fleming, nearing retirement age, toured the world as a modern hero, while the younger Florey returned to his laboratory. On Wright's retirement in 1946, Fleming became head of the newly named Wright–Fleming Institute, but he was often away receiving many and varied accolades. He travelled widely in Europe and through the Americas as further prizes were awarded, honorary degrees by the dozen were conferred, statues unveiled, freedom of cities granted, and streets named in his honour.

3.2.1.3 *The man and his achievements*

Physically, Fleming was short and stockily built with powerful square shoulders, a deep chest, intensely light blue expressive eyes, and, for many years, a good crop of snowy white hair. He had great powers of physical endurance and seemed to stand up astonishingly well to the long travels and junketings he underwent. He was sensitive and sympathetic, enjoyed the simple things in life, and remained humble despite all the honours which were showered upon him. He was not an easy man to know, partly because of his natural reluctance to talk and to express his feelings. He was not a conversationalist and awkward silences were sometimes broken by awkward remarks: as one visitor put it, talking with him was like playing tennis with a man who, whenever you knocked the ball over to his side, put it in his pocket.

Sir Alexander Fleming remains one of the best-known British scientists of the 20th century. He became important for two reasons: first, his role in the development of modern antibiotics, and second, his place as an iconic British scientist. The catalogue of Fleming's published work leaves little room for doubt that he had, to an unusual degree, a faculty for original observation coupled with a high degree of technical inventiveness and skill. He made significant contributions to medical research in several fields and at St Mary's he was a pivotal figure in Wright's department, the influence of which was felt across the hospital and in medical science and clinical practice across the country.

Fleming married twice, first in 1915 to Sarah (Sareen), the daughter of a farmer from Ireland, and herself a trained nurse. They had one son, Robert, who qualified in medicine and entered general practice. Sareen died in 1949 and Fleming subsequently married Amalia Vourekas, a medically qualified Greek bacteriologist, in 1953.

Fleming died suddenly from a heart attack at his home in Chelsea, on 11 March 1955. He was cremated and his ashes interred in St Paul's Cathedral a week later.

3.2.2 Howard Florey

Howard Walter Florey was born in Adelaide, Australia, in 1898, the youngest child and only son of Joseph Florey, an Oxfordshire shoemaker who had emigrated in 1885. He was educated at Kyre College and St Peter's Collegiate School, Adelaide. He was clever, hard-working, and determined, winning six scholarships and many prizes. He was also good at games, representing his school (and later his university) at tennis, football, and athletics. In 1916 he entered Adelaide University medical school. There he was usually first in his class, winning three scholarships, and qualified as MB BS in 1921. He was awarded a Rhodes scholarship and worked his passage to England as a ship's surgeon, arriving in 1922.

3.2.2.1 Move to England

Florey enrolled in the department of physiology at Oxford under Sir Charles Sherrington, who recognized his drive and creative independence of mind, and became his most influential guide and friend. He obtained a first class in the Honour School of Physiology. In 1924 he moved to Cambridge to work as a student in the pathology department under Professor HR Dean, who, like Sherrington, felt that a more experimental approach to pathology could be achieved by an active young physiologist. The following year he was awarded a Rockefeller fellowship to go to the US and spent three months with Dr AN Richards in Philadelphia, a contact that later was to have enormous importance for the penicillin work.

3.2.2.2 Cambridge and early work on lysozyme

While in America Florey accepted the offer of a research fellowship at the London Hospital, where he worked with Paul Fildes. During this time he married Dr Mary Ethel Hayter (d. 1966), whom he had known as a medical student in Adelaide; later they had a son and a daughter. Florey did not enjoy life in London and when offered a lectureship in pathology at Cambridge in 1927, he eagerly accepted. There he appointed a new laboratory boy — the 14-year-old Jim Kent, who was to stay as his indispensable and devoted assistant for the next 41 years, and who contributed so much to the success of his research projects. Florey became a Fellow of Gonville and Caius College and its Director of Medical Studies, and gained a Cambridge PhD for his research on blood and lymph flow. During the next four years he began several fruitful lines of study, one of which had momentous consequences. In 1922 Alexander Fleming had accidentally discovered an agent in mucoid secretions which dissolved certain bacteria. He called it 'lysozyme' and supposed that it might normally prevent infection. Florey took up lysozyme in 1929 because he thought that its presence in mucus might explain its antibacterial action. In 1932 he was appointed Joseph Hunter Professor of Pathology at Sheffield University, where tetanus, gastrointestinal function, and lysozyme were amongst his research interests.

3.2.2.3 *Chair of Pathology in Oxford and the development of penicillin*

In 1934 the Chair of the Sir William Dunn School of Pathology in Oxford became unexpectedly vacant on the sudden death of Georges Dreyer and Florey was appointed, being strongly supported by Edward Mellanby, Secretary of the Medical Research Council. Florey brought his department to life largely by attracting young postgraduates who had their own grants. The quality of his and their research attracted others and within a few years the Oxford School of Pathology was among the best laboratories of its kind in the world. Florey expanded his own lines of research to include these new recruits, forming teams in which each contributed some special expertise, and over which he kept a general but not authoritarian control. The most productive line was that which established the clinical value of penicillin. In 1949 a complete account of the Oxford work done at that time was published as a two-volume book, *Antibiotics*, by Florey and six of his collaborators.[3]

3.2.2.4 *Recognition and its rewards*

In scientific and medical circles the Oxford achievement had been recognized and applauded. Florey was elected a fellow of the Royal

Society in 1941, before the true value of penicillin had been established. Thereafter many other honours followed. He was knighted in 1944, and in 1945 he shared the Nobel Prize with Chain and Fleming. In 1960 Florey was elected President of the Royal Society, and he brought to it a vitality which rejuvenated that rather staid organization and imbued its officers and staff with a new sense of purpose. A major change for which he was largely responsible was the move from the society's elegant but cramped quarters in Burlington House to the far more spacious Carlton House Terrace. He also widened the society's interests to include applied science and demography, and he opened its doors to lively discussion meetings and study groups which extended its already great influence.

In 1962 Florey became Provost of Queen's College, Oxford, and relinquished his Chair of Pathology. In 1965 he was created a life peer as Baron Florey of Adelaide and Marston and a member of the Order of Merit. He had also become a commander of the Légion d'Honneur, and had received the US Medal for Merit and the Royal and the Copley medals of the Royal Society.

In 1966 Ethel Florey died after some years of disabling ill health. The following year Florey married Margaret Augusta Jennings, daughter of the third Baron Cottesloe and formerly wife of Denys Jennings. She had worked in fruitful collaboration with Florey at the School of Pathology since 1936. For some years Florey had suffered from angina and he died suddenly from a heart attack in Oxford on 21 February 1968.

3.2.3 *Ernst Chain*

Ernst Boris Chain was born in 1906 in Berlin, the only son of a Russian-born industrial chemist. Chain's parents were both Jewish, and faith played an important role in the house. He was educated in Berlin at the Luisengymnasium and the University of Berlin from which he graduated in chemistry and physiology in 1930. He then obtained a doctorate for research in the chemical department of the Institute of Pathology at the Charité Hospital. After graduation Chain dabbled with the idea of a musical career, but he was advised that, although a good pianist, he would never be a truly great one.

3.2.3.1 *Move to Britain*

With the rise of Hitler to power in 1933 Chain emigrated to Britain and sought to begin a scientific career. After a few months at University College Hospital, London, he obtained a place in the biochemistry department at Cambridge where he worked under Sir Frederick Gowland Hopkins for a second PhD, believing a Cambridge doctorate would advance an English career.

The election of Howard Florey to the Chair of Pathology at Oxford in 1935 set the scene for Chain's subsequent life. Florey believed that experimental pathology would benefit from the collaboration of pathologists with chemists and invited Chain to develop biochemistry within the Sir William Dunn School of Pathology. In 1936 he became university Lecturer and Demonstrator in Chemical Pathology. At Florey's suggestion he began to study the mode of action of a bacteriolytic enzyme, lysozyme. This led him to read other accounts of the production of anti-microbial substances by micro-organisms, and, during discussions with Florey, he suggested that they should jointly investigate some of these substances. Their decision to do this was motivated by scientific rather than medical interest, but fortunately penicillin was one of three substances chosen for study.

Although Chain was confident that the problem of penicillin's instability could be overcome, little progress with its purification was made until Norman Heatley suggested that it could be transferred from organic solvent into a neutral aqueous solution. In the spring of 1940 Florey, urged by Chain to begin his intended biological experiments, showed that preparations of penicillin less than 1% pure would protect mice from lethal infections with streptococci and staphylococci. This dramatic result entirely changed the focus of research. High priority was given to the laboratory production of enough penicillin for a small clinical trial. With the success of this trial, even using only 3% pure preparations, penicillin suddenly became a substance of major medical importance and of potential value in surgery during the Second World War.

Chain, together with Edward Abraham, showed some bacteria were resistant to penicillin because of their production of a penicillin-inactivating enzyme, penicillinase.[11] They continued their attempts to purify penicillin and, early in 1943, together with Sir Robert Robinson and Wilson Baker, they studied its chemistry. Chain, with Abraham, became a strong supporter of a β-lactam structure for penicillin, which was proposed in 1943 but remained controversial until Dorothy Hodgkin and Barbara Low confirmed it two years later by X-ray crystallography. During these war years Chain played an active part in a major Anglo–American enterprise to produce penicillin by chemical synthesis. Although this collaborative effort threw interesting light on the chemistry of penicillin it failed in its final aim. (The total synthesis of penicillin was only achieved in 1957 by John Sheehan.[12]) In the event, it was the increased yield obtainable by fermentation of *Penicillium chrysogenum* that enabled penicillin to be produced on a large scale.

Chain stimulated Florey and in the early years their relationship was amicable, but it deteriorated when Chain began to complain that he was receiving too little credit for his research, attributing this to his foreign background.

3.2.3.2 *Moves to and from Rome*

In 1948 Chain left Oxford for Rome to become Director of a new international research centre for chemical microbiology at the Istituto Superiore di Sanità. Before leaving he married Dr Anne Beloff, a biochemist, and they had three children; they subsequently collaborated in studies of the mode of action of insulin. In Rome, Chain set up a pilot plant for antibiotic production. He was strongly in favour of collaboration between academic and industrial institutions. He became a consultant to the Beecham Group and suggested that it should explore further the potential of penicillin. Two members of this company, GN Rolinson and FR Batchelor, were seconded to his laboratory in 1956 to become acquainted with penicillin fermentation. During their visit they made observations that later led to the isolation of the nucleus of the penicillin molecule, 6-amino penicillanic acid, and to the chemical synthesis from this nucleus of a series of new and clinically valuable penicillins.

In the 1950s Chain became anxious about the future of the Istituto Superiore di Sanità after its influential director-general, Domenico Marotta, had retired. In 1961 he accepted the Chair of Biochemistry at Imperial College, London, although he retained his position in Rome until 1964.

Chain's role in the initiation of the work on penicillin in Oxford was his major contribution to medicine. He shared a Nobel Prize with Fleming and Florey in 1945 and was elected to the Fellowship of the Royal Society in 1949. He became an Honorary Fellow of the Royal College of Physicians in 1965 and was knighted in 1969. But like Fleming his many honours came predominantly from other countries. He retired from Imperial College in 1973 and died in 1979 in the holiday home he had built in County Mayo, Ireland.

3.3 Steps in the Discovery and Development of Penicillin

In September (probably on the 3rd) 1928 Fleming made the now world-famous observation of a mould inhibiting the growth of bacteria. The details are not clear since the observations were not written up for some weeks. On his return from holiday he noticed, on a discarded plate, that the staphylococcal colonies were absent from an area around a contaminating mould. The contaminant was originally identified as *Penicillium rubrum* but later this was corrected to *Penicillium notatum*, a common mould found across the world. Fleming presumed that the contamination was accidental and that the mould had entered his laboratory through an open window. He worked with the mould and its 'juice' for the next six months, in the first instance determining which pathogenic germs were susceptible. His hopes that he had found a clinically useful natural antiseptic were not fulfilled. One problem was that the action of the mould juice was slow. Also, in animal experiments, Fleming had difficulties in maintaining high enough concentrations around infected areas before the juice lost potency or was excreted. This work suggested that penicillin had little potential as a systemic antibacterial, but would be of limited value in the treatment of local infections. Indeed, in his first recorded clinical use of penicillin, Fleming irrigated an infected surgical wound, using methods similar to those developed by Wright in the First World War.

Fleming first spoke about this work to the Medical Research Club in February 1929. His talk was entitled, 'A medium for the isolation of Pfeiffer's bacillus'. Sir Henry Dale, who was chairman for the meeting, remembers nothing of importance in the talk.[13] There were apparently no questions and no discussion. Fleming published his findings in the *British Journal of Experimental Pathology* on 10 May.[2] The conclusions of this paper make it clear that Fleming regarded penicillin as a new natural antiseptic, whose main properties were its effects on septic and pneumonia germs. Its great advantage was that it did not interfere with white blood cell function, which Wright and his group thought was all-important in natural immunity. Fleming also discussed the use of penicillin in bacteriological laboratories, where he used it in culture media to prevent the growth of unwanted, susceptible organisms. The paper was not received as epoch-making at the time; it was cast within the tradition of Fleming's previous work on lysozyme, Wright's notions of immunity, general scepticism to the use of antiseptics in anything other than local infections, and innovations in bacteriological techniques.

There has been much debate on why the therapeutic potential of penicillin was not recognized in 1929. Some early biographers, perhaps influenced by the Fleming myth, claimed that Fleming immediately saw the value of his mould juice and was prevented from developing it owing to a lack of support and the antagonism of colleagues. However, it now seems that Sir Henry Dale was correct when he wrote that, 'Neither the time when the discovery was made nor, perhaps, the scientific atmosphere of the laboratory in which he worked, was propitious to such further enterprise as its development would have needed.'[13] Through the 1930s Fleming used penicillin in a small number of cases as a local antiseptic and as a laboratory reagent for selective culture. In 1931 he wrote a sceptical review on the value of intravenous germicides and, very significantly, chose not to mention penicillin in this context. However, in the late 1930s, when Chain and Florey began to test antibacterial substances, they used a culture of Fleming's mould that had been maintained at Oxford. By then, however, Fleming was preoccupied with other projects.

In 1935, soon after taking up his Chair in Oxford, Florey engaged a young refugee biochemist, Ernst Chain, and asked him to discover how lysozyme dissolved bacteria. Chain found it was an enzyme which attacks a specific bacterial structure. While reviewing the literature on lysozyme, Chain came across the paper by Fleming, published in 1929, describing the chance discovery of a *Penicillium* mould that apparently dissolved pathogenic bacteria in its vicinity.[2] Chain also found a culture of Fleming's mould in the School of Pathology. Florey had been well aware of many instances in which one micro-organism inhibited another. However, he had not been particularly interested in penicillin, even though Dr CG Paine, who was a junior pathologist in his department in Sheffield, had drawn Florey's attention to his limited success with *Penicillium* culture filtrates in local eye treatments. Paine was a graduate of St Mary's and had worked with Fleming in 1928 and was aware of the penicillin work. Indeed, he had taken a culture to Sheffield and grown it himself. Unfortunately the results of his treatments were not published until much later (by Wainwright[14]) and, like Fleming, he quickly moved to other work.

Florey also noted the fact that Harold Raistrick and his colleagues had abandoned an attempt to purify this labile substance at the London School of Hygiene,[15] but he agreed with Chain that a study of antibacterial substances produced by micro-organisms might widen the research, since that on lysozyme as a therapeutic agent seemed to be reaching a dead end. They decided to work together on three such products, from *Bacillus subtilis*, *Bacillus pyocyaneus*, and *Penicillium notatum*. The project was submitted to the Medical Research Council in 1939 when requests for a special grant yielded £25 and the possibility of £100 later. However, the Rockefeller Institute granted $5,000 (£1,200) per annum for five years, a considerable sum at the time. Preliminary experiments showed that penicillin was the most promising of the substances chosen for study, and might have therapeutic as well as scientific importance. Thereafter the project became a team one. Norman Heatley undertook the production of the mould filtrate and the assay of the active penicillin; Chain, later joined by Edward

Abraham, worked on the purification and chemistry, while Florey and Margaret Jennings (who later became his second wife) carried out the animal work and, with Professor AD Gardner, the bacteriology.

On Saturday 25 May 1940 there was enough penicillin, still less than 1% pure, to discover if it could protect mice from an otherwise lethal infection – a crucial test. Eight mice were injected with virulent streptococci, and an hour later four of these had injections of the crude penicillin. All 4 untreated mice were dead within 16 hours; all the treated mice were alive and well the next day. Florey's remark, 'It looks promising', was a typically laconic assessment of one of the most important experiments in medical history. The results of a large series of such experiments, published in August 1940[7] completely confirmed the initial promise. After reading the results in the *Lancet*, Fleming phoned Florey and arranged to visit Oxford in September to catch up with the work. It is reputed that, on hearing that Fleming was about to visit, Chain said, 'Oh I thought he was dead.'

Florey tried to persuade British drug firms to produce enough penicillin to treat human cases, but they were already hard-pressed by wartime needs and bomb damage. Since, as Florey noted, humans are 3,000 times larger than mice, vastly more penicillin would be needed for human trials. He therefore turned his own department into a small factory. Many physical, chemical, biological, and administrative difficulties were overcome by collaborative perseverance and ingenuity, and by Florey's energy, determination, and personal example. But once again the technical ingenuity of Heatley deserves mention. He was responsible for the design of the ceramic bed pans in which the penicillium cultures were grown by the six penicillin girls specially employed, and for much of the semi-automated apparatus used for the extraction and purification of the antibiotic.

By January 1941, it was considered that there was enough penicillin for a limited trial on patients at the Radcliffe Infirmary under the direction of Charles Fletcher. The first case treated, on 12 February 1941, was Albert Alexander, a 43-year-old policeman, who was moribund with overwhelming staphylococcal and streptococcal infection. He made a dramatic improvement within 24 hours but after 5 days the supply of penicillin was exhausted (4.4 g administered — perhaps

200,000 units). He slowly relapsed and died a month later. Other cases chosen were of similar hopeless infections. Although only six could be treated systematically — and even these with restricted doses — the results were conclusive. Penicillin had been shown to overcome infections which were beyond any other treatment. The results were published in the *Lancet* in August 1941.[8]

In June 1941, with Mellanby's approval but arousing Chain's anger since he had not been consulted, Florey and Heatley went to the US to try to enlist commercial help. Florey's old colleague AN Richards (now chairman of the US Medical Research Committee) promised government support for firms prepared to develop large-scale methods of production, and three accepted. While Heatley remained to assist the US companies, Florey returned to Oxford at the end of September to direct an even greater production effort in his department. This allowed a completely conclusive trial on 187 cases in 1942, largely carried out by Florey's wife, Ethel.[16]

Fleming first made public his proprietorial claims to penicillin in a letter to the *BMJ* on 13 September 1941.[17] He crossed swords in print with the Oxford Group, claiming that as well as having discovered the antibacterial properties of the substance he had recognized its potential as a systemic antibacterial drug. Over the next 12 months work on penicillin continued at Oxford and the government began to take an interest in developing large-scale production. Soon the US government, as well as universities and pharmaceutical companies, became involved. While relations between Fleming and the Oxford Group were not cordial, they did not prevent Fleming obtaining enough penicillin from Oxford in August 1942 to treat an employee of his brother's, who subsequently recovered from severe septicaemia and meningitis.

Over the summer of 1942 press reports about penicillin and its powers increased in number. The differences between Fleming, and Chain and Florey – St Mary's versus Oxford – continued to simmer below the surface. However, on 31 August differences became public when a letter from Wright was published in *The Times*. Never one to shirk controversy or hold back in promoting his St Mary's department, Wright claimed priority for Fleming as both the discoverer of penicillin and for recognizing its value in antibacterial therapy. The following day, a letter from Sir Robert Robinson, Professor of Chemistry at Oxford, was published, stating that if Fleming deserved a 'laurel wreath' for penicillin, then Howard Florey should be given a 'handsome bouquet'. The press descended on both St Mary's and Oxford, but found Fleming more accommodating, and his role in the penicillin story came to dominate. The therapy attracted press attention as it promised good news at a time when the war situation was uncertain. Fleming's life, with his humble background and long road to success, made a romantic story.

In the summer of 1943 Florey and Hugh Cairns went to North Africa to find out how a small amount of penicillin could be used most efficiently for the treatment of war wounds. Six months later Florey went to Russia with information on the new results. Meanwhile commercial production had, at last, begun in Britain, and this revealed that certain technical methods had been patented in America. Florey was criticized for having given away a valuable commercial asset. The information which Florey gave in America had been freely offered earlier in Britain. But in America it was discovered that much larger amounts of penicillin might be obtained by deep fermentation in large aerated vessels and this was to change the whole outlook on penicillin production. It was then considered unethical in Britain for those in medical research to patent medical discoveries. Soon after the end of the war the official attitude to patenting changed completely and this was to have profound consequences for Oxford. Edward Abraham continued the antibiotic work for the rest of his life but his seminal discoveries on the isolation and purification of Cephalosporin drugs were now protected by patents, the proceeds of which have helped to establish trust funds which have benefited research and education in Oxford and beyond enormously.

3.4 The Impact of the Introduction of Penicillin into Clinical Practice

Many claims have been made about the impact of penicillin on mankind. 'Two hundred million lives saved', 'seismic impact', '*the* drug of the 20th century', are typical, but it is impossible to get an accurate or objective view of the true impact. In its early years of use it really seemed like a miracle drug and it transformed the treatment of war wounds (and, incidentally, gonorrhoea and syphilis) during the war years. The lives saved provided a wonderful 'good news story' that did much to improve the morale of the troops and the war effort at home. It became a 'brand' model in the same way as Hoover and Biro had. The mechanism of action of penicillin also fulfilled the criteria for Ehrlich's 'magic bullet'. Penicillin interferes with a specific chemical reaction that is necessary for the synthesis of bacterial cell walls but does not occur at all in mammalian cells. In that sense it is the ideal therapeutic agent since it is not toxic at therapeutic doses.

The 'miracle' antibiotic era probably reached its height of optimism in the late 1960s, when former US Surgeon General William Stewart is credited with stating, when testifying before Congress, that it was 'time to close the book on infectious disease, declare the war against pestilence won'.[18] In 1953 the Nobel Prize-winning Sir Macfarlane Burnet said, 'One can think of the middle of the 20th century as the end of one of the most important social revolutions in history – the virtual elimination of infectious disease as a factor in social life.'[19] These were clearly naive predictions and it is interesting in this context to go back to Fleming's statement in his Nobel lecture that, 'there is the danger that the ignorant man may easily underdose himself and by exposing his microbes to non-lethal quantities of the drug make them resistant'.[20]

3.5 From Triumph to Tragedy?

Robert Bud's 2007 *Penicillin: Triumph and Tragedy* attempts to discuss in a balanced way not only the undoubted benefits bestowed by penicillin — the triumphs — but also the problems it has created. He thinks that the casting of penicillin as a wonder drug has done more harm than good in the long term. The book devotes more space to the tragedies than the triumphs, the development of resistance leading to so-called superbugs, and the flagrant misuse of antibiotics, not only by doctors and patients but also by vets and farmers and those concerned with animals as food. As noted above, Fleming had warned about the possible development of resistance following inadequate treatment in his Nobel lecture.[20] Bud ends on a sombre note: 'Reformulating a global brand trusted for half a century and finding new methods of managing health care is a major challenge. Up to now the Aristotelian progress of a tragedy has been faithfully followed. Will it end with the final dramatic phase: *catastrophe*? At the beginning of the 21st century the prognosis is still uncertain.'[21]

3.6 The Creation of the Fleming Myth

It is easy to see how the myth was created. Firstly, in the early years of the war Britain was in great need of good news and national heroes. As it became obvious that penicillin was indeed a miracle drug which could save the lives of wounded soldiers who previously would have died, anyone associated with that miracle was a potential hero. However, a modest and quiet Scotsman was perhaps a better hero than either a rather gruff, rough colonial or an émigré German Jew. At this time the contribution of Norman Heatley was hardly known by anyone. Fleming may have started with an advantage in this way but that advantage was hugely increased by the second factor working for him: his three St Mary's 'backers'. It is interesting to speculate who was the most important or effective. Might it have been Lord Beaverbrook, the press baron, who was also a generous benefactor and patron of St Mary's Hospital? After Fleming's death he wrote: [22]

> Sir Alexander Fleming was a genius…during his life in his own land recognition of his genius was grudging…. I became indignant on his behalf. I was anxious that justice should be done to this great pioneer. It seemed to me that it was a duty laid on me as the proprietor of newspapers in Britain, the country which gained a measure of reflected glory on account of Fleming's immense achievement.

Another supporter, Charles McMoran Wilson, who became Lord Moran in 1943, Dean of St Mary's Hospital Medical School from 1920 until 1945, President of the Royal College of Physicians from 1941 to 1950, and Churchill's wartime physician, was a man of considerable social standing and influence. He apparently had attracted the nickname 'corkscrew Charlie' for his devious ways! In addition, Fleming's 'boss' was Almroth Wright, also a man of considerable social standing and influence, and naturally keen to enhance the reputation of his own department in which Fleming worked. These three men together mounted an extremely effective campaign to put St Mary's firmly on the 'penicillin map'. Fleming himself did not make unreasonable claims about what he had discovered, but neither did he go out of his way to contradict some of the grossly exaggerated claims made for St Mary's in the popular press. Indeed he apparently kept such press cuttings in a file labelled 'Myths'! Starting in August 1942 with Wright's letter to *The Times* claiming the laurel wreath for Fleming, there were literally hundreds of reports in the press that focused on Fleming and St Mary's with rarely a mention of Florey and Oxford.

Another factor was that Florey wouldn't talk to the press. He was a typical scientist, rather suspicious of the media. But more importantly he feared that if the news that his laboratory was preparing penicillin in Oxford became widely known he would have many sick people or their carers on his doorstep pleading to be given the 'miracle' drug. I think that these factors taken together explain the origins of what I now call 'Medicine's first spin story' but I do not understand how the truth can have been so distorted.

3.7 Allocation of Credit Due and Conclusions

It is interesting that Eric Lax, in his recent book, *The Mould in Dr Florey's Coat: The Remarkable True Story of the Penicillin Miracle*, heads chapters on the three Laureates, 'the quiet Scot', 'the rough colonial genius', and 'the temperamental continental'.[23]

The assignment of the title 'genius' to an individual is a highly contentious and much discussed issue. Fleming has often been called a genius and compared to Galileo, Newton, Pasteur, and Einstein by the media, but rarely by scientists and colleagues who knew and understood his work. However, Sir Paul Nurse, the current President of the Royal Society, and himself a Nobel Prize winner, was one of the presenters of the recent Channel 4 TV series *Genius of Britain*, first screened in June 2010. He stated not only that Fleming was 'a great scientist', but then posed the question, 'So what was the genius of Alexander Fleming?' He replied, 'Well, you know, partly it's as Pasteur said, "chance favours the prepared mind" and Fleming's mind had been prepared during the First World War by seeing people dying of infection.' This treatment of Fleming as a genius is in strange contrast with the view expressed by Professor Ronald Hare in a BBC *Horizon* programme made in the late 1980s. Hare worked with Fleming in St Mary's Hospital and said of him, 'Fleming was a third-rate scientist like me.'

On the question of who was the greater scientist, however, a straightforward examination of the careers of Fleming and Florey and a close examination of each man's papers on penicillin surely indicates that Florey was a better scientist than Fleming. It is also important to note that Florey was a team player and a great leader who inspired the members of his team to follow his example, whereas Fleming was essentially a loner in the laboratory. This was clearly reflected in the attitude towards addressing the difficult problems of extracting and purifying penicillin from culture filtrate, 'juice' — Fleming quickly gave up whereas Florey's team persisted and came up with solutions.

The view from Oxford is naturally subject to charges of bias and prejudice but it is hard not to conclude that the St Mary's Hospital publicity machine was extremely effective. In answer to the question I am frequently asked, 'How would you attribute the credit for the work that resulted in the introduction of penicillin into clinical practice as the world's first antibiotic?', I now say, 'Fleming 10%, Chain 20%, Heatley 30%, and Florey 40%.' This is, of course, extremely simplistic and ignores not only the seven other names on the Oxford memorial (Fig. 3.3) but those Americans who contributed to the upscaling and industrial development of the manufacture of penicillin. However, in the final analysis, like Gwyn Macfarlane,[24,25] I remain pessimistic in that I think it unlikely that the general public will ever comprehend the real truth about the discovery and development of penicillin, 'the 20th century's most important medical discovery'.

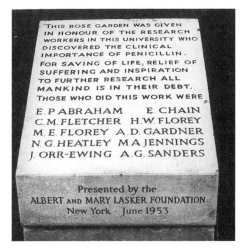

Fig. 3.3. The stone memorial commemorating the work of the Oxford team who isolated and purified penicillin and conducted the first clinical trials (Dunn School archives).

References

1. The Nobel Prize in Physiology or Medicine 1945. Available at: http://nobelprize.org/nobel_prizes/medicine/laureates/1945 [Accessed 18 May 2011].
2. Fleming A. On the antibacterial action of cultures of a penicillium, with special reference to their use in the isolation of B. influenzae. *Br J Exp Path* 1929; 10: 226–236.
3. Florey HW, Chain E, Heathley NG *et al. Antibiotics: a survey of penicillin, streptomycin and other antimicrobial substances from fungi, actinomycetes, bacteria and plants.* Oxford: Oxford University Press; 1949.
4. Burdon Sanderson J. *Appendix 5 in the 13th Report of the Medical Officer of the Privy Council. 1870.* London: HM Stationery Office; 1871; p56–66.
5. Lister J. *Commonplace books.* London: Royal College of Surgeons; 1871; 1: 31–45.
6. Dr Merlin Pryce. Phil Carradice. BBC Radio Wales. 12 July 2010.
7. Chain EB, Florey HW, Gardner, AD *et al.* Penicillin as a chemotherapeutic agent. *Lancet* 1940; ii: 226–228.

8. Abraham EP, Chain EB, Fletcher CM *et al.* Further observations on penicillin. *Lancet* 1941; ii: 177–188.

9. The Nobel Foundation — Special Regulations. Available at: http://nobelprize.org/nobel_prizes/nobelprize_facts.html [Accessed 18 May 2011].

10. Matthew C, Harrison B (general eds). Oxford *Dictionary of National Biography*. Oxford: Oxford University Press; 2004.

11. Abraham EP, Chain EB. An enzyme from bacteria able to destroy penicillin. *Nature* (Lond) 1940; 146. 837.

12. Sheehan JC. *The enchanted ring: the untold story of penicillin*. Cambridge, MA: MIT Press; 1982.

13. Dale HH. Letter. *Br Lib Add*. MSS 56219.

14. Wainwright M, Swan HT. CG Paine and the earliest surviving clinical records of penicillin therapy. *Medical History* 1996; 30: 42–56.

15. Clutterbuck PW, Lovell R, Raistrick H. Studies in the biochemistry of micro-organisms, 26. *Biochem J* 1932; 26: 1907–1918.

16. Florey ME, Florey HW. General and local administration of penicillin. *Lancet* 1943; i: 387–397.

17. Fleming, A. Penicillin. *BMJ* 1941; ii: 386.

18. The Office of the Historian of the Public Health Service http://lhncbc.nlm.nih.gov/apdb/phsHistory/faqs.html.

19. Macfarlane Burnet C. *The Natural History of Infectious Disease*. Cambridge: Cambridge University Press; 1953.

20. Fleming A. *Nobel Lecture* (1945) Available at: http://nobelprize.org/nobel_prizes/medicine/laureates/1945/fleming-lecture.html [Accessed 18 May 2011].

21. Bud R. *Penicillin; Triumph and Tragedy*. Oxford: Oxford University Press; 2007.

22. Lord Beaverbrook. Statement made 5 June 1956. Br. Lib. Add. MSS 56217.

23. Lax E. *The Mould in Dr Florey's Coat*. Boston: Little Brown; 2004.

24. Macfarlane RG. *Howard Florey, The Making of a Great Scientist*. Oxford: Oxford University Press; 1979.

25. Macfarlane RG. *Alexander Fleming: the man and the myth*. London: Chatto and Windus; 1984.

Chapter 4

THE INTRODUCTION OF CARDIAC CATHETERISATION

Tony Seed

4.1 Prologue

During the summer of 1929 a 24-year-old German medical graduate called Werner Forssmann went, in his lunch hour, to the operating room of a small provincial hospital outside Berlin where he was training in surgery, rolled up his left sleeve and infiltrated his antecubital fossa with local anaesthetic. He then made a skin incision, hooked out the antecubital vein with an aneurysm needle, made a small incision in it and inserted the tip of a ureteric catheter (size: Charrière 4/1.3 mm diameter) which had been stored in sterile olive oil. He advanced the catheter proximally into the vein, 'without resistance'[1] and then walked along a corridor and downstairs to the X-ray department in the basement. There, he positioned himself against a fluoroscopic screening apparatus, whilst a nurse held a mirror so that he could watch on the screen as he advanced the catheter. When he had inserted the full 65 cm length of the catheter the tip was lying in the right atrium. He took an X-ray to confirm this (Fig. 4.1), walked back to the operating room, removed the catheter and dressed the incision in his elbow. He reported no complications from the procedure other than slight inflammation at the incision site, which he attributed to inadequate aseptic technique. His account of the experiment was published later that year,[1] by which time, desperate to get a lectureship in a university hospital, he was working as an unpaid assistant to the Professor of Surgery in Berlin. The story goes that when the article appeared, he was sacked — with the comment that he might lecture in a circus but not in a respectable German university.[2]

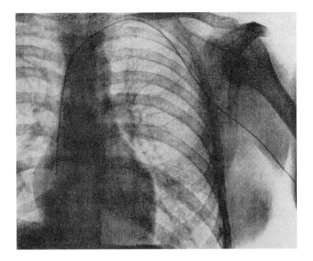

Fig. 4.1. The 1929 radiograph of Forssmann's chest showing the position of the catheter he had inserted from his left forearm. The tip of the catheter is in the right atrium. (Reproduced from ref. 1 with permission from Springer Science and Business Media).

4.2 Introduction

The Nobel Prize in Medicine was awarded to Werner Forssmann, André Cournand and Dickinson Richards in 1956 for their discoveries concerning heart catheterisation and pathological changes in the circulatory system. By the time of the award, right heart catheterisation had been cleared of the many doubts about safety which hindered its early development and had made possible many studies of cardiac and pulmonary function in both normal and disease states.

Forssmann's original contribution, although pioneering and dramatic, did not lead to a general acceptance of the method; prejudice and safety doubts surrounded the method for years, and dispelling them called for resources and collaborators, which he lacked. Cournand and Richards, on the other hand, were career investigative physicians who worked in major American teaching centres and were involved in a long-term programme of research in circulatory and respiratory physiology and pathophysiology. In their hands the technique led to a multiplicity of cardiac and pulmonary insights, both physiological and pathophysiological, during the 20 years preceding the Nobel Prize award and for nearly ten years afterwards. Alongside their work, innovations in technique and equipment by others yielded new diagnostic methods and therapeutic interventions which are still evolving today.

It needs to be emphasised that the work which led to the Nobel Prize was based on catheterisation of the *right* heart and pulmonary circulation. Catheterisation of the left heart, which was only just beginning in the 1950s, lies outside the scope of this chapter.

4.3 Biographical Background of the Laureates

4.3.1 *Werner Forssmann*

Werner Forssmann (Fig. 4.2, left), an only child, was born in Berlin in 1904 and went to school and university there. He lived through the First World War (losing his father) and then in the midst of the subsequent hyperinflation, funded by his mother and inspired by an uncle who ran a country medical practice, went to the University of

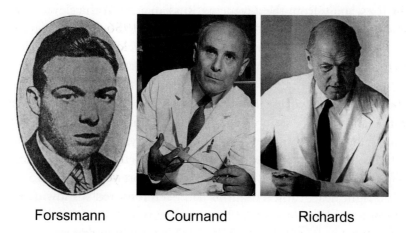

Forssmann   Cournand   Richards

Fig. 4.2.   Werner Forssmann (left) as a young surgeon (reproduced from ref. 3); André Cournand (centre), catheter in hand, photographed on the day the Nobel Prize award was announced (reproduced from ref. 6); Dickinson Richards (right; reproduced from ref. 7, with permission from Elsevier).

Berlin to study medicine. He graduated in February 1929 with the promise of a job in the Academic Department of Internal Medicine, but this fell through and he was faced with the need to earn a living. The reality of the time was that the principal route into academic internal medicine was through long, unpaid assistantships, vying for the few paid posts, and he turned instead to a surgical trainee post, obtained through family contacts, in a small Red Cross Hospital in Eberswalde, a provincial town about 45 miles from Berlin. It was there, some six months later, that he catheterised his own heart and published the account of it.

It did not help his career. Much of the comment and publicity which followed publication was hostile, and although he made several attempts to get back into academic centres in Berlin, working either unpaid or for a pittance, he was considered by the establishment as an ill-disciplined upstart with inappropriate research ideas. So in 1932 he took a surgical post in Mainz, where he married a young surgeon called Elsbet Engel, and began specialising in urology, working in a number of cities before returning to a senior post in Berlin in 1938. Then came the Second World War, and conscription into the army. After a spell in Norway he served on the Eastern Front in Russia, finally escaping from the advancing Russian army at the eleventh hour by swimming across the River Elbe with his shoes strung round his neck and surrendering to the American Army. When he was released at the end of the war his job was gone, his apartment bombed and his possessions lost. But his wife and children had survived by fleeing Berlin for a small village in the Black Forest; there they were reunited and he and his wife set up a family practice until, in 1950, he found a urology post and returned to his old speciality.

Through all these events he was isolated from the world of cardiology, unaware that his work had not been forgotten. By 1945 some 1,200 right heart catheterisations had been reported worldwide without mishap,[4] but almost the first that Forssmann knew about all this was in 1951, when Professor John McMichael invited him to London to contribute to a filmed documentary on cardiac catheterisation being made at the Hammersmith Hospital. Later in the same year Forssmann met André Cournand for the first time — 20 years after his own historic experiment, and ten years after Cournand's influential paper[5] established catheterisation as a clinical method in the US.

When the Nobel Prize award was announced in 1956, he was encouraged by colleagues to return to experimental cardiology but declined; he felt too remote from the subject and too out of date. Instead he continued his surgical career until his retirement in 1969, when he moved back to his old village in the Black Forest. He died there following a myocardial infarct in 1979, aged 74, survived by his wife and six children.

4.3.2 *André Cournand*

André Cournand (Fig. 4.2, centre) was born in 1895, the son of a Paris dental surgeon. He went to school there, and entered first year medical school in the autumn of 1914. Within a year he left to join the army and spent three years in the trenches, winning the Croix de Guerre and ending the war as a patient in a military hospital before returning to Paris to restart his medical course. He qualified in 1925 and spent the next six years training in internal medicine under a succession of distinguished teaching hospital clinicians. He walked and climbed in the Alps and lived in the avant-garde art world of Paris, meeting and later marrying Sybille, whose mother ran an art gallery. He completed his training with an MD dissertation, intending to enter private practice as a chest physician. To prepare for this, and to improve his English, he decided to spend a year in the US and obtained a residency in the Chest Service of Bellevue Hospital in New York, which was affiliated with Columbia University Medical School.

He moved there in 1930, and worked in the Chest Service for some months before being asked to set up a pulmonary function laboratory; he was advised in doing this by Dickinson Richards, a clinical scientist at Presbyterian Hospital. The two became friendly, and shortly afterwards Richards invited him to join in a research collaboration to develop and exploit new methods to investigate cardiopulmonary function in patients with heart and lung disease. This meant a permanent move to the US, but he was excited by the research prospects and liked the egalitarian atmosphere of the US medical research milieu. So in 1932 he moved there permanently and in 1941 became an American citizen. He published the first of many major papers in his new role as Clinical Investigator in 1933, at the age of 38.

He began at Bellevue Hospital in 1932 as Visiting Physician to the Chest Service, and in parallel held a series of posts at Columbia, culminating in an appointment to the Chair of Medicine. At Bellevue Cournand had the facilities — and patients — for cardiac catheterisation, and with Richards was able to set up and direct a laboratory for this purpose. He worked there with Richards, training a succession of distinguished US and European research fellows, until his retirement in 1964.

Apart from the Nobel Prize Cournand received many awards and honorary degrees from universities across North America and Europe. He died of pneumonia in 1988 at the age of 92, survived by his wife and three generations of offspring.

4.3.3 *Dickinson Richards*

Dickinson Richards (Fig. 4.2, right) was born in 1895 in New Jersey. His father was a lawyer; a grandfather and three uncles were doctors. He was educated in Connecticut before entering Yale University to read languages (winning a prize for Greek with the highest grade ever recorded). In 1917, immediately after his degree was awarded, he joined the army and served briefly in France as an artillery lieutenant before the war ended. He then returned to New York and enrolled in medical school at Columbia University. He was awarded a Master's degree in Physiology in 1922 and an MD in 1923. He then joined the staff of Presbyterian Hospital in New York until 1927, when he finished his residency and won a research fellowship to spend a year in England working at the National Institute for Medical Research under Sir Henry Dale on the control of blood flow in the liver. When he returned to the US he re-joined the staff of Presbyterian Hospital and joined the medical faculty of Columbia University — known as the College of Physicians and Surgeons — recently created and renowned for its avant-garde policy of promoting and supporting young medical research talent; the academic unit at Presbyterian Hospital — Columbia-Presbyterian Medical Center — was the model on which the Royal Postgraduate Medical School at Hammersmith Hospital in London was based. Richards remained on the staff of Columbia for the rest of his life. He began research on cardiopulmonary topics, initially under the direction of Lawrence Henderson from Harvard, and in 1931 set up the first cardiopulmonary laboratory in the US. His plan was to study the integrated action of the heart and lungs in respiratory gas exchange; and he invited André Cournand to join him, beginning their long collaboration. In the same year he married his technician, Constance Riley.

In 1945 Richards moved to Bellevue, as Chief and then Lambert Professor of Medicine in the Columbia Medical Center there, leaving the laboratory at Presbyterian Hospital under the supervision of Alfred Fishman. He held these posts until he retired, acting as head of an academic unit, running an acute medical service, teaching, serving on the editorial board of several journals, writing a dozen chapters for medical textbooks and pursuing with Cournand and their staff the research programme, which flowered with the establishment of cardiac catheterisation. He retired in 1961; like Cournand, he was the recipient of many honours apart from the Nobel Prize (though accepting honorary doctorates only from Yale and Columbia); and after his retirement he continued to write on a range of topics — for example, drawing on his early classical education to write a biography of Hippocrates[8] and retranslate his first Aphorism,[9] commenting drily that a physician might bring more insight to the task than a scholar of Greek. Perhaps most notably he collaborated with Alfred Fishman in editing (and contributing to, as did Cournand) a major history of the growth of ideas about circulation which became and remains a classic: *Circulation of the Blood: Men and Ideas.*[10] Looking back on his collaboration with Cournand during his retirement, Richards commented discreetly, '...I have marvelled always to find what a spirited and pleasing interchange there can be between the adventurous flights of the French philosopher and the dogged interrogation of the New England puritan.'[11] He died in 1973 at the age of 77, survived by his wife and 4 daughters.

4.4 The Problem: Cardiopulmonary Physiology and Clinical Investigation of the Heart 80 Years Ago

Until Forssmann, only a handful of experimenters had made invasive studies of the living heart — and then only in animals. The prevailing view amongst cardiologists, which underpinned criticism of Forssmann in Germany and later of Cournand and Ranges in the US[5] and McMichael and Sharpey-Schafer in the UK[12] when they published their first catheter studies, was that invasive study of the heart in man was dangerous and irresponsible. On the other hand, studies on isolated heart and heart muscle preparations in animals and physiological studies of the circulatory and respiratory systems in animals and in man had posed many questions about the human heart: its responses to mechanical, nervous, humoral and therapeutic influences, its interaction with respiratory function and its malfunction in disease. These were pressing issues; in the 1930s, clinical study of the malfunctioning human heart was limited to physical examination, the stethoscope and phonocardiograph, the plain X-ray and the ECG.

One example will suffice to illustrate why Cournand referred to catheterisation as 'the key in the lock' of cardiac investigation.[13] That was the problem of measuring cardiac output in man. In 1870 the German physicist and physiologist Adolph Fick had proposed a method (an English translation of his paper can be found in Fishman and Richards' book)[10] one page in length, and ending with a calculation based on animal data to predict a stroke volume in man of 77 ml. When Cournand and Ranges used the method for the first time in man 70 years later,[5] they measured a stroke volume of 79.5 ml. Fick's principle was simple: if the arterio-venous difference in oxygen content of the blood and the rate of uptake of oxygen from the inspired air could be measured simultaneously, then the blood flow through the lungs — i.e. the cardiac output — could be calculated; the same method could be applied using CO_2 excretion. The idea stimulated a great deal of work. Methods were developed for the measurement of gas content of blood samples, and of respiratory exchange of O_2 and CO_2. Initially the necessary arterial blood gas content could be derived indirectly from end-expiratory (alveolar) air sampling; later, by direct sampling of blood from a peripheral artery. But the venous blood sample had to be representative of the whole body — so-called mixed venous blood — and different organs have different metabolic rates and different blood gas content. Mixing of these venous streams does not take place until the blood has reached the right atrium and ventricle and become inaccessible.

Many ingenious attempts had been made to bypass this problem by using markers other than the respiratory gases. The Fick principle is essentially a dilution method, so it can be applied using infusions or bolus injections of other solutes into the circulation; the markers might be inhaled (nitrous oxide or acetylene), or given intravenously (salt solutions or non-toxic dyes). Another approach, extensively studied by Cournand and Richards as well as others, used exhaled CO_2 but obtained the mixed venous CO_2 content indirectly by a re-breathing method. This depended on there being equilibrium between the carbon dioxide tension in the alveolar air of the lung and in the mixed venous blood in the alveolar wall capillaries. If this is the case, and a steady state is maintained, then the carbon dioxide tension in air re-breathed in a closed circuit will rise to a plateau level equal to that in the alveoli and the mixed venous blood; this can be measured and the CO_2 content calculated. This 'indirect Fick' method could be made to work in man, but it was technically demanding and subject to a number of errors; in particular it is vitiated in patients with lung pathology because ventilation and perfusion are not uniform in the lung, so equilibrium is not reproducibly attainable.[14] As a result of all these problems, published figures for normal cardiac output in man during this era were not only below those accepted today, but varied between laboratories by 50% or more.

This difficulty of measuring cardiac output, particularly serially, was frustrating the study of one aspect of cardiopulmonary physiology; but there were other cardiovascular problems which had not been explored at all. For example, little was known of the pressures and flows in cardiac chambers and the pulmonary circulation, or of the applicability to man of physiological mechanisms like Starling's Law of the heart. Neural and humoral influences on the heart were recognised but unexplored, and electrophysiology of the heart was unknown (in Forssmann's memoirs[2] he describes unsuccessfully advocating catheterisation as a means of recording electrocardiograms directly from the heart at a meeting with Wilhelm His, who was at that time Professor of Medicine in Berlin. That was in 1929; it was 40 years before a catheter-based method of recording His' bundle activity in man was reported). The pathophysiology of cardiac failure and the influence of pulmonary disease on the heart were ill-understood, and physiological and clinical investigation of the human pulmonary circulation was in its infancy. Similarly, measurement of cardiac functions other than pulse rate and blood pressure had little place in the acute management of cardiopulmonary disease.

4.5 Description of the Research

The initiating event in the evolution of catheterisation — Forssmann's contribution in 1929[1] — has been described above. Despite the negative atmosphere in which his work was received, he continued for a time to experiment with the method. He demonstrated, first in animals and then again on himself,[15] that injection of radio-opaque material into the circulation and its imaging was feasible; but he was working with basic and old-fashioned equipment and minimal resources, and in 1931 had to give up and turn to a career in surgery. Elsewhere the method was not wholly abandoned; isolated reports of the procedure came from Czechoslovakia, France, Spain and Latin America, mainly for angiography. However, it was Cournand and Richards who first exploited the method in a sustained and well-resourced programme. In this chapter the emphasis will be on their joint work, but as the technique of catheterisation spread many other groups made contributions, in particular McMichael and his collaborators in London. Nor could the work have succeeded on the scale it did without the use of fast-responding metal membrane manometers modified from the original design of Hamilton.[16] These became the standard tool for Cournand and Richards.

They had begun their long-term collaboration in New York shortly after Forssmann's paper appeared. Like other groups they were having difficulties using the re-breathing method to measure mixed venous CO_2 content, particularly in patients with lung disease. So in 1936 they decided to examine cardiac catheterisation and the direct Fick method to estimate cardiac output. Cournand visited Paris where one of his erstwhile teachers, Ameuille, was using the technique to visualise the right heart and pulmonary artery angiographically.[17] Cournand studied their method and then explored it extensively for several years in his own laboratory. After mastering the technique in human cadavers and then dogs, and satisfied with its safety, he and Richards began studies on patients and later on normal volunteers. They developed suitable equipment and techniques of catheterisation and methods for right atrial blood sampling and pressure measurement, and demonstrated that the catheter could be left in place for up to an hour without complications and that cardiac output could indeed be measured by the direct Fick method. In 1941 they published their first account of right heart catheterisation in man[5] (acknowledging in the first sentence Forssmann's prior claim to the method, and probably thereby rescuing him from permanent obscurity). This landmark study initiated a sustained torrent of work; by the time of the Nobel Prize award, Cournand and Richards had, between them, published approximately 140 papers based on their work together.

They began with exploration of the reliability and limitations of the direct Fick method for measuring cardiac output,[4] making comparisons with other methods[18] and establishing normal ranges. Measurements of cardiac output in disease soon followed.[19] They examined the applicability to man of the concepts elucidated in animal experiments by Frank, Starling and others on the control of cardiac output. The importance of right atrial filling pressure (used in clinical work rather than diastolic volume because it was easier to measure) as a determinant of cardiac output was established, and the influence on it of posture, circulating volume and respiratory manoeuvres examined.[12,20]

Early in the work, America entered the Second World War, and for almost three years Cournand and Richards put a major effort into cardiovascular studies of shock. It is illuminating to consider what these involved; they would probably be impossible to undertake today. Cournand and his team (up to six physicians and a similar number of technicians) were on call 24 hours a day, including weekends. When trauma cases were admitted to the Emergency Room at Bellevue, they were immediately treated and transferred to an adjacent cardiopulmonary lab. There, treatment and research went on simultaneously; patients were either unconscious or sedated. An indwelling arterial needle was inserted into one femoral artery, and a venous cannula into an arm vein. Then the cardiac catheter was introduced into the other arm. The X-ray equipment was wheeled in and the lab lights switched off whilst the catheter was guided into the right atrium — image intensifiers had yet to be invented, and the image of the catheter was visualised by the dim green glow of fluoroscopy. The catheter was attached to pressure manometers and sampling taps, a face mask fitted to the patient for measurement of ventilation and gas exchange, and baseline measurements made. Simultaneous samples of arterial and mixed venous blood and expired air were collected; these were analysed and cardiac output calculated whilst recordings of arterial and cardiac blood pressures were made and dye injected intravenously for blood volume measurement. The haematocrit was measured; in many cases renal clearance also, necessitating a bladder catheter. Then came the research interventions — perhaps blood volume expansion with saline, plasma or blood; perhaps alterations of venous return by posture changes; perhaps vasopressor agents or oxygen. And all the measurements were repeated. These studies were done on control subjects — trauma victims who were not in shock — as well as shock cases; typically a study took four to six hours. In all, over a three-year period, Cournand and Richards studied more than a hundred patients, and mapped out the pathophysiology of shock. This was new knowledge; they showed the falls in right atrial pressure, cardiac output, blood volume and arterial pressure that accompany shock, the importance of right atrial filling pressure in maintaining output, and demonstrated the almost linear relation between blood volume and cardiac output. They showed that blood loss prompts reductions of blood flow to many organs, particularly the kidney, due to vasoconstriction as well as to a fall in arterial pressure, and also prompts a shift of extracellular fluid into the vascular space. Their findings[21,22] still guide the management of shock today.

During this period, cardiac catheterisation was being taken up in other centres as well as Bellevue, and topics like heart failure and its treatment examined. The mode of action of cardiac glycosides in both the normal and the failing heart attracted attention; prior studies in animals and the normal heart had given results which conflicted with clinical observations in heart failure. The new methodologies resolved many of these inconsistencies, demonstrating that increases in contractile force, leading to increased ventricular emptying and stroke volume, and falling diastolic pressures, followed acute administration of cardiac glycosides in the dilated failing v-entricle, but not in the normal heart.[23-25] Cardiac function in congestive heart failure was also studied;[26,27] the essential feature was shown to be a failure of cardiac emptying, leading to high diastolic pressures in the left heart which acted back on to the pulmonary circulation to generate oedema and pulmonary hypertension, which in turn led to right ventricular failure and systemic venous congestion. The beneficial effect of lowering right atrial pressure in heart failure, and the existence (in anaemia, hypoxia, fever and cor pulmonale, for example) of forms of cardiac failure in which the output is actually high were confirmed, and the relevance of the Frank–Starling mechanisms explored.

In his acceptance speech at the Nobel ceremony, Richards commented that both he and Cournand had originally seen themselves as respiratory physiologists, and their prior work bears that out — in the 1930s they were devising new ways to explore pulmonary function, and studying gas mixing in the lung. They worked on causes of breathlessness, and first described the hypoventilation and CO_2 retention which follows high inspired oxygen therapy in exacerbations of chronic obstructive pulmonary disease. So it was natural for them to study the pulmonary circulation with their new catheter techniques. This was particularly true for Cournand, interested primarily in the physiology, whilst Richards, the physician of the two, leaned more to pathophysiology, though neither lost sight of possible therapeutic outcomes. Once dynamic methods of pressure measurement through catheters had been established, they began to examine pressure waveforms, not only in the atrium but in the right ventricle[28] and the pulmonary artery.[29] In the latter study they deployed for the first time a double-lumen catheter which allowed simultaneous measurements at different sites. This provided information on the sequence of events during a cardiac contraction and the pressures and pressure gradients generated. Another outcome of studies of the pulmonary arteries was the recognition that pressure in the *left* atrium could be measured through a catheter wedged in a distal branch of the pulmonary artery.[30,31] The immense value of this became clear in later years when balloon-tipped catheters came into use which could be 'floated' without X-ray visualisation into the pulmonary artery,[32] making it possible in intensive and coronary care units and operating theatres to monitor left heart function by measuring this 'wedge pressure'.

This work demonstrated the complexity of pressure-flow relations in the pulmonary circulation. In health, the pulmonary microcirculation is extremely distensible (as was shown, for example, by the absence of any rise in pulmonary artery pressure at rest, despite a maintained cardiac output, after pneumonectomy),[33] and the effective distending (transmural) pressure in pulmonary capillaries is highly influenced by the pressure in the lung airways, as Cournand and his colleagues demonstrated by studying the effects of respiratory manoeuvres and positive pressure ventilation on pulmonary pressure and flow. During deep inspiration,[20] the negative intrathoracic pressure causes an increase in venous return to and therefore output from the right ventricle, but also expands the pulmonary capillaries, which act as a sponge. So venous return to the left heart diminishes, as does left ventricular output; the arterial pressure falls. During expiration, the reverse happens: the airway pressure becomes positive, reducing systemic venous return, compressing the pulmonary capillaries and transiently increasing left ventricular output. This reduction in venous return by positive airway pressure has important practical consequences in positive pressure ventilation,[34] which causes a marked fall in cardiac output. The same effect, as every schoolchild knows, can be achieved by the Valsalva manoeuvre.[35]

These studies of the pulmonary circulation included a crucially important observation on the effects of chronic pulmonary disease — he profound effect of hypoxia on the pulmonary microcirculation. A fall in alveolar oxygen tension was shown to cause a marked rise in pulmonary artery pressure in normal subjects[36] and patients with obstructive lung disease;[37] since blood flow was little changed, the inference was that hypoxia caused pulmonary vasoconstriction. This proved to be an important key to understanding the evolution of right heart failure. As chronic lung disease progresses and destroys pulmonary capillaries, right ventricular work and systolic pulmonary artery pressure have to rise in order to maintain blood flow, at first on exercise but later also at rest.[37] If hypoxia accompanies the lung disease it further increases the pulmonary vascular resistance[38] as well as causing polycythaemia and blood volume expansion. Finally, as had been shown in an earlier study,[39] the right ventricle reaches a point where it fails to support this load; it dilates, diastolic pressure and therefore atrial pressure rises and cor pulmonale follows.[40] It was this sequence of studies, highlighting the need for correction of hypoxia and blood volume in the management of cor pulmonale,[41] which occupied Cournand and Richards and their co-workers in the period leading up to the award of the Nobel Prize in 1956.

4.6 Impact of Cardiac Catheterisation on Medical Science

Cardiac catheterisation has changed both the science and the practice of acute medicine. The application of the method established much of what we know of the normal and abnormal function of the heart and pulmonary circulation. This knowledge, acquired in the heyday of the physiological study of entire systems — and illustrating the value of such work — now guides the management of cardiac and respiratory failure and contributes to the resuscitation and care of many other acutely ill patients. Cardiopulmonary physiological measurements are in use in the ward, theatre and intensive and coronary care units, and facilitate clinical procedures ranging from ventilatory support and dialysis to cardiopulmonary bypass. All this knowledge is nowadays so familiar that it seems we always had it; but in reality it stems from the work of these few pioneers, who took methods from animal work and shaped them, in the face of hostility and prejudice, to study man.

But there is much more; there is the contribution of the catheter itself. Catheterisation techniques drove the evolution of a host of advances for years. Specialised types of radio-opaque catheter and means of introducing them, safe contrast media, rapid film changers and then image intensifiers were all developed to facilitate the study and imaging of the pulmonary circulation, so that pulmonary angiography became the diagnostic method of choice in pulmonary vascular disease. The use of catheter-tip electrodes to record electrical events in the conducting system of the heart and the myocardium became a cardiological speciality in its own right. External and implanted pacemakers connected to the right atrium or ventricle by transvenous leads, and balloon-tipped catheters capable of measuring cardiac output and right atrial and wedge pressures, evolved. Finally, within a few years of the award of this Nobel Prize, and supported by proof of the safety of catheterisation and the technical achievements in access and imaging, angiographic studies of the left heart and coronary circulation began, to be followed by a wave of advances in cardiac surgery, angioplasty and stenting procedures. Both acute and cardiopulmonary medicine have been transformed.

Acknowledgements

I wish to thank Professor Jochen Schaefer, of the Institute for Theoretical Cardiology, Kiel, Germany, for helpful comments and for a translation of Forssmann's original paper.[1]

References

1. Forssmann W. Die Sondierung des rechten Herzens. *Klin Wochenschr* 1929; 8: 2085–2087.
2. Forssmann W. *Experiments on Myself: Memoirs of a Surgeon in Germany.* Trans Davies H. New York: St Martin's Press; 1974.

3. Hart FD. Werner Forssmann (1904–1979), auto-experimenter/medical martyr. The original cardiac catheterization. *J Med Biogr* 1997; 5: 120–121.

4. Cournand A. Measurement of the cardiac output in man using right heart catheterization. Description of technique, discussion of validity and of place in the study of the circulation. *Fed Proc* 1945; 4: 207–212.

5. Cournand AF, Ranges HA. Catheterization of the right auricle in man. *Proc Soc Exp Biol Med* 1941; 46: 462–466.

6. Cournand AF. *From Roots to Late Budding: The Intellectual Adventures of a Medical Scientist.* New York: Gardner Press Inc; 1986.

7. Symposium on the lung and pulmonary circulation. *Am J Med* 1974; 57: 311–328.

8. Richards DW. Hippocrates of Ostia. *JAMA* 1968; 204: 1049–1056.

9. Richards DW. The first Aphorism of Hippocrates. *Perspect Biol Med* 1961; 5: 61–64.

10. Fishman AP, Richards DW (eds). *Circulation of the Blood: Men and Ideas.* Oxford: Oxford University Press; 1964.

11. Richards DW. Acceptance of the 1970 Kobler Prize. *Trans Assoc Am Physicians* 1970; 83: 43.

12. McMichael J, Sharpey-Schafer EP. Cardiac output in man by a direct Fick method. *Br Heart J* 1944; 6: 33–40.

13. *Nobel Lectures: Physiology or Medicine 1942–1962.* Amsterdam: Elsevier Publishing Co; 1964.

14. Richards Jr DW, Cournand A, Bryan NA. Applicability of rebreathing method for determining mixed venous CO_2 in cases of chronic pulmonary disease. *J Clin Invest* 1935; 14: 173–180.

15. Forssmann W. Über Kontrastdarstellung der Höhlen des lebenden rechten Herzens und der Lungenschlagader [On contrast demonstration of the chambers of the living right heart and the pulmonary artery]. *Munch Med Wochenschr* 1931; 78: 489–492.

16. Hamilton WF, Brewer G, Brotman I. Pressure pulse contours in the intact animal: I. Analytical description of a new high-frequency hypodermic manometer. *Am J Physiol* 1934; 107: 427–435.

17. Ameuille P, Ronneaux G, Hinault V *et al.* Remarques sur quelques cas d'artériographie pulmonaires chez l'homme vivant. *Bull Mem Soc Med Hop Paris* 1936; 52: 729–739.

18. Cournand A, Ranges HA, Riley RL. Comparison of results of the normal ballistocardiogram and a direct Fick method in measuring the cardiac output in man. *J Clin Invest* 1942; 21: 287–294.
19. Richards DW. Cardiac output by the catheterization technique in various clinical conditions. *Fed Proc* 1945; 4: 215–220.
20. Lauson HD, Bloomfield RA, Cournand A. The influence of respiration on the circulation in man, with special reference to pressures in the right auricle, right ventricle, femoral artery and peripheral veins. *Am J Med* 1946; 1: 315–336.
21. Cournand A, Riley RL, Bradley SE *et al.* Studies of the circulation in clinical shock. *Surgery* 1943; 13: 965–995.
22. Richards Jr DW, Cournand A. Circulation in shock: mechanical and vasomotor factors. *Trans Assoc Am Physicians* 1944; 58: 111–118.
23. McMichael J, Sharpey-Schafer EP. The action of intravenous digoxin in man. *Q J Med* 1944; 13: 123–135.
24. Harvey RM, Ferrer MI, Cathcart RT *et al.* Some effects of digoxin upon the heart and circulation in man. I. Digoxin in left ventricular failure. *Am J Med* 1949; 7: 439–453.
25. Bloomberg RA, Rapoport B, Milnor JP *et al.* The effects of the cardiac glycosides upon the dynamics of the circulation in congestive cardiac failure: I. Ouabain. *J Clin Invest* 1948; 27: 588–599.
26. Richards DW. Contributions of right heart catheterization to the physiology of congestive cardiac failure. *Am J Med* 1947; 3: 434–446.
27. Richards DW. Dynamics of congestive heart failure. *Am J Med* 1949; 6: 772–780.
28. Cournand A, Lauson HD, Bloomfield RA *et al.* Recording of right heart pressures in man. *Proc Soc Exp Biol Med* 1944; 55: 34–36.
29. Cournand A, Bloomfield RA, Lauson HD. Double lumen catheter for intravenous and intracardiac blood sampling and pressure recording. *Proc Soc Exp Biol Med* 1945; 60: 73–75.
30. Hellems HK, Haynes FW, Dexter L. Pulmonary 'capillary' pressure in man. *J Appl Physiol* 1949; 2: 24–29.
31. Dexter L, Haynes FW, Burwell CS *et al.* Studies of congenital heart disease: II. The pressure and oxygen content of blood in the right auricle, right ventricle and pulmonary artery in control patients, with

observations on the oxygen saturation and source of pulmonary 'capillary' blood. *J Clin Invest* 1947; 26: 554–560.

32. Swan HJC, Ganz W, Forrester J *et al.* Catheterization of the heart in man with use of a flow-directed balloon-tipped catheter. *N Engl J Med* 1970; 283:447–451.

33. Cournand A, Riley RL, Himmelstein A *et al.* Pulmonary circulation and alveolar ventilation-perfusion relationships after pneumonectomy. *J Thorac Surg* 1950; 19: 80–116.

34. Cournand A, Motley HL, Werkö L *et al.* Physiological studies of the effects of intermittent positive pressure breathing on cardiac output in man. *Am J Physiol* 1948; 152: 162–174.

35. Richards Jr DW, Cournand A, Motley HL. Effects on circulatory and respiratory functions of various forms of respirator. *Trans Assoc Am Physicians* 1946; 59: 102–109.

36. Motley HL, Cournand A, Werkö L *et al.* The influence of short periods of induced acute anoxia upon pulmonary artery pressures in man. *Am J Physiol* 1947; 150: 315–320.

37. Riley RL, Himmelstein A, Motley HL *et al.* Studies of the pulmonary circulation at rest and during exercise in normal individuals and in patients with chronic lung disease. *Am J Physiol* 1948; 152: 372–382.

38. Harvey RM, Ferrer MI, Richards DW *et al.* The influence of chronic pulmonary disease on the heart and circulation. *Am J Med* 1951; 10: 719–738.

39. Bloomfield RA, Lauson HD, Cournand A *et al.* Recording of right heart pressures in normal subjects and in patients with chronic pulmonary disease and various types of cardiocirculatory disease. *J Clin Invest* 1946; 25: 639–664.

40. Cournand A. Some aspects of the pulmonary circulation in normal man and in chronic cardiopulmonary diseases. *Circulation* 1950; 2: 641–657.

41. Fishman AP, Richards DW. The management of cor pulmonale in chronic pulmonary disease, with particular reference to the associated disturbances in the pulmonary circulation. *Am Heart J* 1956; 52: 149–160.

Chapter 5

THE DISCOVERY OF THE STRUCTURE OF DNA

James Scott and Gilbert Thompson

5.1 Introduction

Arguably the most famous and best publicised of the Nobel Prizes in this book was the award in 1962 of the Prize in Physiology or Medicine to Crick, Watson and Wilkins, 'for their discoveries concerning the molecular structure of nucleic acids and its significance for information transfer in living material'. The discovery of the double-helical structure of DNA in 1953 was the start of something entirely novel and has been described as the greatest achievement of science in the 20th century.[1] In his account of that discovery, *The Double Helix*, James Watson relates how his co-worker Francis Crick burst into The Eagle, a pub in Cambridge, one lunchtime and announced to all and sundry that, 'they had found the secret of life'.[2] In his foreword to the book Sir Lawrence Bragg, head of the Cavendish Laboratory where they both worked, described the discovery as an explosion which transformed biochemistry. He also remarked that those who figure in the book should read it in a very forgiving spirit, the reason being illustrated by its opening sentence, 'I have never seen Francis Crick in a modest mood'. That lack of modesty must have been infectious because Watson persuaded his sister to type the manuscript of his and Crick's renowned Letter to *Nature* by telling her that their discovery was the most famous event in biology since Darwin's *The Origin of Species*. Now, almost 60 years later, this astonishing claim still holds true.

One of the major participants in the events leading up to the discovery of the structure of DNA was the physicist Rosalind Franklin.

Had she lived long enough it is possible that she, rather than her colleague Maurice Wilkins, would have shared the Nobel Prize with Crick and Watson. Her X-ray diffraction data on DNA provided them with the pivotal clue to its structure but her premature death from cancer in 1958 ruled her out of contention — Nobel Prizes are never awarded posthumously.

5.2   Brief Biographies of the Major Protagonists

5.2.1   *Francis Crick*

Francis H.C. Crick was born in Northampton in 1916. He was educated at Mill Hill and then got a second class honours BSc in physics at University College, London. The war interrupted his research for a PhD but after it was over he went to work in Cambridge, first at Strangeways Research Laboratory and then with the Medical Research Council (MRC) in Max Perutz's Molecular Biology Unit at the Cavendish. While there he re-commenced working for a PhD and obtained this degree in 1953 with a thesis on 'X-ray diffraction: polypeptides and proteins'. Subsequently he spent a postdoctoral year at the Brooklyn Polytechnic in New York. He was elected an FRS in 1959 and, together with Watson and Wilkins, received a Lasker Award in 1960 and the Nobel Prize in 1962. That same year he and Sydney Brenner became joint heads of the Molecular Genetics division of the MRC Laboratory of Molecular Biology in Cambridge. He remained there until 1979 when he was made a Distinguished Research Professor at the Salk Institute. He was appointed to the Order of Merit in 1991 and died in California in 2004.

Crick and Watson first met in the autumn of 1951 when Watson started work at the Cavendish. He relates that Crick talked louder and faster than anyone else and his laugh was a 'shattering bang', traits which irritated Bragg and caused him to avoid him.[2] However, Watson was not bothered by these mannerisms and thoroughly enjoyed conversing with Crick. He often had dinner with him and his wife and recalls that, 'There was no restraint in Francis' enthusiasms about young women'. Watson comments that although Bragg was unconvinced of Crick's value to the Cavendish there was a growing acceptance both within and outside Cambridge that Francis' brain was a genuine asset. For his part Crick says that Watson was regarded as too bright to be really sound.[3] Erwin Chargaff, the well-known American biochemist and authority on DNA, once described the two of them as 'scientific clowns',[2] a comment one imagines he later regretted.

5.2.2 *James Watson*

James D. Watson was born in 1928 in Chicago where he grew up and went to school. He got a BSc in zoology at the University of Chicago in 1947 and a PhD in the same subject at Indiana University three years later. This was followed by a year spent in Copenhagen as a post-doctoral fellow working on bacteriophage. In 1951 he attended a symposium in Naples at which Maurice Wilkins presented his X-ray diffraction data on crystalline DNA. This caused Watson to change the direction of his research and led to his going to Cambridge to work with John Kendrew in Max Perutz's unit at the Cavendish. There he met Francis Crick, an event which initiated one of the most productive collaborations in the history of science and culminated in their discovery of the structure of DNA. Subsequently Watson returned to the US to spend two years at the California Institute of Technology in Pasadena.

Judging from *The Double Helix*, Watson and Crick got on remarkably well with each other while they were at Cambridge but later on the relationship had its ups and downs. In a letter from Pasadena dated October 1953 Watson criticised Crick's intention to give a talk on the BBC: 'You are the one to suffer most from your attempts at self-publicity.... If you need the money that bad, go ahead. Needless to say I shall not think any higher of you and shall have good reason to avoid any further collaboration with you.'[4] Despite this threat Watson returned to Cambridge from Pasadena in 1955 where he spent a further year working with Crick.

On his return to the US he was appointed to the Biology Department at Harvard and made a Professor in 1961, the year before he got the Nobel Prize. From 1968 onwards he was Director of the Cold Spring Harbor Laboratory on Long Island, New York, and became its President in 1994. Subsequently he was its Chancellor until 2007, when he resigned following the controversy provoked by an interview in which he claimed that black Africans were less intelligent than white people.

5.2.3 *Maurice Wilkins*

Maurice H.F. Wilkins was born in New Zealand in 1916 but was brought up in England from the age of six. He was educated at King Edward's School, Birmingham, and took a degree in physics at Cambridge in 1938 followed by a PhD in 1940 at the University of Birmingham. During the war he worked in Berkeley, California, on the Manhattan Project to build the atomic bomb. Returning to Britain after the war he became a lecturer in Physics at St Andrew's University and worked with Professor J. Randall, moving with the latter to King's College, London in 1946 and becoming a member of his MRC Biophysics Research Unit. That marked the start of his X-ray diffraction studies of DNA.

Wilkins became Assistant Director of the MRC Unit in 1950, which was when Rosalind Franklin joined it. He was elected FRS in 1959 and was made a CBE in 1962, the year in which he received the Nobel Prize. In his Nobel lecture Wilkins commented that several lines of evidence showed that DNA, a pure chemical substance, was imbued with a deeply significant biological activity[5] but pointed out that only X-ray diffraction studies could provide an adequate description of its three-dimensional configuration.

Letters from Wilkins to Crick show that he was on good terms with both of his Cambridge collaborators but not with his junior colleague at King's, Rosalind Franklin, with whom he had a difficult working relationship. In one letter to Crick he says, 'Franklin barks often but doesn't succeed in biting me',[6] and in another, 'Rosie's colloquium made me a bit sicker. God knows what will become of all this business.'[7] His sense of relief is evident in a third letter to Crick where he writes, 'Our dark lady leaves us next week and much of the three-dimensional data is (sic) already in our hands.'[8] However, after her death he acknowledged how valuable was her contribution to the X-ray analysis of the structure of DNA.[5]

5.2.4 *Rosalind Franklin*

Rosalind Elsie Franklin (Fig. 5.1) was born in London in 1920 and educated at St Paul's Girls' School. She went on to Cambridge where she obtained a BA in physical chemistry in 1941. This was followed by wartime research on the colloidal properties of coal, which led to a PhD in 1945. Franklin then went to work in Paris at the Laboratoire Central des Services Chimiques de l'Etat where she undertook X-ray diffraction studies of carbons. She returned to Britain in 1951 to start a three-year fellowship in Randall's MRC Biophysics Research Unit at King's College, London. In a letter written to her while she was still in Paris Randall proposed that she focus on X-ray diffraction studies of DNA when she joined the unit, mentioning that Maurice Wilkins and Ray Gosling, a postgraduate student, had made some preliminary findings in that respect.[9] However, as already discussed, a clash of personalities prevented any collaboration between her and Wilkins with the result that, assisted by Gosling, she conducted her studies of DNA separately.

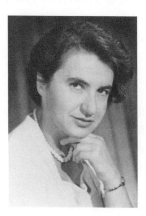

Fig. 5.1.   Rosalind Franklin in 1956 (National Library of Medicine http://profiles. nlm.nih.gov/KR/B/B/J/N/_/krbbjn.jpg).

In 1953, at the end of her fellowship at King's, Franklin moved to John D. Bernal's laboratory at Birkbeck College to conduct X-ray diffraction studies of tobacco mosaic virus, together with Aaron Klug. Sadly she developed ovarian cancer and died, aged 37, in 1958. Unlike her relationship with Wilkins she was on good terms with Francis Crick and his wife and convalesced with them post-operatively a few months before she died. Twenty years later, in a letter to the President of the New York Academy of Sciences, who wished to give her a posthumous award, Aaron Klug described her as an outstandingly good experimental scientist with acute powers of observation and a clear powerful mind.[10] He considered that her work contributed crucially to the discovery of the structure of DNA but denied Watson's claim[2] that she was an active feminist. Klug later became Director of the Laboratory of Molecular Biology in Cambridge and President of the Royal Society.

5.3 Early Discoveries that Paved the Way to Unravelling the Structure of DNA

DNA was first isolated from the pus of discarded surgical bandages by the Swiss chemist Friedrich Miescher in 1869. Miescher subjected purified cell nuclei to an alkaline extraction followed by acidification, resulting in a precipitate now known as DNA. He found that it contained phosphorus and nitrogen, but not sulphur. He recognised it as a unique macromolecule quite unlike anything else at the time. He called it nuclein, since it was located in the nucleus of the cells. The significance of the discovery was not at first apparent. A German doctor, Albrecht Kossel, made the initial investigations into its chemical structure, and described the four DNA bases, for which he received the 1910 Nobel Prize in Physiology or Medicine. In 1928 Fredrick Griffiths noticed that a rough type of pneumococcus bacteria changed to a smooth type when an unknown 'transforming principle' from the smooth type was present. Sixteen years later, in 1944, Oswald Avery identified that 'transforming principle' as DNA. In 1929 at the Rockefeller Institute Phoebus Levene, who had worked with Kossel, discovered the sugar deoxyribose, and showed that in DNA the components were linked together in the order phosphate–sugar–base to form units. Andrei Belozersky isolated DNA in the pure state in 1935, and in 1937 William Astbury produced the first X-ray diffraction patterns — an approach used first by Lawrence Bragg in 1912 — proving that DNA had a regular structure. In 1950 Chargaff found that in DNA the amounts of adenine and thymine are about the same, as are the amounts of guanine and cytosine. These relationships were later known as 'Chargaff's Rules' and served as a key principle for Watson and Crick in assessing various models for the structure of DNA. That DNA might be a helical structure was suggested by the Nobel Prize-winning discovery made by Linus Pauling in 1951 of the right-handed α-helix as a key structure in proteins.

5.4 Complementary Approaches to Analysing the Structure of DNA in the 1950s

Watson states that his interest in DNA was triggered when he attended a conference in Naples in 1951 at which Wilkins presented an X-ray diffraction image of DNA.[2] The idea that genes could crystallise excited him because it meant they must have a regular structure that could be determined. Later that year he started work at the Cavendish where Crick was working on X-ray diffraction analysis of proteins under the supervision of Max Perutz. Watson soon discovered that Crick shared his interest in DNA and the two of them decided to try to determine its configuration by emulating the American chemist Linus Pauling, who had used molecular modelling to study protein structure.

A more direct approach was employed at King's College by Maurice Wilkins and Rosalind Franklin, both of whom used X-ray diffraction to analyse the structure of DNA. Wilkins was happy to cooperate with Watson and Crick but Franklin refused them access to her data. This situation continued until 1952 when, unknown to her, Wilkins showed Watson, who was on a visit to King's, one of her unpublished X-ray photographs of the B (hydrated) form of DNA. For Watson it was a transformative moment. Later he wrote in *The Double Helix*, 'The instant I saw the picture my mouth fell open and my pulse began to race. The pattern was unbelievably simpler than those obtained previously (of the A form). Moreover, the black cross of reflections which dominated the picture could only arise from a helical structure.'[2] Subsequently Perutz showed Crick a summary of Franklin's results, which he'd been sent in his role as a member of the MRC committee reviewing the work of Randall's Unit. Her data provided the Cavendish workers with crucial experimental evidence regarding the validity of a helical model of DNA.

5.4.1 *Model building at the Cavendish and X-ray diffraction at King's*

Watson recounts[2] the excitement caused within the scientific community by Pauling *et al*'s paper proposing that proteins had an α-helical structure, which was published in the *Proceedings of the National Academy of Sciences* in April 1951.[11] Based upon accurate determination of the crystal structure of amino acids and peptides Pauling obtained detailed information on inter-atomic distances and the angles of chemical bonds in polypeptide chains. This enabled him to predict that they were helical structures containing either 48 residues in every 13 turns or 41 residues in every 8 turns. He proposed that the latter configuration was the important structural feature of proteins like haemoglobin and myoglobin, noting that Bragg, Kendrew and Perutz had earlier rejected this concept on the basis of their X-ray diffraction data. Pauling and his colleagues followed up this coup by publishing a further seven papers on the same topic in the May issue of *PNAS*, a scientific *tour de force*.

Enthused by these findings, Watson and Crick decided to try to determine the structure of DNA in an analogous manner, although Wilkins cautioned them that his X-ray diffraction data indicated that DNA was a more complex molecule than the proteins studied by Pauling. Although Perutz and Kendrew were nominally supervising Crick and Watson at the Cavendish, they were mainly involved in the X-ray diffraction analysis of haemoglobin and myoglobin respectively, work for which they shared the Nobel Prize in Chemistry in 1962.

At that time all X-ray diffraction studies of DNA were being performed in Randall's unit at King's by Wilkins and Franklin, Watson's own attempts to get X-ray diffraction photos of DNA being unsuccessful. Hence Crick and Watson's early attempts at model building lacked a sound foundation. That all changed at the end of 1952 when Watson paid the now historical visit to King's and Wilkins showed him the crucial X-ray diffraction photo taken by Franklin of the B form of DNA, which clearly indicated a helical structure and led to Watson's decision to build a double-helix model. While Franklin and Wilkins believed the purine and pyrimidine bases were at the centre of DNA and the sugar–phosphate backbone outside, they lacked any real structural hypothesis that would allow them to pack the bases regularly inside the helix. In his detailed account of the events leading up to the discovery of the structure of DNA Robert Olby states that before 1953 all the proposed models for DNA were single or triple helices.[12] Mathematical calculations by Griffiths in Cambridge of the electrostatic interaction between two bases in apposition suggested that adenosine would attract thymine and guanine would attract cytosine, in keeping with Chargaff's Rule that the percentage of adenosine in DNA equals that of thymine and the percentage of guanine equals that of cytosine[13] and implying complementary pairing of the bases. At this stage, however, there was uncertainty as to which tautomeric form the bases existed in DNA — enol or keto, imino or amino?

5.4.2 *The wrong model*

At the end of 1952 Watson and Crick received the news that Pauling had solved the structure of DNA and was due to publish his results the following February. Pauling sent a copy of his manuscript to his son, Peter, who was working in Cambridge at that time and the latter showed it to Watson and Crick. Pauling's proposed model was a three-chain helix with its phosphate groups on the inside.[14] However, the phosphates in Pauling's model were un-ionised, which Watson and Crick immediately perceived to be a major flaw in the model and Pauling later admitted his mistake.[12]

5.4.3 *The correct model*

After Wilkins showed Franklin's X-ray diffraction photograph of the B form of DNA to Watson, which the latter immediately interpreted as indicative of a helical structure (Fig. 5.2), the question remained as to how many helices comprised each DNA molecule. Existing data regarding the density of its sodium salt suggested there were not less than two and not more than three helices and Watson opted for two, basing his assumption on the premise that, 'important biological objects come in pairs'.[2]

The next question needing to be resolved was the location of the sugar–phosphate backbone in each helix. Franklin's data suggested that the phosphate groups were exposed and therefore on the outside of the helix whereas Watson and Crick's initial model had the backbone inside and the purine and pyridimine bases on the outside. However, their model looked 'awful', and they soon came to the conclusion that the bases probably formed the core and the sugar–phosphate backbone the circumference of the helix.[15]

Early in 1953 Max Perutz showed Crick the report which Randall's group had produced for the MRC Biophysics Research Committee. This contained unpublished calculations by Franklin which enabled Crick to deduce that the helices in DNA were anti-parallel, i.e. they

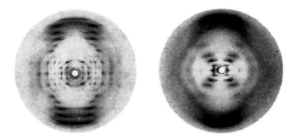

Fig. 5.2. X-ray diffraction patterns of the A and B forms of the sodium salt of DNA obtained by RE Franklin and RG Gosling in 1953. The A form occurs under non-physiological conditions in partially dehydrated samples of DNA. It lacks the ordered base-pairing and base-stacking interactions of the B form. The B form is most common at the high hydration levels present in living cells. (Reprinted with permission from Macmillan Publishers Ltd: *Nature*, 219: 808–844, ©1968).

went in opposite directions. Watson then examined the question of how the bases were paired and initially came to the conclusion that like went with like. However, he used the wrong tautomeric forms of guanine, thymine and cytosine in his calculations, enol instead of keto, so had to reject this solution. Luckily Jerry Donohue, an American crystallographer with whom Watson shared an office, had an intuition that the bases were in the keto form. Subsequently, while shuffling the base pairing possibilities, Watson suddenly realised, in a 'Eureka' flash of insight, that the molecular footprint of adenine and thymine, held together by two hydrogen bonds, was identical to that of guanine and cytosine hydrogen bonded in a similar manner. This complementary pairing of the bases not only looked correct but was also in accordance with Chargaff's Rule. Hence the sequence of bases on one helical chain determined the sequence of bases on the opposite one.

Watson and Crick worked feverishly during March 1953 perfecting their model. Their double-helix concept soon gained the approval of both Wilkins and Franklin, who, for once, were in agreement. Both groups of workers at King's declared that they would publish their X-ray diffraction studies at the same time as Watson and Crick published their model of DNA and the three Letters to *Nature* appeared together on 25 April 1953.[16–18] These were followed by two further Letters to *Nature*, one from Watson and Crick[19] on the genetic implications of their findings and the other from Franklin and Gosling[20] containing X-ray diffraction data on the A form of DNA, corroborating its double-helical structure. As mentioned earlier, these findings caused Pauling to concede that he was wrong and to acknowledge that, 'The formulation of their structure by Watson and Crick may turn out to be the greatest development in the field of molecular genetics in recent years.'[12] The two of them with their model of DNA at the Cavendish are shown in Fig. 5.3.

The respective contributions to this discovery made by the Cambridge workers and the two groups at King's, especially Franklin, have been assessed retrospectively by Crick[3] and by Klug.[21] Both acknowledge the significance of her observation that the phosphate groups were on the outside of the DNA backbone and the importance of her X-ray diffraction studies in confirming its helical

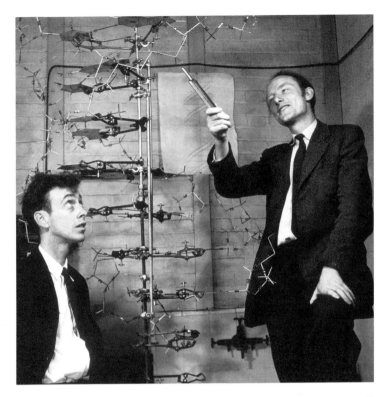

Fig. 5.3.   Watson and Crick with their DNA model (A Barrington Brown/Science Photo Library).

conformation. Whether she would have solved the structure of DNA on her own, as has been suggested,[22] seems unlikely but she undoubtedly played a vital role in Watson and Crick's achievement.

5.5 Impact of the Discovery of the Structure of DNA on Medical Science

In their seminal 1953 *Nature* letter Watson and Crick wrote, 'It has not escaped our notice that the specific pairing we have postulated immediately suggests a possible copying mechanism for genetic material'[16] (Fig. 5.4). They had indeed found the secret of life. Their discovery explained the storage, replication and transmission of genetic

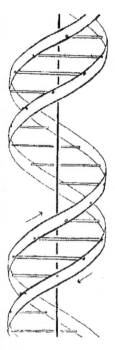

Fig. 5.4. Diagrammatic representation of the double-helical structure of DNA. The two ribbons symbolise the two phosphate–sugar chains and the horizontal rods the pairs of bases holding the chains together. The vertical line marks the axis of the right-handed anti-parallel double helix. (Reprinted with permission from Macmillan Publishers Ltd: *Nature*, 171: 737–738, ©1953).

material. A dozen or so gene-orientated Nobel Prizes later, we routinely clone, manipulate and sequence DNA. From the mid-1960s until the turn of the millennium a cornucopia of discovery revealed the genes for numerous Mendelian diseases. New forensic methods for DNA fingerprinting were to revolutionise forensic science. Concepts of human evolution underwent radical revision. The genome sequences of *E. coli*, yeast, fruit flies and flatworms were determined.

On Monday 26 June 2000 the US President Bill Clinton announced to the world the completion of the rough draft sequence of the human genome with the words: 'Today, we are learning the language in which God created life. With this profound new knowledge humankind is on the verge of gaining immense, new power to heal.'[23]

In this endeavour Watson played a key facilitating role. It was realised because of new strategies for DNA sequencing and major advances in sequencing technology. It ushered in an intense decade of DNA sequencing, allowing large-scale comparative genomics of organisms, detection of the huge amount of variation in the human genome and profound insights into the origins of human traits and disease.[24-26]

5.5.1 *Mendelian genetics*

The identification of the defective genes responsible for the more frequent Mendelian diseases was the theme of the 1980s and 1990s. A significant step was the development of strategies for positional cloning, using family-based linkage analysis with DNA polymorphisms that span the genome and disease gene identification by comparison of DNA sequences in patients and controls. Huntington's chorea, Duchenne muscular dystrophy and cystic fibrosis genes were identified in the late 1980s. In 1994 the breast cancer gene *BRAC1* was cloned. The human genome sequence has greatly facilitated the discovery of genes causing Mendelian disease. Three thousand such genes have now been discovered, and sequencing will reveal the remainder.

5.5.2 *The HapMap Project*

The 2003 HapMap Project was designed as a resource to find genetic variants affecting human health. Variation within genomes takes a variety of common forms: single nucleotide polymorphisms or SNPs (allele frequency greater than 1%) are overwhelmingly the commonest form of variation; small insertion deletions, called indels and copy number variation (CNVs) are less common forms. CNVs correspond to relatively large regions of the genome that have been deleted or duplicated. This variation accounts for roughly 12% of human genomic DNA and each variation may range from about a kilobase to several megabases in size. Most are ancient variants that are tightly correlated with SNPs, which can be used as a proxy. Unrelated humans differ at millions of SNPs in the genome. A typical person has about 100 heterozygous CNVs.

Nearby SNPs on a single chromosome are correlated because each SNP arose surrounded by other, earlier SNPs. A sequence of consecutive SNPs in a block on a chromosome is known as a haplotype, where SNPs are said to be in linkage disequilibrium (LD). SNPs separated by large distances are not very well correlated because of recombination at hotspots during gamete formation.

Analysis of African, European and East Asian populations showed that haplotypes are generally shared between populations. Africans, the oldest ethnic group, have the shortest LD blocks and probably evolved from a small founder modern human group in East Africa some 200,000 years ago. Migrations out of Africa between 125,000 and 60,000 years ago formed other ethnic groups. Development of genotyping arrays (often called SNP chips), with up to two million variants, allows comparisons between populations.

5.5.3 *Human history*

Early in the 1970s Marie-Claire King and Wilson showed that the human and chimpanzee genomes were only 1% different, and postulated that the differences resided in the non-coding regulatory region of genes.[27] Several hundred loci called human accelerated regions (HARs) have now been identified at which the rate of mutation since our divergence from the chimpanzee is exceptionally high. HAR1 is next to a non-coding RNA expressed in a markedly expanded brain region in humans. HAR2 includes a transcriptional enhancer that may have contributed towards the evolution of the opposable thumb in humans. The *FOXP2* gene has undergone accelerated amino acid substitution in human evolution, and is implicated in language. Compared to great apes and monkeys humans also lack about 500 short stretches of non-coding DNA, which regulate traits such as facial whiskers, penile spines — absence of which is thought to favour monogamous sex — and brain cell growth. These sequences were also lost in Neanderthals.

SNP analysis and whole genome sequencing (WGS) reveal a rich picture of population mixing and natural selection during human evolution. Europeans and Asians, but not Africans, all inherit 1–4% of the

Neanderthal genome, indicating interbreeding on the way out of Africa. Moreover, around 300 regions show evidence of positive selection in the past 5,000–30,000 years, often around a single gene, and sometimes a single variant. These genes encode proteins related to skin colour, infection, metabolism, nutrition and sensory perception. Even the origins of art and sacred practice may have been under positive selection.

5.5.4 *The genomic basis of common diseases and traits*

Common diseases are polygenic, and we now know that each contributing gene has a very small effect, which cannot be mapped by linkage in families. The common disease, common variant (CD/CV) hypothesis was posited to explain the aetiology of common disease. To evaluate this, the strategy of genome-wide association studies (GWAS) was conceived, which involves testing a comprehensive catalogue of common genetic variants in cases and controls from a population to find those variants associated with a given disease. The HapMap Project, genotyping arrays and rigorous statistical methods allowed the CD/CV hypothesis to be tested and validated in very large populations numbering from tens to hundreds of thousands.

Over a thousand loci are now associated with some 150 common diseases and traits. Most diseases are influenced by many loci, but the majority of the common disease variants have modest effects, increasing risk by 10–50% (like many environmental risk factors). Many genes previously found by linkage have been rediscovered. There are many new ones, which highlight new disease pathways and possible new treatment approaches. While many GWAS disease associations are attributed to amino acid variants, more are non-coding variants.

The power of this approach is illustrated by studies on the genetic control of height and lipid levels. Height is an archetypal polygenic trait with high heritability. A recent analysis of 180,000 individuals identified 180 loci, many with multiple distinct alleles, but only explaining 10% of the heritability.[28] Lipid levels are a major risk factor for coronary heart disease. In a study of 100,000 individuals 95 loci (including most of the 18 genes previously implicated in rare Mendelian lipid disorders) were associated with 1 or more major lipid or lipoprotein classes (low-density lipoprotein (LDL) cholesterol, high-density lipoprotein (HDL) cholesterol, triglycerides).[29] Although all loci are of moderate effect collectively they explain 25% of the genetic variance for LDL and HDL. Furthermore the study emphasises that genes of modest effect may have major therapeutic implications. The *HMGCR* locus (the product of which is the target of statins) has a variant with a frequency of 40%, which only alters LDL by 0.07 mmol/L, and no known rare mutations of large effect. The biology of several of the new genes has been elucidated by transgenic mouse and human clinical studies. For example, the sortilin gene (*SORT1*) harbours a common allele that alters a transcription factor binding site and expression of the gene.

Despite the great success of GWAS the results have only explained a fraction of human heritability. Where is the missing heritability? Already the larger GWAS have explained 20–25% of the heritability for various diseases and traits such as lipid metabolism. However, present estimates underline the contribution of low frequency and small effect size alleles. Limited sample size and stringent statistical methods have put some of them just out of reach. Other variants with still smaller effects (as expected with Darwinian evolution) may be too small to ever be detected with reasonable cohort sizes, but collectively explain a significant fraction of heritability. Indeed, it is inferred that tiny effects of common variants account for 55% of heritability for height and 33% for schizophrenia.

Rare variants of large effect also play an important part in common diseases, but their contribution to heritability will be small because of their low frequency. For example, only 0.0025% of heritability is explained by rare alleles at three loci affecting blood pressure. New genotyping arrays based on the 1000 Genomes Project should be able to capture many of the more frequent rare alleles of strong effect. Also, the estimates of heritability are inflated by genetic interactions or gene environment interactions, and through mis-interpreting shared environment as genetic. Epigenetic factors that sit between genes and the environment may make important contributions, and these can be transgenerational in their effects.

5.5.5 *Somatic cell genomics and cancer*

Some 80 cancer-causing genes had been identified by the year 2000. Whole genome sequencing and whole exome sequencing (WES) and GWAS have yielded another 150 solid tumours' genes.[24–26,30,31] These studies have revealed that recurrent mutations and CNV occur in cancer, as well as mutations favouring epigenetic change. Early focus on genes such as kinases in signalling pathways underlying cell growth led, for example, to the finding of Epidermal Growth Factor Receptor (EGFR) mutations in 15% of lung cancers and predicted which patients would respond to gefitinib and erlotinib, drugs which have been shown to extend life. WES of glioblastomas found a new class of cancer gene involved in basic cellular metabolism: recurrent mutation alters the active site of isocitrate dehydrogenase, causing it to generate an 'oncometabolite', 2-hydroxygluterate. Pharmaceutical companies are working to develop inhibitors of the neo-enzyme.

Gene expression profiling has allowed the biological classification of tumours, the identification of prognostic markers and therapeutic predictors. For example, over-expression and amplification of *HER2* (Human Epidermal growth factor Receptor 2), a marker of aggressiveness in breast cancer, is a strong predictor of benefit from treatment with a monoclonal antibody directed against *HER2*, which is a highly effective treatment of *HER2*-amplified metastatic breast cancer.

Small interfering RNAs have been developed that interfere with the function of all genes in living cells, and are being used in myriad ways, for example, to determine which genes are required for cancer cells to survive and which confer sensitivity to particular drugs. In cancer, as in genetics, the research tools of today are becoming the diagnostic and therapeutic tools of the future.

5.5.6 *Diagnosis and treatment*

DNA-based approaches are being used in numerous ways for the diagnosis, prevention and treatment of disease. Cancer and Mendelian disease mutations (e.g. familial hypercholesterolaemia and cystic fibrosis) are routinely identified. These lead to key decisions about disease management. The genome sequences for numerous pathogenetic viruses, bacteria and parasites have been catalogued. In a matter of hours or days the hepatitis C virus can be detected, a virulent form of the tuberculosis bacillus identified or the genome of a new strain of influenza virus sequenced, and a vaccine prepared. Limited gene expression profiling is used in cancer therapeutics and prediction of the risk of transplant rejection and, perhaps, of acute coronary syndromes.

Recombinant DNA technology through genome projects and engineering of proteins such as antibodies has led to a substantial array of protein therapeutics including antibodies for the treatment of rheumatoid arthritis and breast cancer. Antisense strategies are in trial as therapeutics. One antisense drug, fomivirsen, has been FDA approved as a treatment for cytomegalovirus retinitis. Similar approaches are in development for the lethal haemorrhagic fever viruses, Ebola and Marburg viruses, and there has been some success with HIV. Mipomersen, an antisense oligonucleotide against apolipoprotein B mRNA, which encodes the main cholesterol transport protein in blood, has successfully completed phase-3 trials for treating familial hypercholesterolaemia.

Pharmacogenetic association studies have revealed genetic factors underlying hypersensitivity to the antiretroviral drug abacavir, drug induced myopathies associated with cholesterol-lowering drugs, cardiovascular risks in patients receiving the antiplatelet drug clopidogrel and variations in metabolic clearance of the anticoagulant warfarin, screening for which is entering routine usage.

5.6 The Future

Medical revolutions require many decades to achieve their promise. The decade after the draft sequencing of the genome has been spectacular for progress in understanding its biology and the genetic basis of common diseases. Future genomic research will greatly enhance understanding of disease mechanisms, disease-risk prediction and new advance treatments. GWAS and massively parallel sequencing will need to be applied to well-annotated patient samples from many diseases — an international 'One Million Genomes Project'. Similarly in oncology the complete genome sequence of multiple samples of all cancer types (including primary, secondary and relapsing) will be determined, along with GWAS, to find adjuvant genes. There will be increased integration of epigenetic, transcriptomic, metabonomic and microbiomic analyses. Intensive functional studies — as well as human studies — will be required to characterise genes and pathways, and to construct animal models that mimic human physiology. Such studies will define new drug targets, chemical screens and clinical trials.

Special attention has been drawn to modular cell biology, cell re-programming (as in stem cells) and chemical biology and therapeutic science, in conjunction with high throughput strategies to discover new therapeutics, enhancing the efficacy of existing medicines through genomics-guided patient selection, or targeted drug improvement. Attention will also need to be turned to regulatory approval and clinical trials, in particular to the genomic basis of side effects and understanding of the pathways concerned so as to avoid these. There will need to be major advances in bioinformatics and computational biology. The computational challenges around data analysis, display and integration are now rate limiting. New approaches and methods are needed for data analysis and integration, visualisation, computational tools and infrastructure as well as training.

To realise the benefits of genomics the public needs to be educated. For this, genomics needs to be built into primary and secondary education, public outreach conducted, the genomic competency of healthcare providers built and the next generation of genomics researchers trained. Genomics also has great implications for society. To effectively examine the societal implications of genomic advances requires collaborations involving individuals with expertise in genomics, clinical medicine, ethics, law, economics and health services research.

We are warned not to promise the public a pharmacopoeia of quick pay-offs.[24] At the same time the ultimate impact of genomic medicine will be to transform the health of our children and our children's children. Importantly, complete explanation of a disease is not required for success. Good progress is being made on the long march from 'base pairs to bedside',[23] which started nearly 60 years ago in Cambridge with that remarkable Anglo-American discovery of the structure of DNA.

References

1. Unsigned editorial. Twenty-one years of the double helix. *Nature* 1974; 248: 721.
2. Watson JD. *The Double Helix*. London: Weidenfeld and Nicolson; 1968.
3. Crick F. The double helix: a personal view. *Nature* 1974; 248: 766–769.
4. National Library of Medicine. *Letter from James D Watson to Francis Crick (October 9, 1953)*. Available at: http://profiles.nlm.nih.gov/SC/ Views/AlphaChron/date/10003/10005/10003/ [Accessed 27 May 2011].
5. Wilkins MHF. The molecular configuration of nucleic acids. *Nobel Lectures, Physiology or Medicine 1942–1962*. Amsterdam: Elsevier Publishing Company; 1964.
6. National Library of Medicine. *Letter from Maurice Wilkins to Francis Crick* [ca. 1948–1953]. Available at: http://profiles.nlm.nih.gov/SC/ B/B/W/T/_/scbbwt.pdf [Accessed 27 May 2011].
7. National Library of Medicine. *Letter from Maurice Wilkins to Francis Crick* [ca. 1948–1953] (Thursday). Available at: http://profiles.nlm. nih.gov/SC/B/B/W/V/_/scbbwv.pdf [Accessed 27 May 2011].
8. National Library of Medicine. *Letter from Maurice Wilkins to Francis Crick* [ca. 1948–1953] (Saturday). Available at: http://profiles.nlm. nih.gov/SC/B/B/W/W/_/scbbww.pdf [Accessed 27 May 2011].
9. National Library of Medicine. *Letter from JT Randall to Rosalind Franklin (4 December 1950)*.Available at: http://profiles.nlm.nih.gov/ KR/B/B/B/B/_/krbbbb.pdf [Accessed 27 May 2011].
10. National Library of Medicine. *Letter from Aaron Klug to Philip Siekevitz (14 April 1976)*. Available at: http://profiles.nlm.nih.gov/KR/B/B/ C/X/_/krbbcx.pdf [Accessed 27 May 2011].

11. Pauling L, Corey RB, Branson HR. The structure of proteins: two hydrogen-bonded helical configurations of the polypeptide chain. *Proc Natl Acad Sci USA* 1951; 37: 205–211.

12. Olby R. *The Path to the Double Helix.* New York: Dover Publications Inc.; 1994.

13. Chargaff E. Chemical specificity of nucleic acids and the mechanism of their enzymatic degradation. *Experentia* 1950; 6: 201–209.

14. Pauling L, Corey RB. A proposed structure for the nucleic acids. *Proc Natl Acad Sci USA* 1953; 39: 84–97.

15. Crick FHC, Watson JD. The complementary structure of deoxyribonucleic acid. *Proc R. Soc* 1954; 223A: 80–96.

16. Watson JD, Crick FHC. Molecular structure of nucleic acids; a structure for deoxyribose nucleic acid. *Nature* 1953; 171: 737–738.

17. Wilkins MHF, Stokes AR, Wilson HR. Molecular structure of deoxypentose nucleic acids. *Nature* 1953; 171: 738–740.

18. Franklin RE, Gosling RG. Molecular configuration in sodium thymonucleate. *Nature* 1953; 171: 740–741.

19. Watson JD, Crick FHC. Genetical implications of the structure of deoxyribonucleic acid. *Nature* 1953; 171: 964–967.

20. Franklin RE, Gosling RG. Evidence for 2-chain helix in crystalline structure of sodium deoxyribonucleate. *Nature* 1953; 172: 156–157.

21. Klug A. Rosalind Franklin and the discovery of the structure of DNA. *Nature* 1968; 219: 808–844.

22. Klug A. Rosalind Franklin and the double helix. *Nature* 1974; 248: 787–788.

23. Clinton W. *New York Times,* 27 June 2000.

24. Green ED, Guyer MS. Charting a course for genomic medicine from base pairs to bedside. *Nature* 2011; 470: 204–13.

25. Lander ES. Initial impact of the sequencing of the human genome. *Nature* 2011; 470:187–197.

26. Mardis ER. A decade's perspective on DNA sequencing technology. *Nature* 2011; 470: 198–203

27. King MC, Wilson AC. Evolution at two levels in humans and chimpanzees. *Science* 1975; 188:107–116.

28. Lango Allen H, Estrada K, Lettre G *et al.* Hundreds of variants clustered in genomic loci and biological pathways affect human height. *Nature* 2010; 467: 832–838.

29. Teslovich TM, Musunuru K, Smith AV *et al.* Biological, clinical and population relevance of 95 loci for blood lipids. *Nature* 2010; 466: 707–713.

30. McDermott U, Downing JR, Stratton MR. Genomics and the continuum of cancer care. *N Engl J Med* 2011; 364: 340–350.

31. Berger MF, Lawrence MS, Demichelis F *et al.* The genomic complexity of primary human prostate cancer. *Nature* 2011; 470: 214–220.

Chapter 6

THE INTERPRETATION OF THE GENETIC CODE

John MacDermot and Ellis Kempner

6.1 Introduction

The unravelling of the genetic code was undoubtedly among the most important scientific events of the 20th century, with huge implications for the understanding and practice of medicine. It came as the climax to a revolution in medicine that followed the introduction of scientific method.

6.2 The Scientific Revolution in Medicine 1770–1970

Effective and rational medical practice requires an understanding of both human biology and the processes that underpin disease. It involves also a systematic approach to the diagnosis and investigation of individual patients, families or populations, and finally the capacity to recommend appropriate treatment to prevent, cure or palliate disease. There are quite accurate descriptions of disease that date back to antiquity, but in this chapter we will argue that the fundamental processes of biology, namely growth, metabolism, reproduction and evolution were demystified by the introduction of scientific method from about 1770, culminating in the elucidation of the genetic code 200 years later.

There was certainly little understanding before the 17th century of how the body worked, and a strong case can be made that William Harvey, who discovered the circulation of the blood,[1] led medical knowledge into the new age. The truth is, however, that there was very limited progress in the understanding of human physiology during the next 150 years. Religious dogma, deference to beliefs dating back to ancient Greece and Rome and sometimes pure invention provided a most unreliable background to biology and medical practice. Human dissection and accurate anatomical drawings had been published since the Renaissance, and there is good evidence that surgical techniques improved from that time. Nevertheless, physiological processes were not clearly defined, much less understood, and there was confusion about the functions of the various organs.

The 18th century was a period of great change in scientific thought, and the scientific revolution in biology, which started towards the end of the century, can arguably be dated back to Antoine-Laurent Lavoisier in about 1770. His interest in chemistry was focused on what we now recognise as oxidative reactions.[2] In just a few years, he demonstrated the errors inherent in the phlogiston theory, and showed also that air is not an element (a belief dating back to Aristotle), but is comprised of at least two separate gases (reviewed[3]). The greater part of systems physiology is now known to be underpinned by a very simple concept, which was first introduced by Lavoisier. Metabolic processes involve a series of controlled oxidative reactions, and the terminal electron acceptor of all such oxidative pathways is molecular oxygen. The purpose of the lungs and circulatory system is simply to deliver oxygen in sufficient amounts throughout the body to permit such reactions to occur.

The impact of the application of scientific method to biology was seen in the ensuing 200 years. Extraordinary advances followed the discoveries made by Gregor Mendel, Louis Pasteur, Charles Darwin, Robert Koch, Hans Krebs, Alexander Fleming and many others, and by the 1940s it was appreciated that the greatest barrier to a complete understanding of how biological systems worked was the very limited knowledge of how proteins are made, and how their structures are inherited from generation to generation. Proteins or polypeptides may serve as enzymes, cytoskeletal elements, molecular carriers, agents to combat specific invading pathogens, inflammatory mediators, hormones and many others, and it is the conserved structure of these molecules in all their complexity that enables the characteristics of one cell to be replicated in another during cell division. The characteristics of a particular animal or plant are also replicated from generation to generation during reproduction. As discussed in the previous chapter, genetic information is carried in DNA during both cell division and reproduction, and the nucleotide sequence of DNA encodes the amino acid sequence of the many proteins found in any particular species.

6.3 Discovery of the Genetic Code

The Nobel Prize in Physiology or Medicine was awarded in 1968 to three scientists for their contribution to the elucidation of the genetic code. They were Marshall W. Nirenberg, Har Gobind Khorana and Robert W. Holley. Khorana and Holley were outstanding chemists who worked on the structure and synthesis of oligonucleotides and transfer RNA. In the present chapter, however, we have concentrated primarily on the contributions made by Nirenberg (Fig. 6.1) and those scientists

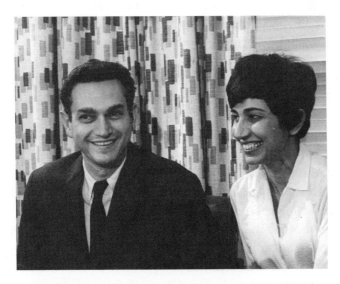

Fig. 6.1. Marshall Nirenberg and his wife Perola on the day of the announcement of the 1968 Nobel Prize in Physiology or Medicine. (Photo courtesy of the National Institutes of Health, USA).

who worked on protein synthesis and how the amino acid sequence of a protein is coded within the sequence of DNA. The focus of the present chapter relates to the relevance of their discoveries to clinical medicine, and in that context we have concentrated on the elucidation of the code.

Many scientific discoveries are rightly attributed to just one or two scientists, while all acknowledge the important early contributions made by others who took up the challenge, but never quite made the breakthrough. This was certainly true in the elucidation of the genetic code. The events surrounding the discovery, and the personalities of those involved, combine to make a compelling story. The field of biochemistry was firmly established during the first half of the 20th century, and the chemical nature of cellular contents was revealed by the 'grind and find' approach. Tissues were disrupted and their cellular contents released. Thereafter, a variety of techniques were applied to identify the different classes of chemicals, especially the macromolecules. The most numerous among these were the proteins, while smaller amounts of polysaccharides and lipids were also observed. The least abundant group was the nucleic acids, although they comprised the largest individual molecules.

All proteins were found to be linear polymers with molecular weights usually in the range 20000 to 300000 Da. The monomeric subunits comprised 18–20 different amino acids, and each individual protein had a specific sequence of amino acids and a precisely defined length. The structures of carbohydrates and lipids were much simpler, and their biosyntheses were catalysed by specific enzymes. The biosynthesis of proteins, however, was far more complicated. The first clue came in 1941 when Torbjörn Caspersson reported[4] that cells with the largest amount of nucleic acids were those that synthesised proteins most rapidly. By that time, both DNA and RNA had been identified, although their structures were unknown. Soon thereafter Oswald Avery, Colin MacLeod and Maclyn McCarty showed that DNA contained genetic information.[5]

Workers at the time attacked the problem of DNA structure from widely different angles. Erwin Chargaff focused on its chemistry, and established that in DNA the amounts of adenine- and thymidine-containing nucleotides were equal, and furthermore that the amounts of cytosine- and guanosine-containing nucleotides were also the same. X-ray crystallographers, most notably Maurice Wilkins and Rosalind Franklin, addressed the issue of the three-dimensional structure of the molecule, but struggled at first to obtain DNA crystals of sufficient quality. They went on, however, to establish in their pivotal experiments that DNA was a linear polymer in a helical configuration. Linus Pauling and others proposed various structural models, all of which proved incorrect, and finally James D. Watson and Francis Crick re-interpreted the earlier results (principally those of Chargaff and Franklin) and proposed the famous double helix with base pairing. At that point, the structure of DNA was known and its metabolic role seemed certain. The mechanism(s) of its action, however, and how it coded for the structure of proteins, presented a mighty challenge.

Two key discoveries were made a few years later. First, Elliot Volkin and Lazarus Astrachan[6] reported in 1956 that the synthesis of new viral particles from DNA involved the transient synthesis of RNA. Secondly, the primary sequence of amino acids in a protein (insulin) was determined for the first time. The sequence of amino acids in other proteins soon followed, and the scene was set to try and match the structure of DNA with its corresponding protein(s). The experimental strategy to elucidate the genetic code did not, however, involve a direct comparison of the structures of DNA and proteins. The approach adopted was based on the realisation that protein synthesis involved an unstable RNA intermediate,[7] whose sequence is complementary to genomic DNA. Thereafter, the mechanisms whereby amino acids are assembled into proteins were studied by correlating the structure of the RNA intermediate with the growing polypeptide chain.

Attempts to unravel the mechanisms of protein synthesis had been actively, but unsuccessfully, pursued for several decades. The general approach was to find a cell-free system that was able to synthesise polypeptides. Two different methods were usually involved. The first was to monitor the appearance of increasing amounts of a specific protein, usually an enzyme, whose increasing catalytic activity could readily be measured. In the second approach, the appearance of new virus particles, which contain protein, was also tried. After 1950, the ready availability of radionuclides permitted measurement of the incorporation of radioactive amino acids into newly synthesised proteins, and the method was increasingly applied. Many different laboratories were actively engaged on this problem, the most notable of which were Ernest Gale and Joan Folkes in England, Jacques Monod in France, and David Novelli, Sol Spiegelman, Paul Zamecnik and Severo Ochoa in the US.

There was wide acceptance that protein synthesis required nucleic acids, a pool of the necessary amino acids and probably specific enzymes. Some form of energy source, perhaps ATP, might also be required. Electron microscopy of mammalian cells revealed large lipoprotein plates containing electron-dense 'lumps', which were named microsomal particles, and were believed to be the sites of protein synthesis. In bacteria, the plates could not be identified microscopically, but the 'lumps' were readily found in bacterial extracts. There was a degree of confusion at first among scientists working on these intracellular organelles, and in the report of a symposium on protein synthesis in 1958, the organiser Richard Roberts recorded[8]:

> During the course of the symposium a semantic difficulty became apparent. To some of the participants, microsomes mean the ribonucleoprotein particles of the microsome fraction contaminated by other protein and lipid material; to others, the microsomes consist of protein and lipid contaminated by particles. The phrase 'microsomal particles' does not seem adequate, and 'ribonucleoprotein particles of the microsome faction' is much too awkward. During the meeting the word 'ribosome' was suggested; this seems a very satisfactory name, and it has a pleasant sound. The present confusion would be eliminated if 'ribosome' were adopted to designate ribonucleoprotein particles in the size range 20 to 100 S.

By the second half of the 1950s, many different 'cell-free systems' that contained these materials were developed. Most were unstable or not reproducible, and the yields of new protein were always quite small. Around this time, the discovery of a new type of RNA was reported (ribosomal RNA was the only one that had been known previously). These newly-found RNA molecules ('soluble RNA') were quite small and were found free in cell extracts. A short while later Nirenberg and his colleagues showed that soluble RNA molecules attach to amino acids, and serve a role in delivering the amino acids to the evolving polypeptide chain (see below).

Great excitement surrounded research on protein synthesis and the mystery of the genetic code, and particular efforts were directed to confirming which molecules (presumably nucleic acids) specified which amino acids were incorporated, and how the specific sequence of amino acids in proteins might be controlled. Several theories were put forward, most assuming that a particular sequence of nucleic acid bases specified each amino acid. George Gamow had predicted as early as 1954 that since there were 18–20 different amino acids and only 4 nucleic acid bases, it would require a minimum of 3 bases to specify a particular amino acid.[9]

Marshall Nirenberg at the National Institutes of Health in the US had been working in other areas of biochemistry, but considered working on the problem of protein synthesis. When he mentioned this to colleagues, their reaction was not always supportive. Bruce Ames said it was 'suicidal'! One of the present authors, who had worked in this area, discouraged Nirenberg, reminding him of all the futile attempts made by others. Nirenberg's reaction was, 'I think with modern biochemistry it could be done.' (Nirenberg, personal communications, 1959–1960.)

It was clear by this time that protein synthesis required three discrete RNA species, namely messenger RNA (mRNA), transfer or soluble RNA (tRNA) and ribosomal RNA (rRNA). The functions of the different RNAs emerged quite quickly, and in an important paper François Gros and colleagues provided good evidence[10] from experiments with *E. coli* that ribosomal RNA does not itself carry the genetic information, but appears to provide a stable surface on which transfer RNAs can bring their specific amino acid to the messenger RNA template.

A critical discovery and a key technical advance were reported shortly thereafter by Heinrich Matthaei and Marshall Nirenberg.[11,12] They described a new cell-free system from *E. coli* for measuring protein synthesis. The incorporation of radioactive amino acids was greatly increased in the presence of ribosomal RNA, independent of the presence of DNA.[11] The major difference between Nirenberg's new procedure and all others used previously was the inclusion of β-mercaptoethanol, a reducing agent. No one, not even the most distinguished Nobel Prize-winning biochemists, had previously considered the simple device of maintaining enzymes in a reduced state. Nirenberg's prediction about modern biochemistry seemed fully justified!

This was the first time that Nirenberg's name had been heard in this area of research. The paper appeared at about the same time as the 1961 International Biochemistry Congress in Moscow. Nirenberg presented a ten-minute report, in which he revealed that in his cell-free system phenylalanine incorporation (and only phenylalanine) was greatly increased in the presence of polyuridylic acid (polyU, a synthetic RNA containing only one base, uracil). Francis Crick had organised a special symposium on protein synthesis a few days later, and immediately made room for Nirenberg to speak to a much larger audience. The news that 'polyU in RNA codes for phenylalanine' spread rapidly. The first element of the genetic code had been broken — at least in *E. coli*. Shortly thereafter, Nirenberg showed that before incorporation AMP-phenylalanine attached to 'soluble RNA', which identified the role of what is now called transfer RNA.[13]

Many scientists immediately shifted their efforts to Nirenberg's cell-free system, including Severo Ochoa. Ochoa had a large research group, and had also been trying unsuccessfully to develop a cell-free system (from *Alcaligenes faecalis*). He quickly adopted Nirenberg's system to extend his own research to determine which 'code letters' of RNA specified which amino acid. Many others also adopted the method to explore other aspects of protein synthesis. One of the most important developments appeared only four months after Nirenberg's announcement, when Crick and colleagues presented a remarkable study.[14] They showed that the code probably involves nucleotide triplets (or multiples of triplets), that it is degenerate with more than one triplet code for each amino acid and that it is not overlapping. They inferred that, 'The sequence of bases is read from a fixed starting point.' In a very clever experiment a short while later, François

Chapeville and colleagues demonstrated the specificity of the recognition site between a particular tRNA molecule (complexed to its specific amino acid) and the mRNA encoding the particular polypeptide.[15] Their approach was to modify the structure of the amino acid after it had been complexed to tRNA by reduction with the catalyst Raney nickel. They reduced cysteine to alanine, following which alanine was incorporated into the growing polypeptide chain at a site that encoded cysteine. They inferred correctly that the specificity of the code was dependent on the recognition by mRNA of the corresponding tRNA and not the amino acid.

From about 1961, an important and very challenging series of experiments was reported by Robert Holley and colleagues at Cornell University on the structure of alanine-transfer RNA (reviewed in Holley's Nobel lecture[16]). Their experimental approach involved a series of cleavage reactions, with structural analysis of the corresponding fragments. Their results revealed the sequence of a nucleic acid for the first time, and more importantly (with appropriate modification to the corresponding bases of the DNA encoding the tRNA) they revealed the first nucleotide sequence of a gene. In later experiments, the group went on to demonstrate the classical 'cloverleaf' three-dimensional structure of tRNA.

The chemical synthesis and sequential analysis of short-chained oligonucleotides was undertaken by Har Gobind Khorana and his colleagues working at about the same time at the University of Wisconsin. They devised methods for the polymerisation reactions required to generate polynucleotides in the laboratory, and for the synthesis of polynucleotides with specific sequences (reviewed in Khorana's Nobel lecture[17]). While the work of Khorana and Holley is not discussed further here, their key contributions to the field were acknowledged in their share of the 1968 Nobel Prize with Marshall Nirenberg.

At the National Institutes of Health, the significance of Nirenberg's work was immediately noticed. New research positions were made available to him, and scientists from many different laboratories gave up their own research to help him. It was a shining moment in the history of the Institutes. Most notable were Robert Martin and Maxine Singer.

Martin provided dimers of nucleotides and Singer's expertise was in nucleic acid enzymology. Many new postdoctoral students came to work with Nirenberg, among the first of whom were Oliver W. Jones, Samuel Barondes, Brian Clark, William Sly, Philip Leder and Sidney Pestka.

Creating synthetic RNA-like polymers with repeating pairs and triplets of nucleic acid bases became paramount; this was initiated by Martin. For each specific nucleotide sequence, all amino acids were tested for incorporation. Each polymer was added to the Nirenberg system together with radioactive amino acids. After incubation, trichloroacetic acid was added to precipitate any new polypeptides. These were trapped on a filter, dried and the radioactivity was counted — tedious, but effective. Leder then designed a manifold on which multiple filters could be placed, increasing substantially the speed of the assays. It was by the application of these methods that the 'words' of the genetic code were eventually revealed.

There was still much work to be done, however. Many laboratories worldwide began working on the problem, and publications soon appeared reporting 'new' code words. Most notable were the many papers from the laboratory of Severo Ochoa. He had already received a Nobel Prize (1959) and had a large laboratory, certainly much larger than Nirenberg's. There developed a feeling of unfair competition, which was seen by some at the time as almost unethical: an older and powerful competitor was usurping the line of research from a young, previously unknown scientist. This attitude caused many scientists to rush to Nirenberg's side to help him in any way they could. Surprisingly, Nirenberg did not view Ochoa's entry as hostile. He felt it was helpful as it stimulated him to work harder. Indeed, some years later, Nirenberg and Ochoa (and their wives) were at a foreign meeting and were housed in the same small guest house where they ate their meals together. Nirenberg said he got to know Ochoa and liked him (Nirenberg, personal communication, 2008). Nirenberg had one of the most unassuming and humble personalities. Indeed, many years later, Crick advised Nirenberg that he did not spend enough time on public relations, but Nirenberg felt one's published work should speak for itself.

While reflecting on Nirenberg's personality and his way of working, the present authors were reminded of his extraordinary enthusiasm for scientific discovery, which extended far beyond his own area of research. He was a voracious reader of the scientific literature, and the floor of his study at home had to be specially strengthened from the cellar to prevent his collection of journals disappearing through it. He was a very hard worker, but kept unusual hours, particularly for someone employed in the government sector. He would usually arrive at work shortly after midday, and undertake a tour of the laboratory. Bursting with ideas for new experiments and avenues of research, his postdocs needed a measure of self-discipline and a firm focus on the task in hand in order not to be diverted on to some new line of research before the previous one had been completed. In one area of activity, however, namely the writing of scientific papers, Nirenberg was a stickler for detail, highly focused, exasperating to his collaborators and totally ungoverned by the clock. He was not a prolific writer (his whole contribution to the literature on the genetic code was contained in less than 30 papers), but he wanted everything he wrote to be as clear, accurate and generally perfect as he could make it. The problem was that Nirenberg could never stop tinkering with a manuscript he was writing, unless he worked to a deadline. There were those in his laboratory who maintained that he would never publish another paper if the office of the *Proceedings of the National Academy of Sciences* ever abandoned its practice of imposing each month a closing date and time for the submission of papers. The journal did eventually revoke the 'deadline' policy, and Nirenberg continued to publish there, but indeed more slowly.

One element of the code proved particularly elusive, namely that of lysine. It was finally established that the product, polylysine, was soluble in trichloroacetic acid and was thus not precipitated and trapped on a filter. This was overcome by including tungstic acid.[18] Over the course of several years, code words were established for each of the amino acids,[19] although a few code words did not stimulate the incorporation of any amino acids and were termed 'nonsense'. The 'nonsense' code words were shown[20] to code for 'stop', and the RNA sequence AUG, which codes for methionine, was also shown to serve

Table 6.1.   The genetic code. The code comprises triplets of
RNA bases along a chain of mRNA. The four bases in RNA are uracil
(U), cytosine (C), adenine (A) and guanine (G). The order shown in
the table is read in the following order: (i) left hand column, (ii) top
row, (iii) right hand column. An example would be the amino
acid histidine (His), for which the RNA code is either CAU or
CAC. The three STOP codons are shown, and AUG serves as
both the code for methionine (Met) and as the START codon.
Consequently, all proteins (when first translated, and before any
subsequent modification) start with the amino acid methionine at
the N-terminal end.

	U	C	A	G	
U	Phe	Ser	Tyr	Cys	U
	Phe	Ser	Tyr	Cys	C
	Leu	Ser	STOP	STOP	A
	Leu	Ser	STOP	Trp	G
C	Leu	Pro	His	Arg	U
	Leu	Pro	His	Arg	C
	Leu	Pro	Gln	Arg	A
	Leu	Pro	Gln	Arg	G
A	Ile	Thr	Asn	Ser	U
	Ile	Thr	Asn	Ser	C
	Ile	Thr	Lys	Arg	A
	Met	Thr	Lys	Arg	G
G	Val	Ala	Asp	Gly	U
	Val	Ala	Asp	Gly	C
	Val	Ala	Glu	Gly	A
	Val	Ala	Glu	Gly	G

Note: The abbreviations for the amino acids are phenylalanine (Phe), leucine
(Leu), isoleucine (Ile), methionine (Met), valine (Val), serine (Ser), proline
(Pro), threonine (Thr), alanine (Ala), tyrosine (Tyr), histidine (His), gluta-
mine (Gln), asparagine (Asn), lysine (Lys), aspartate (Asp), glutamate (Glu),
cysteine (Cys), tryptophan (Trp), Arginine (Arg), glycine (Gly).

as the start codon. In *E. coli*, newly synthesised polypeptides were
already known to begin with formyl-methionine. Within a decade all
the code words were deciphered (see Table 6.1), and the basic mechanisms of protein synthesis were established. The momentous leaps in
molecular biology were about to begin.

6.4 Implications of the Genetic Code for Clinical Medicine

Anyone working in medicine or a related field today will recognise the extraordinary developments that have led from the discovery of the structure of DNA and the elucidation of the genetic code. None of the methods of molecular biology can be said to rely solely on a single discovery, but the determination of the primary structure of polypeptides and proteins by genomic or cDNA sequencing has been a major development in biochemistry. cDNA is generated in the laboratory using a viral enzyme (reverse transcriptase), which enables a DNA sequence to be generated from the corresponding RNA. This indirect method of determining the sequence of a protein depends on an understanding of the genetic code, and the sequencing of DNA is certainly very much quicker and less expensive than direct sequencing of proteins by either N-terminal analysis or mass spectrometry. Once methods had been developed for the rapid determination of DNA and protein sequence, it was possible within a very short time to:

(i)   Synthesise chemically small fragments of known proteins, which are required in a whole variety of diagnostic and experimental protocols.

(ii) Incorporate foreign DNA into bacteria and generate large amounts of the corresponding protein.

(iii) Transfect wild-type or structurally modified DNA into cultured eukaryotic cells, or whole organisms, for the purposes of unravelling or altering particular cellular processes.

These and many other techniques of molecular biology have been applied widely in the development of diagnostic procedures, vaccines, pharmaceuticals, drug screening systems, enzyme replacement protocols and gene therapy. It is in the field of human genetics, however, that the many applications of molecular biology, and quite specifically a knowledge of the genetic code, have provided some of the most striking advances into our understanding of human disease, and where future developments appear particularly promising. Single gene disorders that are inherited according to Mendelian laws have been recognised for many years, and were the first to receive attention in the early days of molecular genetics. Examples would include sickle cell disease, haemophilia, cystic fibrosis, Huntington's chorea, Duchene muscular dystrophy and many others. The investigation of human disease changed substantially in the year 2003, however, with the completion of the human genome project. In the years that followed, the techniques for yet more rapid DNA sequencing were developed, and the extent of the variability of the human genome became apparent. Much of the variability is based on single-nucleotide polymorphisms (SNPs), in which a single base within a strand of DNA from one individual is found to be different from the base at the same position in other individuals. Very rapidly, it became possible in genome-wide association studies to test hundreds of thousands of SNPs for an association with a particular disease in hundreds or even thousands of affected individuals. Clearly, the presence or absence of a particular SNP in a gene of a single individual is not necessarily predictive of disease. On the other hand, if a disease is indeed associated with the presence of one or more SNPs in a particular gene, that association will eventually come to light when the SNP is identified more frequently in a sufficiently large number of affected individuals when compared to a control population.

One of the benefits of genome-wide association studies has been the possibility to investigate for the first time the genetic influence in complex (multi-gene) disorders.[21] It is now possible to study the contribution of combinations of multiple or rarer alleles to the heritability of a particular disease. An example would be Crohn's disease, in which there is a fairly low level of heritability; one in five patients has an affected first-degree relative. Genome-wide association studies have demonstrated more than 30 DNA variants (SNPs) in patients with Crohn's disease, of which 3 are quite common (in the order of 9% in the population), and are accompanied by a 1.5 to 4-fold increase in the risk of disease. The remaining DNA variants are, however, very much less common, and require very large studies for their detection.[22] Similar results were obtained in studies on Type 1 diabetes, in which more than 40 DNA variants have been identified to date. Of these, only a few contribute in a major way to the heritability of Type 1 diabetes, while the majority contribute very little.[23]

It is a relatively straightforward matter now to analyse the DNA strands in which SNPs are identified during genome-wide association studies. The proteins that are encoded by those particular DNA sequences are revealed by the genetic code, and there have been several interesting and very unexpected discoveries. Certain inherited disorders have associations with genes not thought previously to have any role in the condition. An example would be age-related macular degeneration (AMD), which is an important cause of impaired vision in the elderly. The condition is associated with SNPs in the complement factor-H (*CFH*) gene,[24] which is located on chromosome 1 and encodes a protein that is involved in an important pathway of inflammation. The DNA variant yields a change of a tyrosine to a histidine at amino acid 402 in CFH, which is in a region of the CFH molecule that binds heparin and C-reactive protein. CFH is part of the alternative pathway of complement activation, and has a role (in combination with other proteins) in inhibiting the cascade. The abnormal regulation of the complement pathway in patients with AMD is accompanied by an uncontrolled inflammatory response within Bruch's membrane and the adjacent retinal pigment epithelial cells, which leads eventually to impaired sight. Until this association was reported, age-related macular degeneration was thought (as the name implies) to be a degenerative condition, with little or no inflammatory component.

Other examples of unexpected gene-disease associations have been found, including both coronary heart disease[25] and Type 2 diabetes,[26] which are associated with genes implicated in cell-cycle regulation (the *CDKN2A/B* and *CDKAL1* genes respectively). The significance of these discoveries in the development of either coronary heart disease or Type 2 diabetes has yet to be determined, but will no doubt emerge in due course.

Another unexpected benefit of genome-wide association studies has been the finding that SNPs may occur in genes that are shown subsequently to be associated with more than one disease. For years clinical observation has led physicians to recognise that several conditions with some degree of heritability may be found in association with each other — an example would be coeliac disease and dermatitis herpetiformis. Genome-wide association studies have now revealed, however, that there are numerous disease associations that physicians had not even considered in the past. Among the more striking and least expected were the findings:

(i)   That SNPs in a single gene (*LRRK2*) are associated with both Parkinson's disease and Crohn's disease.

(ii) That SNPs in another gene (*KITLG*) are associated with testicular cancer and blond or brown hair.

(iii) That SNPs in a gene associated with Type 2 diabetes and prostate cancer (*JAZF1*) are also predictive of adult height (reviewed[21]).

There is no requirement for conditions that are inherited together to be related in every case to an SNP in a single gene, but in the cases cited above they probably are. The frequency of quite unrecognised associations of particular diseases, or sometimes associations of diseases with normal physical attributes (hair colour, height, etc.), has certainly come as something of a surprise. Furthermore, these findings may in future have important clinical implications. Screening programmes are already in place for many conditions such as cancer, in which an early diagnosis may have a significant impact on prognosis. Populations are generally screened for particular diseases on the basis of a perceived increased risk of that condition. Until such time, therefore, that everyone is screened for everything, it seems likely that the future selection of patients for screening will rely increasingly on recognised associations of the particular disease with any number of inherited features or associated pathological conditions.

Genome-wide association studies do not initially yield the cause of a disease in strictly pathological terms. They may, however, trigger a line of research which would not have been undertaken in other circumstances, and which elucidates the cause of the disease. An example would be the association described above of SNPs in the *CFH* gene with age-related macular degeneration. Genome-wide studies have also indicated that our knowledge of how inherited diseases are carried in genomic DNA remains incomplete. The vast majority of SNPs associated with disease are located in untranscribed sequences of DNA that are either buried within a gene (intronic) or are located in the sometimes lengthy regions of DNA between genes (intergenic). The genetic code identifies these regions unequivocally as being remote from DNA that encodes a protein. Furthermore, the great majority are not related to those DNA domains which bind any of the many regulator proteins involved in the control of transcription. Genome-wide association studies will certainly lead to further avenues of research with implications for both basic cell biology and clinical medicine.

We have argued in this chapter that the discovery of the genetic code was the final step in a series of discoveries that led to an understanding in general terms of the processes that drive living organisms, namely growth, metabolism, reproduction and evolution. Over a period of 200 years from about 1770, scientific method was introduced into biology and medicine. In the 40 years since the discovery of the genetic code, we have seen only the first hint of its likely impact.

References

1. Harvey W. *Exercitatio Anatomica de Motu Cordis et Sanguinis in Animalibus*. Frankfurt am Main: W Fitzer; 1628.
2. Lavoisier AL, Kerr R. *Elements of Chemistry, in a New Systematic Order, Containing All the Modern Discoveries*. Trans Kerr R. Printed for William Creech, and sold in London by GG and J Robinson; and in Edinburgh by T Kay; 1799.
3. Hunter GK. *Vital Forces: the Discovery of the Molecular Basis of Life*. London: Academic Press; 2000.
4. Caspersson T. Studien über den Eiweissumsatz der Zelle. *Die Naturwissenschaften* 1941; 29: 33–43.
5. Avery OT, MacLeod CM, McCarty M. Studies on the chemical nature of the substance inducing transformation of Pneumococcal types: induction of transformation by a desoxyribonucleic acid fraction isolated from Pneumococcus type III. *J Exp Med* 1944; 79: 137–158.
6. Volkin E, Astrachan L. Phosphorus incorporation in Escherichia coli ribonucleic acid after infection with bacteriophage T2. *Virology* 1956; 2: 149–161.

7. Brenner S, Jacob F, Meselson M. An unstable intermediate carrying information from genes to ribosomes for protein synthesis. *Nature* 1961; 190: 576–581.

8. Roberts RB. *Microsomal Particles and Protein Synthesis*, Roberts RB (ed.). New York: Pergamon Press; 1958: vii–viii.

9. Gamow G. Possible relation between deoxyribonucleic acid and protein structures. *Nature* 1954; 173: 318.

10. Gros F, Hiatt H, Gilbert W *et al.* Unstable ribonucleic acid revealed by pulse labelling of *Escherichia coli. Nature* 1961; 190: 581–585.

11. Matthaei JH, Nirenberg MW. The dependence of cell-free protein synthesis in E. coli upon RNA prepared from ribosomes. *Biochem Biophys Res Commun* 1961; 4: 404–408.

12. Matthaei JH, Nirenberg MW. Characteristics and stabilization of DNAase-sensitive protein synthesis in E. coli extracts. *Proc Natl Acad Sci USA* 1961; 47: 1580–1588.

13. Nirenberg MW, Matthaei JH, Jones OW. An intermediate in the biosynthesis of polyphenylalanine directed by synthetic template RNA. *Proc Natl Acad Sci USA* 1962; 48: 104–109.

14. Crick FHC, Barnett L, Brenner S *et al.* General nature of the genetic code for proteins. *Nature* 1961; 192: 1227–1232.

15. Chapeville F, Lipmann F, von Ehrenstein G *et al.* On the role of soluble ribonucleic acid coding for amino acids. *Proc Natl Acad Sci USA* 1962; 48: 1086–1092.

16. Holley RW. Alanine transfer RNA. In: *Nobel Lectures, Physiology or Medicine 1963–1970*, Lindsten J (ed.). Amsterdam: Elsevier Publishing Co.; 1972: 324–338.

17. Khorana HG. Nucleic acid synthesis in the study of the genetic code. In: *Nobel Lectures, Physiology or Medicine 1963–1970*, Lindsten J (ed.). Amsterdam: Elsevier Publishing Co.; 1972: 341–369.

18. Gardner RS, Wahba AJ, Basilio C *et al.* Synthetic polynucleotides and the amino acid code, VII. Proc *Natl Acad Sci USA* 1962; 48: 2087–2094.

19. Matthaei JH, Jones OW, Martin RG *et al.* Characteristics and composition of RNA coding units. *Proc Natl Acad Sci USA* 1962; 48: 1588–1602.

20. Caskey CT, Tompkins R, Scolnick E *et al.* Sequential translation of trinucleotide codons for the initiation and termination of protein synthesis. *Science* 1968; 162: 135–138.

21. Manolio TA. Genomewide association studies and assessment of the risk of disease. *N Engl J Med* 2010; 363: 166–176.

22. Barrett JC, Hansoul S, Nicolae DL *et al.* Genome-wide association defines more than 30 distinct susceptibility loci for Crohn's disease. *Nature Genet* 2008; 40: 955–962.

23. Barrett JC, Clayton DG, Concannon P *et al.* Genome-wide association study and meta-analysis find that over 40 loci affect risk of Type 1 diabetes. *Nature Genet* 2009; 41: 703–707.

24. Klein RJ, Zeiss C, Chew EY *et al.* Complement factor H polymorphism in age-related macular degeneration. *Science* 2005; 308: 385–389.

25. Helgadottir A, Thorleifsson G, Manolescu A *et al.* A common variant on chromosome 9p21 affects the risk of myocardial infarction. *Science* 2007; 316: 1491–1493.

26. Scott LJ, Mohlke KL, Bonnycastle LL *et al.* A genome-wide association study of Type 2 diabetes in Finns detects multiple susceptibility variants. *Science* 2007; 316: 1341–1345.

Chapter 7

THE DISCOVERY OF NEUROPEPTIDES AND RADIOIMMUNOASSAY OF PEPTIDE HORMONES

Jaimini Cegla and Stephen Bloom

7.1 Introduction

1977 was the year that the Queen celebrated her Silver Jubilee, *Star Wars* fever gripped the world and the rock and roll 'king' Elvis Presley died. It was also the year that the Nobel Prize in Physiology or Medicine was awarded to three distinguished American scientists: one half jointly to Roger Guillemin and Andrew Schally for their discoveries concerning 'the peptide hormone production of the brain', and the other half to Rosalyn Yalow for 'the development of radioimmunoassays of peptide hormones'.

In his presentation speech, Professor Rolf Luft described the mystique that had long since been associated with the term hormone: 'These were chemical substances with often very powerful actions at concentrations which for a long time seemed so low that they were impossible to measure. Once one learned to identify the active chemical substances — in this case hormones — and to measure their rate of synthesis, only then did one establish a firm basis for turning fantasy and mystery into reality.'[1] The three Nobel Laureates (Fig. 7.1) did exactly this.

Roger Guillemin and Andrew Schally worked independently towards the same goal: to extract and isolate substances from the hypothalamus and then demonstrate the ability of these substances to

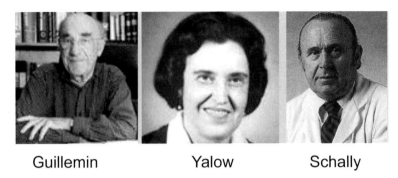

Guillemin   Yalow   Schally

Fig. 7.1.   The winners of the 1977 Nobel Prize in Physiology or Medicine (image of Professor Guillemin reproduced with his permission).

cause release of pituitary hormones. Their discovery of these neuropeptides led to the ground-breaking knowledge that there was indeed a link between the hypothalamus and the pituitary gland. They went on to sequence and synthesise several of these neuropeptides and thus helped to establish the chemical link between the brain and visceral systems.

Rosalyn Yalow, together with her late co-worker, Solomon Berson, addressed the associated challenge of measuring these hormones in blood. Because of their extremely low concentrations, peptide hormones could not be measured quantitatively and this led to a real stagnation in this field of research. Through the discovery that patients receiving insulin therapy developed anti-insulin antibodies, Yalow was able to use these antibodies with isotope-labelled insulin to determine plasma levels of insulin. Her work combined the fields of immunology, isotope research, mathematics and physics and has had a profound impact on medical and biological research.

7.2 Background of the Laureates

7.2.1 *Roger Guillemin*

Roger Guillemin was born in 1924 in Dijon, France. Here he did his schooling and entered medical school, but later transferred to the Faculté de Médecine in Lyon where he obtained his MD in 1949.

Guillemin's interest in endocrinology prevailed early on in his career, having been inspired by a lecture he attended in Paris on the endocrinology of the general adaptation syndrome by Hans Selye. He followed Selye back to Canada where he performed experimental work towards a PhD at the Institute of Experimental Medicine and Surgery at the University of Montreal. Selye's laboratory was prolific and the perfect place for the young Guillemin to gain experience in experimental endocrinology. It was here that he became more involved in research of hypothalamic hormones and their involvement in pituitary control during the acute stress response.

In 1953, he took up an Assistant Professor post at Baylor University College of Medicine in Houston, Texas, teaching physiology and living there for 18 years. Schally came to Houston and together they began their quest to characterise the corticotrophin-releasing factor. In 1970, Guillemin moved to the Salk Institute where he set up the Laboratories for Neuroendocrinology and his work on hypothalamic hormones really gained momentum. He was seminal in the isolation and synthesis of thyrotropin-releasing hormone (TRH), luteinizing hormone-releasing hormone (LHRH), somatostatin and also the endorphins. For this work, he was honoured with numerous awards, including the Lasker Award in Basic Sciences (1975) and the National Medal of Science presented by the President of the US (1976).[2] He retained his Gallic outlook and was always the perfect gentleman.

7.2.2 *Andrew Schally*

Andrew Schally was born in Wilno, Poland, in 1926, of mixed ancestry including Polish, Austro–Hungarian, French and Swedish roots. His childhood was far from idyllic, growing up first in war-torn Poland and then moving to a Jewish–Polish settlement in Romania. After the Second World War he made his way to the UK, which must have seemed like paradise compared to the harsh conditions to which he had been accustomed; the latter probably explained an occasional tendency to crudeness of behaviour. In 1946, Schally completed his schooling in Scotland and then moved down to London where he studied chemistry at undergraduate level.

Schally joined the National Institute of Medical Research (NIMR, MRC) Mill Hill, UK, as a young scientist in 1949 and here his true appetite for scientific research began to reveal itself. This was certainly helped by exposure to several very high-calibre scientists, including Dr Rodney Porter, Dr Archer Martin and Dr John Cornforth, who went on to become Nobel Prize Laureates for Chemistry, or Physiology or Medicine themselves. His three years at the Institute taught him technical skills as well as a basic approach to science that was both logical and ethical. In 1952, Schally moved to Montreal, Canada, to take up a PhD at McGill University. He developed an interest in endocrinology through the stimulating lectures of Professor David Thomson and experimental work with Dr Murray Saffran looking at the relationship between ACTH and adrenocortical steroids. He found this potential connection between brain function and endocrine activity intriguing and was determined to demonstrate this experimentally.

In 1955, Schally and Saffran became the first scientists to show that corticotrophin-releasing factor (CRF) was present in the hypothalamus and neurohypophyseal tissue. This was a real breakthrough in the field of neuroendocrinology as, prior to this, many had looked on with scepticism. Schally completed his doctoral studies and moved to Baylor in 1957 to continue his work on CRF with Guillemin. The five years that followed were a time of real frustration and dissatisfaction. Failure to isolate CRF from hypothalamic tissue cast doubt on Schally's original findings; however, his determination did not waiver and in 1962 he moved to New Orleans to set up and lead a Veterans Administration laboratory and continue his hypothalamic studies.

Schally was rewarded for his tenacity in 1969 when his group was able to discover the structure of TRH and two further hypothalamic hormones, LHRH in 1971 and porcine somatostatin in 1975. Having elucidated its structure and synthesised somatostatin, Schally set about collaborating with other groups around the world to further underpin the physiology and clinical importance of the hormone. It was this work that saw a collaboration between Schally and one of the authors (Stephen R. Bloom) at Hammersmith Hospital, London.

Schally has been the recipient of numerous awards for this work, notably the William S. Middleton Award, which is the highest award of the Veterans Administration, and the Lasker Award in Basic Medical Research.[2]

7.2.3 *Rosalyn Yalow*

Rosalyn Yalow was born in 1921 in New York, where she spent most of her life. Her mother was of German origin and her father of mixed Eastern European descent — neither had the opportunity to complete a secondary school education and were therefore determined that their children were given every chance to make it to university. Yalow's love for physics started at school and when she later attended Hunter, the all-women college of the City University of New York, it was nuclear physics that particularly attracted her. She was inspired by the biography of Marie Curie and was gripped by a lecture that she attended by Dr Enrico Fermi on the 'hot' topic of nuclear fission.

Yalow's family were keen for her to settle into a stable job as a primary school teacher on graduating from Hunter. However, Yalow had other ideas. She was determined to continue her studies in physics but her financial circumstances were a limiting factor. Therefore, in 1940, she took up a post as a part-time secretary to Dr Rudolf Schoenheimer, an eminent biochemist at Columbia University in order to pave her route into graduate studies. This came to fruition the following year as she was offered a teaching assistant-ship in physics at the University of Illinois. It was only when she arrived that Yalow learnt that she was the only woman of the 400 members of the faculty and the first since 1917. This did not deter her and by January 1945 she had completed her PhD in nuclear physics, picking up experimental skills in the creation and use of techniques to measure radioactive isotopes. It was also during this time that she met Aaron Yalow and they were married in 1943.

After completing her doctoral studies, Yalow returned to New York where she taught physics at Hunter. In 1947 she was offered a unique opportunity to set up a radioisotope service at the Bronx Veterans Administration Hospital. She was joined there by Dr Solomon Berson in 1950, with whom she worked closely for the next 22 years. Yalow's knowledge of physics and Berson's clinical experience enabled them to use radioisotopes for medical applications so far unexplored. Their work led them to the challenge of the measurement of small peptides such as hormones and it was for this work that Yalow was awarded the Nobel Prize in Medicine, becoming only the second woman to receive this prize and the sixth to receive any Nobel Prize. Yalow was also the first woman, and the first nuclear physicist, to win the Albert Lasker Basic Medical Research Award in 1976. Berson's premature death in 1972 meant that he did not receive these accolades as neither award is given posthumously. However, Yalow renamed her laboratory the Solomon A. Berson Research Laboratory so that Berson's name would appear on all her future publications.[2] Despite the seriousness with which she tackled her work, and her perceived arrogance, Yalow was often light-hearted about life and society. A particular anecdote: 'You know, we are strict Orthodox Jews. We obey all the laws and the traditions. When we walk down the street, I walk behind my husband. Of course, when I go to pick up my Nobel Prize, he can walk behind me!'[3]*

7.3 Discoveries Concerning the Peptide Hormone Production of the Brain

7.3.1 *The elusive link between the hypothalamus and pituitary*

By the early 1950s, it had been reported by various groups on both sides of the Atlantic that the anterior lobe of the hypophysis was involved in the control of target endocrine organs and that this in turn may be regulated by neuronal elements in the hypothalamus. How the hypothalamus was involved in this process was less clear. The curious anatomy of the junction between the hypothalamus and hypophysis connected by small blood vessels was postulated to be key to the link and this was demonstrated by tissue culture experiments by Guillemin and Rosenberg in 1955.[4] However, the neuronal factors were yet to be identified. These were likely to be small peptides and

* Unfortunately Professor Rosalyn Yalow passed away on 30 May 2011.

therefore difficult to characterise. Novel techniques of purification and assays to test these fractions were urgently needed. In addition, it was estimated that massive numbers of hypothalamic fragments would be necessary as each fragment contained only a thousand millionth of a gram of these substances. This mammoth task was undertaken by two independent groups led by Guillemin and Schally in what was to become a formidable race.

7.3.2 Identification of the first hypothalamic hormone: Thyrotropin-releasing hormone (TRH)

In a major effort to characterise TRH, the Guillemin group collected over 300,000 sheep hypothalamic fragments and by late 1968, they successfully isolated the elusive factor that controlled the thyroid gland via the pituitary.[5] Concurrently, Schally and his colleagues had collected 100,000 porcine hypothalami and managed to isolate 2.8 mg of TRH.[6] After overcoming considerable technical challenges, Guillemin went on to establish the primary structure of sheep (ovine) TRH by mass spectrometry as a simple tripeptide: pGlu-His-Pro-NH$_2$.[7] Schally's group confirmed these findings and their characterisation of porcine TRH gave an identical structure.

The characterisation of TRH was no mean feat. Once the hormone had been isolated, a combination of spectrometric techniques, including ultraviolet, infrared and nuclear magnetic resonance, were used to determine that TRH was likely to be a tiny polypeptide. Furthermore, the spectra were consistent with the presence of three particular amino acids: His, Pro and Glu. Both groups went on to examine analogues containing equimolar ratios of the three amino acids, looking for TRH activity; however, neither groups' analogues showed biological activity.[8] Schally, disheartened by his lack of positive findings, turned his attention to LHRH but returned to the TRH problem a couple of years on. Meanwhile Guillemin pursued the analogues and proposed to treat them with acetic anhydride in order to protect the N-terminus. He found that one of these analogues, H-Glu-His-Pro-OH, had biological activity qualitatively similar to native TRH and confirmed that this was indeed the major reaction product by mass spectrometry.[9] However, the two did not behave identically during chromatographic processes and Guillemin's group delved further. They proposed the structure pGlu-His-Pro-NH$_2$, based on the similarity of its structure to other naturally occurring hormones such as oxytocin and their deduction proved correct: they demonstrated that its specific activity was identical to TRH *in vitro* and *in vivo*.[10] The work of Guillemin's group was paralleled by that of Schally's and porcine TRH was shown to be identical to ovine TRH around the same time.[11] Schally's group was subsequently the first to show that porcine TRH stimulated TSH release in humans.[12] Today, TRH is widely used to differentiate between TSH and TRH deficiency and also between a TSH-secreting tumour and thyroid hormone resistance.

7.3.3 *Luteinizing hormone-releasing hormone (LHRH)*

Early in the 1960s, it was reported that a factor, able to stimulate secretion of luteinizing hormone from the pituitary, had been isolated from the hypothalamus.[13] Because of this ability, it was named luteinizing hormone-releasing hormone (LHRH). Intrigued by this find, Guillemin rapidly purified LHRH so that it was active at 1 µg in an animal bioassay and this was later confirmed by Schally.[14,15] In 1971, Schally's group successfully isolated porcine LHRH and through a series of experiments using around 200 nmol of the peptide, by enzymatic hydrolysis, they elucidated the sequence of LHRH, a decapeptide.[16] Four weeks later, Guillemin reported that this decapeptide had the same *in vivo* and *in vitro* activity as ovine LHRH.[17]

The clinical significance of the discovery of LHRH was profound. Both groups realised that it could have a real impact on the two spectrums of reproductive medicine: fertility and contraception. And so began the race to design agonists and antagonists of the molecule. In 1972, Guillemin published the structure of the first antagonist of LHRH, a potentially new contraceptive agent.[18] Also in search for potent agonists, the term 'super LHRHs' was coined to describe a group of analogues that was able to stimulate ovulation 150 times more potently than native LHRH. Guillemin's group was key in determining the modifications that gave the super LHRHs this property and their potential as ovulatory stimulating agents was realised.[19]

The discovery of LHRH also had far-reaching implications in the field of oncology. Between 1972 and 1978, Schally developed numerous agonistic LHRH analogues and became the first to demonstrate that they inhibited prostate cancer cell proliferation in rats. He was instrumental in the first clinical trials using LHRH agonists in patients with prostate cancer and sustained-release versions of these are now widely used in treatment of the disease.

7.3.4 *Somatostatin*

Hypothalamic hormones that released TSH and LH had been discovered and it followed that a peptide that stimulated growth hormone (GH) should also be in existence. Variances in assays and inaccuracies in methodology meant that this peptide was not discovered by the time the Nobel Prize of 1977 was awarded. However, in the search, it was observed that the addition of hypothalamic fragments to rat pituitary cells led to a decrease in resting secretion of GH. This was dose-dependent and specific; it was not seen by the addition of cerebellar extract nor by adding a host of other peptides including vasopressin, oxytocin and serotonin.[20] The factor responsible for this effect was named 'somatostatin'. The Guillemin group was able to extract somatostatin from sheep hypothalami and purify it by gel filtration.[21] By 1973, they had elucidated its structure by mass spectrometry.[22] Schally confirmed the structure of somatostatin in pigs was identical to that of the ovine peptide[23] and went on to demonstrate its presence in rat pancreas, intestine and stomach.[24]

Through his collaboration with several groups and people in England (including the author Stephen R. Bloom), Schally demonstrated that somatostatin suppressed glucagon and insulin release from the pancreas in healthy and diabetic individuals, indicating its involvement in the regulation of carbohydrate metabolism.[25] Later he observed the anti-tumour effects of somatostatin and its analogues in animal models. These are now widely used in the treatment of acromegaly and carcinoid tumours.

7.3.5 *Endorphins*

In 1973, the demonstration of opiate receptors in the brain led to a search for endogenous ligands. These were termed 'endorphins', combining the words 'endogenous' and 'morphine'. Guillemin hypothesised that endorphins were involved in GH and prolactin secretion as these hormones were known to be released after morphine injection. It took the group only a few months to isolate a substance with morphine-like activity from whole ox, pig and rat brains. The highest concentration was found in the hypothalamic region and by gel filtration, Guillemin was able to isolate several oligopeptides that he termed endorphins.[26]

To test his hypothesis, Guillemin injected beta-endorphin intraventricularly in rats and demonstrated GH and prolactin release. However, endorphins were not active directly at the level of the pituitary, indicating that this function was mediated elsewhere in the central nervous system (CNS).[27] The role of endorphins as neurotransmitters in the brain was also examined by the group and they showed the differential excitation of regional neurones in the CNS when exposed to endorphins.[28] Lastly, it was observed that beta-endorphin induced catatonia in animal models and Guillemin proposed that disturbance in its regulation may be important in mental illness.[29] Our knowledge and understanding of the structure and physiology of the endorphins has moved forwards tremendously thanks to the work of Guillemin and his colleagues.

7.4 The Development of Radioimmunoassays of Peptide Hormones

7.4.1 *Challenges of peptide hormone measurement*

By the mid-1950s, chemical quantitation of hormones had become commonplace and was routinely being used in the diagnosis and management of disease. However, it was not possible to use these methods in particular fields such as endocrinology as the peptide hormones to be studied were of too low a concentration in the blood. In fact, it was estimated that using conventional methods of that time, in order to measure basal levels of plasma ACTH (circa 1×10^{-12} mol/l), one would have needed 250 ml blood! Stagnation in research and inaccuracies in measurement leading to dubious assertions in the literature meant that the need for an accurate technique to determine peptide hormone concentration was pivotal to progress.

7.4.2 *The basis of radioimmunoassay*

Yalow and Berson's development of radioimmunoassay was not by directed design but more by serendipitous discovery through working on an independent project. In their quest to work out whether Type 2 diabetes mellitus was related to rapid metabolism of insulin, they studied the pharmacokinetics of ^{131}I-labelled insulin in healthy and diabetic subjects. Both were intrigued by what they observed: the radiolabelled insulin disappeared more quickly in patients who had received insulin previously as a treatment for their disease. Yalow and Berson hypothesised that these patients had developed antibodies to their insulin therapy, thus the labelled insulin was being bound, promoting its clearance. Using electrophoresis, they showed the presence of insulin–antibody complexes in the serum of patients treated previously with insulin. However, their work was against prevailing immunological theory and was met with much scepticism. In fact, their initial paper describing their findings was rejected by the *Journal of Clinical Investigation*. After conceding not to use the words 'insulin antibody' in the title, the work was finally published.[30] It is now widely recognised that peptides much smaller than insulin, such as vasopressin, can raise an immunological response and lead to antibody production; Yalow and Berson's work was certainly instrumental in propagating this view. However, it was the following observation that formed the basis of radioimmunoassay: that the percentage binding of added labelled insulin to a small fixed quantity of added antibody was proportional to the original amount of insulin present.

7.4.3 *The development of radioimmunoassay*

The principle of radioimmunoassay is straightforward in theory. An antigen (or analyte such as a peptide hormone) in a sample competes with an added small known quantity of radiolabelled antigen, e.g. ^{131}I-Insulin, to bind to a small fixed amount of added antibody which was raised to the antigen in question, e.g. insulin. The greater the unknown concentration of the non-radioactive antigen in the test sample, the less free antibody is left to bind to the radioactive antigen, so percentage radioactive binding falls. The extent of binding is then compared to test tubes with similar samples with added known amounts of the antigen. When you get a binding match then the unknown sample must have the same antigen concentration as the sample with a known concentration of added antigen. Though simple to grasp in theory, it was quantitating the kinetics of the reaction that took Berson and Yalow several years to optimise.[31,32] Issues regarding species specificity of the antibody also needed to be addressed. However, in 1959 they announced that they were successfully able to measure insulin levels in a rabbit given exogenous insulin. Shortly after, they optimised the assay to accurately measure insulin levels in humans.[33] By 1960, radioimmunoassay was born as a novel technique for peptide hormone measurement.

The sensitivity of radioimmunoassay was very impressive; for example, gastrin could now be measured at concentrations as low as 0.05 pmol/l. Another great advantage was that the technique was not limited to use with antibodies but competitive binding to receptors or binding proteins was also possible. This was exploited by Victor Herbert in the measurement of vitamin B12 using intrinsic factor (for which B12 is an endogenous ligand) as binding material.[34] Similarly, Roger Ekins used thyroxine-binding globulin to measure serum thyroxine levels.[35]

7.4.4 *Application of radioimmunoassay*

The advent of radioimmunoassay allowed the possibility of measuring peptide hormones in hundreds of samples batched together, with very small sample volumes necessary. Between the late 1950s and the 1970s, when Yalow received her prize, the rise in the number of hospitals using radioimmunoassay was exponential. Insulin had been the first peptide hormone to be measured as it was readily available in a purified form. In the years to come, all manner of peptide and non-peptide hormones were measured including those arising from the pituitary, pancreas, gut, thyroid, adrenal glands and gonads. This allowed more accurate diagnosis and monitoring of endocrine disorders.

Radioimmunoassay has also enabled the discovery of many novel hormones, particularly prohormones such as proinsulin and 'big'-ACTH.[36,37] It also brought forth the concept of heterogeneity, whereby hormones may exist in their intact or fragmented form. Yalow's group described an inactive PTH fragment, thus increasing our understanding of the biosynthesis and metabolism of these hormones.[38] Furthermore, they exploited the technique to examine the physiology and pathophysiology of hormone secretion. A great example of this was in their work on gastrin secretion. It was known that food was a powerful stimulant of gastrin and this increased gastric acidity, which in turn had a negative feedback on gastrin secretion. In both Zollinger–Ellison syndrome and non-tumorous hypergastrinaemic hyperchlorhydria, patients have high basal gastrin levels; however, the treatment of the two conditions is quite distinct. Yalow was able to use measurement of gastrin levels after provocation with secretin in order to accurately differentiate the two and so was born the concept of dynamic function testing, which is now commonplace in endocrinology.[39]

Endocrinology saw the first use of radioimmunoassay but the technique's applicability spans many fields. Drugs, enzymes and viruses can all be readily detected by the technique. In toxicology and therapeutic drug monitoring, differentiation and identification of drug metabolites may also be possible, depending on the specificity of the antibody. Enzyme concentration can potentially be measured at lower concentrations than catalytic techniques, without the influence of cofactors or inhibitors. In the field of infectious diseases, Yalow's group used radioimmunoassay for the detection of hepatitis viruses as well as tuberculin purified protein derivative.[40,41]

Radioimmunassay is still used widely today, particularly in the measure of steroid hormones. However, its real legacy is its founding principles which have been adapted and used with alternative non-radioactive labels such as enzymes, fluorescence and chemiluminescence. This has enabled automation of immunoassay and its routine use in most hospital laboratories today.

7.4.5 *Radioimmunoassay and peptides of the brain*

The topics for which the Nobel Prize was awarded to Guillemin and Schally (50%) and Yalow (50%) are intrinsically linked. It was through Yalow's radioimmunoassay that the neuropeptides that Guillemin and Schally had isolated could be accurately measured and their physiology studied. The discoveries of all three Laureates show that meticulous work and determination do pay off and that one scientific question, once answered, usually raises another. It was Yalow who once noted, 'The excitement of learning separates youth from old age. As long as you're learning you're not old.'[42]

References

1. Odelberg W. *Les Prix Nobel. The Nobel Prizes* 1977. Stockholm: Nobel Foundation; 1978.
2. Lindsten J. *Nobel Lectures, Physiology or Medicine 1971–1980*. London: World Scientific Publishing Co; 1992.
3. Patton DD. Three nobelists who paved the way. *J Nucl Med* 2002; 43 (3): 25N–28N.
4. Guillemin R, Rosenberg B. Humoral hypothalamic control of anterior pituitary: a study with combined tissue cultures. *Endocrinology* 1955; 57: 599–697.
5. Guillemin R, Yamazaki E, Jutisz M *et al*. Présence dans un extrait de tissue hypothalamiques d'une substance stimulant la sécrétion de l'hormone hypophysaire thyréotrope (TSH). Première purification par filtration sur gel Sephadex. *C R Acad Sci (Paris)* 1962; 255: 1018–1020.
6. Schally AV, Bowers CY, Redding TW *et al*. Isolation of thyrotropin-releasing factor (TRF) from porcine hypothalamus. *Biochem Biophys Res Commun* 1966; 25: 165–169.

7. Guillemin R, Burgus R, Vale W. The hypothalamic hypophysiotropic thyrotropin-releasing factor. *Vitamins and Hormones* 1971; 29: 1–39.

8. Schally AV, Arimura A, Bowers CY *et al*. Hypothalamic neurohormones regulating anterior pituitary function. In: *Recent Progress in Hormone Research*, Astwood EB (ed.). New York: Academic Press; 1968: 497–590.

9. Gillessen D, Felix AM, Lergier W *et al*. Syntheses of thyrotropin-releasing hormones (TRH) (Schaf) and related peptides. *Helv Chim Acta* 1970; 53, 63.

10. Burgus R, Dunn TF, Desiderio D *et al*. Characterization of ovine hypothalamic hypophysiotropic TSH-releasing factor. *Nature (London)* 1970b; 226: 321.

11. Bowers CY, Schally AV, Enzmann F *et al*. Porcine thyrotropin releasing hormone is (Pyro)Glu-His-Pro(NH2). *Endocrinology* 1970; 86: 1 1143–1153.

12. Bowers CY, Schally AV, Hawley DW *et al*. Effect of thyrotropin-releasing factor in man. *J Clin Endocrinol Metab* 1968; 28: 978–982.

13. McCann SM, Taleisnik S, Friedman HM. LH-releasing activity in hypothalamic extracts. *Proc Soc Exp Biol Med* 1960; 104: 432.

14. Guillemin R, Yamazaki E, Card DA *et al*. *In vitro* secretion of thyrotropin (TSH): stimulation by a hypothalamic peptide (TRF). *Endocrinology* 1963; 73: 564.

15. Schally AV, Arimura A, Bowers CY *et al*. Hypothalamic neurohormones regulating anterior pituitary function. *Rec Progr Horm Res* 1968; 24: 497–588.

16. Matsuo H, Arimura A, Nair RMG *et al*. Synthesis of porcine LH- and FSH-releasing hormone by solid-phase method. *Biochem Biophys Res Commun* 1971a; 45: 822–827.

17. Monahan M, Rivier J, Burgus R *et al*. Synthese totals phase solide d'un decapeptide qui stimule les secretions des gonadotrophines hypophysalires e.g. LH, FSH. *C R Acad Sci (Paris)* 1971; 273: 205.

18. Vale W, Grant G, Rivier J *et al*. Synthetic polypeptide antagonists of hypothalamic luteinizing hormone-releasing factor. *Science* 1972c; 176: 933–934.

19. Monahan M, Amoss M, Anderson H, Vale W. Synthetic analogs of hypothalamic luteinizing hormone-releasing factor with increased agonist or antagonist properties. *Biochemistry* 1973; 12: 4616–4620.

20. Vale W, Grant G, Amoss M *et al.* Culture of enzymatically dispersed anterior-pituitary cells: functional validation of a method. *Endocrinology* 1972a; 91: 562–572.
21. Burgus R, Butcher M, Amoss M *et al.* Primary structure of ovine hypothalamic luteinizing hormone-releasing factor (LRF). *R Proc Nat Acad Sci USA* 1972; 69: 278–282.
22. Burgus R, Ling N, Butcher M *et al.* Primary structure of somatostatin, a hypothalamic peptide that inhibits secretion of pituitary growth-hormone. *Proc Nat Acad Sci USA* 1973; 70: 684–688.
23. Schally AV, DuPont A, Arimura A *et al.* Isolation and structure of growth hormone-release inhibiting hormone (somatostatin) from porcine hypothalami. *Biochemistry* 1976; 15: 509–514.
24. Arimura A, Sate H, DuPont A *et al.* Abundance of immunoreactive somatostatin in the stomach and the pancreas. *Science* 1975; 289: 1007–1009.
25. Mortimer CH, Tunbridge WMG, Carr D *et al.* Effects of growth-hormone release-inhibiting hormone on circulating glucagon, insulin, and growth hormone in normal, diabetic, acromegalic and hypopituitary patients. *Lancet* 1974; 1: 697–701.
26. Guillemin R, Ling N, Burgus R. Endorphins, hypothalamic and neurohypophyseal peptides with morphinomimetic activity. Isolation and primary structure of alpha-endorphin. *C R Acad Sci (Paris)* 1976a; 282: 783–785.
27. Rivier C, Vale W, Ling N *et al.* Stimulation *in vivo* of secretion of prolactin and growth-hormone by beta-endorphin. *Endocrinology* 1977b; 100: 238–241.
28. Nicoll R, Siggins G, Ling N *et al.* Neuronal actions of endorphins and enkephalins among brain-regions: a comparative microiontophoretic study. *Proc Nat Acad Sci USA* 1977; 74: 2584–2588.
29. Bloom F, Segal D, Ling N *et al.* Endorphins: profound behavioral-effects in rats suggest new etiological factors in mental-illness. *Science* 1976; 194: 630–632.
30. Berson SA, Yalow RS, Bauman A *et al.* Insulin-I metabolism in human subjects: demonstration of insulin binding globulin in the circulation of insulin-treated subjects. *J Clin Invest* 1956; 35: 170–190.

31. Berson SA, Yalow RS. Kinetics of reaction between insulin and insulin-binding antibody. *J Clin Invest* 1957; 36: 873.

32. Berson SA, Yalow RS. Quantitative aspects of reaction between insulin and insulin-binding antibody. *J Clin Invest* 1959; 38: 1996–2016.

33. Yalow RS, Berson SA. Assay of plasma insulin in human subjects by immunological methods. *Nature* 1959; 184: 1648–1649.

34. Herbert, V. Studies on the role of intrinsic factor in vitamin B12 absorption, transport, and storage. *Am J Clin Nutr* 1959; 7: 433–443.

35. Ekins RP. The estimation of thyroxine in human plasma by an electrophoretic technique. *Clin Chim Acta* 1960; 5: 453–459.

36. Steiner DF, Cunningham D, Spigelman L, Aten B. Insulin biosynthesis: evidence for a precursor. *Science* 1967; 157: 697.

37. Yalow RS, Berson SA. Size heterogeneity of immunoreactive human ACTH in plasma and in extracts of pituitary glands and ACTH-producing thymoma. *Biochem Biophys Res Commun* 1971; 44: 439–445.

38. Berson SA, Yalow RS. Immunochemical heterogeneity of parathyroid hormone in plasma. *J Clin Endocrinol Metab* 1968; 28: 1037–1047.

39. Yalow RS, Berson SA. Radioimmunoassay of gastrin. *Gastroenterology* 1970; 58: 1–14.

40. Walsh JH, Yalow RS, Berson SA. Detection of Australia antigen and antibody by means of radioimmunoassay techniques. *J Inf Dis* 1970; 121: 550–554.

41. Straus E, Yalow RS. Radioimmunoassay for tuberculin purified protein derivative. *Clin Res* 1977; 25: A384.

42. Kahn CR, Roth J. Berson, Yalow, and the JCI: the agony and the ecstasy. *J Clin Invest.* 2004; 114(8): 1051–1054.

Chapter 8

THE DEVELOPMENT OF COMPUTER-ASSISTED TOMOGRAPHY

Adrian M. K. Thomas

8.1 Introduction

The Nobel Prize in Physiology or Medicine for 1979 was awarded jointly to Allan M. Cormack and Godfrey N. Hounsfield for their development of computer-assisted tomography. James Bull, the pioneer British neuroradiologist, reviewed the history of computed tomography and said that seldom in the history of medicine has a new discovery swept the world quite so quickly.[1] The CT scanner has not only transformed medical care but has also changed the way we look at the body. The same could also be said for the original discovery of X-rays by Wilhelm Conrad Röntgen in 1895. The discovery of the X-rays swept the world even more rapidly than the invention of CT scanning and also changed the way we look at ourselves, with its demonstration of living anatomy. Both the discovery of X-rays and the invention of computer-assisted tomography resulted in the award of a Nobel Prize, with Wilhelm Röntgen receiving the first Nobel Prize in Physics in 1901.

8.2 Brief Biographical Sketches of the Laureates

8.2.1 *Allan MacLeod Cormack (1924–1998)*

Allan Cormack[2,3] was born in February 1924 in Johannesburg, South Africa. He matriculated from Rondebosch Boys High School in Cape

Town in 1941. He initially studied electrical engineering at the University of Cape Town but switched to physics and graduated in 1944. He completed his Master's thesis in 1945, taking the subject of X-ray crystallography. Following this he moved to St John's College, Cambridge, in the UK, where he worked at the Cavendish Laboratory as a research student under Otto Frisch. Following his marriage he needed a job and so he returned to Cape Town as a Lecturer in Physics at the university. Cormack described his work as being lonely because of the paucity of nuclear physicists in South Africa. It is also worth noting that Cormack never received a doctoral degree in physics.

In 1956 Cormack was working at Groote Schuur Hospital with the radiotherapist Dr James Muir Grieve. He became interested in the absorption of radiation in the body and this initiated his interest in the basis of what became computed tomography. In 1958 he took a sabbatical from his post in South Africa and worked at the Harvard University Cyclotron. Cormack was then offered a position as Assistant Professor in the Department of Physics in Tufts University, Massachusetts, US, which he accepted. Cormack moved to the US and became a US citizen in 1966. He continued to work on CT but his main interest for most of this time was in nuclear and particle physics and he pursued the CT scanning problem only intermittently. By 1963 he had developed his ideas on CT to such an extent that they were published in the *Journal of Applied Physics*.[4] Cormack had tested his ideas using phantoms; however, when his paper appeared there was little response from the scientific community so he continued his normal course of research and teaching. He was appointed Chairman of the Physics Department at Tufts University from 1968 to 1976 and retained his interest in nuclear physics and the interaction of sub-atomic particles. In the period 1970–1972 Cormack became aware of developments related to CT scanning and following this he devoted much of his time to these problems. He was a member of the American Academy of Arts and Sciences. He was awarded the Nobel Prize in Physiology or Medicine jointly with Godfrey Hounsfield in 1979, retired in 1980 and died in Winchester, Massachusetts, on 7 May 1998.

8.2.2 *Sir Godfrey Newbold Hounsfield FRS (1919–2004)*

Godfrey Hounsfield[2,5] was born in Newark in Nottinghamshire in the UK on 28 August 1919. He went to school at the Magnus Grammar School in Newark. He grew up on a farm and from his earliest days was interested in how things work, performing many practical experiments. He was always interested in aeroplanes and when the Second World War started he joined the Royal Air Force as a volunteer reservist. He became interested in radar and radio communications and worked as a radar mechanic instructor. In the RAF he attended the Royal College of Science in South Kensington, which was then occupied by the RAF, and then he went to the Cranwell Radar School and passed the City & Guilds examination in Radio Communications. After the war Hounsfield attended the Faraday House Electrical Engineering College in London, and received their diploma. He was never an undergraduate at a university and the only university degrees he received, and there were six of them, were honorary.

Hounsfield joined EMI in Middlesex in 1951 where he worked on guided weapons and on radar. He was involved with computers, which were only in their infancy, and from 1958 he led a design team that built the first all-transistor computer constructed in Britain, the EMIDEC 1100. Following this, his next project was to design a thin-film computer store. When this project was abandoned he started the work that was to result in the CT scanner. By 1972 he was Head of the Medical Systems Research Department.

Godfrey Hounsfield received many honours for his work on CT scanning. In 1972, when he was given the prestigious MacRobert Award, the referee said, 'No comparable discovery has been made in this field since Röntgen discovered X-rays in 1895.' He was elected to the Fellowship of the Royal Society and in 1974, together with James Ambrose, he received the Barclay Prize of the British Institute of Radiology, followed by the honorary membership of the Institute in 1980. In 1979 he received the Nobel Prize in Physiology or Medicine jointly with Allan Cormack. Godfrey Hounsfield was knighted by Her Majesty Queen Elizabeth in 1981.

Until his death after a long illness on 21 August 2004 Hounsfield remained interested in the development of CT and in MRI. He was involved with the Department of Radiology at the Royal Brompton Hospital and regularly attended meetings at the British Institute of Radiology including the annual Hounsfield Lecture, the eponymous lecture given each year in his honour.

8.3 The Medical Problem or Scientific Question

The questions posed by Cormack and Hounsfield were different and neither was initially related to medical imaging.

When Allan Cormack[2,3,6] was a lecturer in physics in Cape Town in 1955 the hospital physicist at Groote Schuur Hospital resigned. The law in South Africa required that a qualified physicist should supervise the use of radioactive isotopes. As he was the only nuclear physicist in Cape Town Cormack therefore spent a day and a half at the hospital. He became interested in radiotherapy treatment planning and in the use of isodose charts. The isodose charts in use at that time described the passage of radiation through homogenous materials and showed the distribution of the dose of radiation. The body is, of course, not homogenous and contains tissues of varying densities including gas-filled tissues, solid organs and bone. Cormack realised that treatment planning could be facilitated if the distribution of attenuation coefficients in the body could be determined. This distribution of attenuation coefficients could be determined by external measurements. At some point later it occurred to Cormack that this data might have diagnostic significance. How to determine this distribution of attenuation coefficients was the problem that Cormack set himself.

The situation for Godfrey Hounsfield[2,5,6] was rather different. When the EMI project to design a thin-film computer store was abandoned Godfrey Hounsfield was not immediately assigned another task. Instead he was allowed to suggest his own ideas for research so he put forward a project for automatic pattern recognition which had no medial implications. It was in 1967 that it occurred to Hounsfield that it did have medical implications and the EMI-Scanner and computed tomography were born. This illustrates the value of research that is undertaken with no immediate commercial benefit. Hounsfield had two problems to solve. The first was similar to that of Cormack and was one of automatic pattern recognition using external measurements. The second was to build a functioning and practical scanner having realised the medical possibilities.

8.4 A Description of the Research that was Undertaken to Provide the Solution

The history of the development of computerised axial tomography is complex.[6-9] The need for tomography, either mechanical or computerised, lies in the fact that in conventional radiography a three-dimensional object is displayed as a two-dimensional image with no depth data. The X-rays come from a point source and the object radiographed appears on photographic film as a shadow of varying densities depending on differences in absorption. Classical tomography was well-developed by the 1950s, the pioneer work having been done by Bernard Zeides des Plantes and published in the 1930s. In classical tomography the X-ray source and the detector both move and the points of pivot all lie in the same plane. Objects out of the plane are blurred and those at the level of the pivot are in focus. This tomographic image gives information in one plane and helps in diagnosis.

Whilst Allan Cormack and Godfrey Hounsfield received the Nobel Prize there were others who had worked in the field that became CT scanning. The mathematical basis for reconstruction started with Johann Radon (1887–1956). Between 1912 and 1919 he was the Assistant Professor for Mathematics at the Department for Mathematics at the Technische Hochschule, Wien (Technical University Vienna, Austria). Johann Radon applied the calculus of variations to differential geometry, and this led to various applications in number theory. In 1917 he published his fundamental work on the 'Radon transform', which mathematically transforms two-dimensional images with lines into a domain of possible line parameters, where each line in the image will give a peak positioned at the corresponding line parameters. This idea of reconstructing a function from a set of projections therefore plays a significant role in the development of computed tomography.

There were a number of workers over the years who looked at developing tomography from its mechanical form.[8] In the mid-1940s Shinji Takahashi in Japan had worked on the principles underlying rotational radiography and developed what we would now call sinograms. In 1957 Boris Korenblyum and his co-workers built a medical CT scanner in Kiev in the then USSR. In 1960 William Oldendorf made experiments to demonstrate the feasibility of CT scanning using a rotating phantom made of nails and mounted on a track.[10] In the early 1960s David Kuhl and Roy Edwards developed an apparatus for emission CT scanning (radioisotope section imaging). It is interesting to observe the number of unconnected workers tackling the same problem but coming at it from quite different directions.

8.4.1 *Mathematical basis of CT scanning*

Allan Cormack developed the mathematical basis of what became CT scanning[4] and worked quite independently from others. He developed a mathematical approach to looking at the problems of variations in body tissues that are important in radiotherapy. The exponential attenuation of radiation through material had been known and used for over 60 years when Cormack considered the problem; however, the attenuation was determined for parallel-sided blocks of material. Cormack found out, rather to his surprise, that the generalisation had not been transferred to inhomogeneous materials. He initially considered a fine beam of radiation passing through a body with circular symmetry. In 1957 he made experiments using a phantom that had circular symmetry. By 1963 he was ready to make experiments on a phantom that did not have circular symmetry. The apparatus consisted of two cylinders containing a detector and a gamma ray source. The phantom lay between the two cylinders and the work was done in the summer of 1963. Cormack then considered how many measurements need be made since only a finite number of measurements can be made with beams of a finite width. The results were presented for publication in graphical form and were published in 1964.[4] There was almost no response to the publications although Cormack related that the most interesting reprint request was from the Swiss Centre for Avalanche Research since the method he had described could be used for examining snow on a mountain, assuming that the source or detector could be placed in the mountain under the snow. There was certainly no commercial interest in his work. He became aware of the pioneering work of Radon only in the late 1970s.[11] Radon had stated that if the line integrals of a particular property of an object, such as its density, could be known for all lines intersecting a slice of an object and coplanar with the slice then the density can be reconstructed exactly. Cormack had developed the mathematics of line integrals independently.

In the 1960s Godfrey Hounsfield was working at EMI Ltd in Hayes, Middlesex.[12-14] He was interested in pattern recognition and also in computers which were in an early stage of development. He had worked on radar with the RAF in the Second World War and had built the first solid-state electronic computer in the UK. Hounsfield was looking at internal structure and considered a closed box with an unknown number of items inside. The box could be looked at from multiple directions using an X-ray source and a radiation detector. The results of the transmission readings could then be analysed by the computer and presented, sliced, in a single plane. Hounsfield developed a mathematical approach to determine the nature of the objects in the box in a process of reconstruction. The original apparatus was very simple and resembled that used by Cormack. The basis of the apparatus was an uncomplicated lathe holding the object to be examined (Fig. 8.1). On opposite sides were a radiation source (initially an americium radioisotope source) and a radiation detector. The early experiments were made using Perspex phantoms of varying complexity. Figure 8.2 is from an album made by Hounsfield and is scanned directly from the original Polaroid photograph. It was labelled by Hounsfield as 'first picture ever' and is the first CT image ever taken by him. The readings were taken using a scintillation counter which counted the gamma ray photons. It took nine days to take the picture and fifteen minutes' computing time to reconstruct it. Following the use of Perspex phantoms a section of human brain

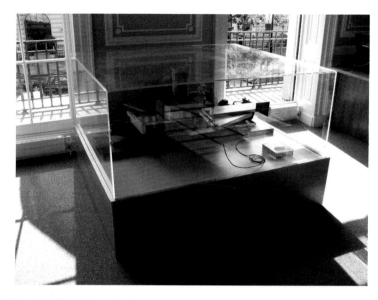

Fig. 8.1.   Godfrey Hounsfield's lathe bed scanner at the British Institute of Radiology.

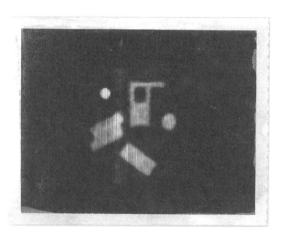

Fig. 8.2.   Polaroid image of the first CT scan made by Godfrey Hounsfield of a Perspex phantom.

in formalin in a Perspex box was used as a phantom. Most of the pictures from the lathe bed were scanned in 1969 and 1970. The original apparatus may be viewed in the library of the British Institute of Radiology in Portland Place in London.

8.4.2 *Roles of EMI and the Department of Health*

Hounsfield looked at practical applications of the technique and approached the Department of Health in London in 1968. If a medical use could be found then this would stimulate the development of the project. Hounsfield met Cliff Gregory and Gordon Higson, who were scientific advisers at the then Department of Health and Social Security (DHSS). Hounsfield was then introduced to Evan Lennon, a radiological adviser to the DHSS. Lennon knew that Frank Doyle from the Hammersmith Hospital was working on the problem of bone density measurements. Doyle gave Hounsfield two lumbar vertebrae of different densities. Hounsfield examined the vertebrae and returned with computer printouts of numbers in the coronal plane of the vertebral body. He had already worked out a scale of numbers and Doyle was impressed with the result. It was a recurring theme with Hounsfield, even after the development of the EMI scanner, that he preferred the computer printout of numbers to a pictorial presentation of the data. Lennon also made contact with two other radiologists — James Ambrose and Louis Kreel. Ambrose was a neuroradiologist from Atkinson Morley's Hospital in south London and Kreel was from the Royal Free Hospital, subsequently moving to Northwick Park Hospital in Harrow, north London, where he did pioneer work using the EMI body scanner. Ambrose later discovered that Hounsfield had been previously dismissed by an eminent radiologist as a crank.

It became apparent that EMI would not spend any more money on developing the new technique without the support of and a contribution from the DHSS. Lennon and Higson reported to the Department of Health, who agreed to the necessary support. The three radiologists then worked more closely with EMI. Doyle supplied bone specimens, Ambrose supplied brain specimens and Kreel supplied abdominal specimens. Work continued on specimen radiography and then on 14 January 1970 there was a meeting at the Department of Health between the three radiologists and Dr Lennon, Mr Gregory and Mr Higson. The initial results were very promising and it was agreed to produce a prototype machine. Because of the difficulties of abdominal scanning it was agreed that the prototype would be a brain machine and that this was to be at Atkinson Morley's Hospital.[3] Atkinson Morley's Hospital had several advantages: it was quite close to EMI, the scanner could be placed in a discreet location so patients could be examined without too much advertisement and the department had an innovative approach to radiological practice. During this period James Ambrose developed a close relationship with Godfrey Hounsfield.

8.4.3 *Neuroradiological applications of CT scanning*

James Ambrose (1923–2006)[15] is a key figure in the development of CT scanning and in neuroradiology. Ambrose was born in Pretoria, South Africa, on 5 April 1923. He initially studied science at Johannesburg and during the Second World War he joined the Royal Air Force. After the war he studied medicine at Cape Town and came to the UK in 1954 to study radiology, initially at the Middlesex Hospital and then at Guy's Hospital. Ambrose became interested in neuroradiology and in 1959 went to work at Atkinson Morley's Hospital, where he spent his working life. Atkinson Morley's was in Wimbledon in south London and by 1948 it had become the busiest neurosurgical unit in London. Neurosurgery at Atkinson Morley's Hospital had been developed by Wylie McKissock, who had visited Stockholm and been very impressed by the close collaboration between the surgeon Herbert Olivecrona and the radiologist Eric Lysholm. McKissock disliked the current invasive neuroradiological techniques of angiography and pneumoencephalography and James Ambrose shared his concerns. The department at Atkinson Morley's Hospital actively investigated alternative imaging techniques including cranial ultrasound and nuclear medicine brain scans with the support of the physics department at St George's Hospital. Ambrose presented his work on cranial ultrasound in 1969 to the meeting of the British Medical Association in Leicester, and although the paper was well received Ambrose would admit that the technique was not generally useful. He was therefore well prepared to respond positively to Godfrey Hounsfield and to his novel ideas regarding cranial imaging. In 1974 James Ambrose and Godfrey Hounsfield jointly received the Barclay Prize of the British Institute of Radiology, and Ambrose received honorary membership in 1993.

The prototype scanner was installed at Atkinson Morley's Hospital on 1 October 1971. It is quite remarkable that Hounsfield went in one move from the primitive lathe bed apparatus to the prototype CT scanner. This prototype CT scanner (Fig. 8.3) looks very similar to modern CT scanners and is on display in the Science Museum in South Kensington, London. The scanning time was 4 minutes per slice with a slice thickness of a little over 1 cm. There was no computer attached to the machine and the data had to be taken by car on magnetic tape to be analysed by EMI at Hayes. The data was reconstructed using an ICL 1905 mainframe computer and a picture with an 80×80 matrix took 20 minutes to reconstruct. The software was written by Stephen Bates who made major contributions to the early CT computing at EMI. It would have been possible to have reconstructed the data using a 160×160 matrix but that would have taken

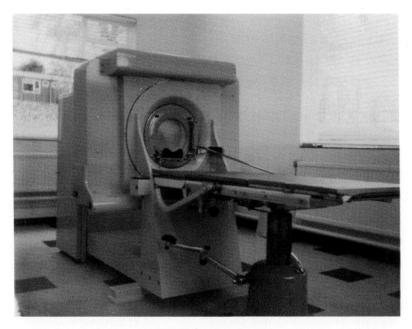

Fig. 8.3.   The first clinical CT scanner at Atkinson Morley's Hospital.

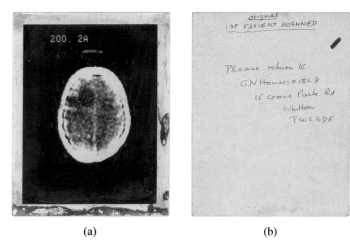

(a)   (b)

Figs 8.4a & b.   Polaroid image of the first clinical CT scan, showing a large cystic lesion in the left frontal lobe, and Hounsfield's comment on the reverse.

considerably longer. Ambrose had felt that at least six months of work would be needed to build up an appreciation of the normal and abnormal. The first patient scanned on the new machine was a 41-year-old lady with a possible frontal lobe tumour. The data was acquired and the tapes were sent to EMI. The results were returned after two days. The cystic tumour in the left frontal lobe was clearly shown (Figs 8.4 a & b), and Ambrose said the result caused Hounsfield and himself to jump up and down like football players who had just scored a winning goal. Radiology was changed forever. The scan is presented in the opposite direction from modern scans and is viewed as a neurosurgeon would look, which is from above. Modern scans are viewed as looking from below upwards. The reverse of the Polaroid print has Hounsfield's words, 'original 1st PATIENT SCANNED', with his request for it to be returned to him.

The preliminary results were presented at the 32nd Annual Congress of the British Institute of Radiology, which was held at Imperial College, London, in April 1972. The session was held on the afternoon of Thursday 20 April, chaired by the neuroradiologist George du Boulay, and was entitled 'New Techniques for Diagnostic Radiology'. The paper presented by Ambrose and Hounsfield was entitled 'Computerised axial tomography (a new means of demonstrating some of the soft tissue structures of the brain without the use of contrast media)'. As might be expected the paper produced a sensation and the first press announcement was in *The Times* on 21 April 1972. The presentation appeared as an abstract in the *British Journal of Radiology*[16] with three papers appearing later that year. The first paper by Hounsfield[17] described the technical background, the second paper was by Ambrose[18] and described the clinical findings, and the third paper by Perry and Bridges[19] looked at radiation doses. EMI then started the production of a brain machine and made five: one for the National Hospital, Queen Square, one for Manchester, one for Glasgow and two for the US — one for the Mayo Clinic and the other for the Massachusetts General Hospital. All machines were installed in the summer of 1973. James Bull described the new machine to Dr Fred Plum, a leading American neurologist. Plum said that the US would need at least 170 brain machines to cover the neurology departments and that it would soon become unethical for a neurologist to practise without access to a brain machine since it saved many patients from unnecessary suffering from the currently available techniques. Ambrose also looked at the use of the new scanner in orbital lesions which were previously difficult to image.[20]

Whilst the new scanner was obviously effective it was also very expensive. EMI had various problems, which Melvyn Marcus outlined in the *Sunday Telegraph* of 30 July 1978 in an article entitled 'It's crisis time for scanners'. The difficulties that EMI experienced came from two directions. Firstly, competition from other companies: there were several court cases for patent infringements, including a suit filed by EMI against Ohio-Nuclear in 1976 and Pfizer in 1977. However, more significant was the clampdown on hospital expenditure in the US under the administration of President Jimmy Carter. America was the largest market for the EMI scanner and hospitals had to meet very rigorous conditions to be able to undertake any major capital expenditure. However, in spite of the problems experienced by EMI and the EMI scanner, CT has continued to develop. The award of the Nobel Prize in Physiology or Medicine to Godfrey Hounsfield and Allan Cormack in 1979 emphasised the arrival of the new technique.

8.5 The Nature and Scale of the Impact of these Discoveries on Medical Science

It is difficult to overestimate the impact that the EMI or CT scanner has had on investigative medicine. The neuroradiologist James Bull introduced the book based on the 1977 First European Congress on Computerised Axial Tomography in Clinical Practice (edited by Boulay and Mosley) and said that Hounsfield's revolutionary radiological technique was the most important advance in X-ray photography since Wilhelm Röntgen radiographed his wife Bertha's hand in November 1895 in Würzburg.[21] Within five years of the introduction of the CT scanner there were machines in major centres on all continents and the technique was rapidly adopted into clinical practice. It is now difficult to imagine how medicine was practised before the introduction of CT scanning. The CT scanner followed by the widespread use of ultrasound and MRI has resulted in the blossoming of the radiological sciences since the 1970s. As an example, the diagnosis of cerebral haemorrhage following a head injury was difficult and uncertain. Internal injury was inferred from a fracture of the skull or a shifted pineal gland revealed on the plain film. Haemorrhage was diagnosed more certainly using the invasive technique of cerebral angiography but doctors were obviously reluctant to perform invasive diagnostic examinations unless the chances of finding an abnormality were high. Patients with head injury were commonly admitted for neurological observations after undergoing a skull X-ray and were observed in hospital with a 'wait and see' policy. Patients with significant trauma to the head now have an early CT scan and appropriate medical intervention can be undertaken with confidence, and many lives have been saved as a consequence. Figure 8.5 shows the brochure cover for the EMI1010 scanner, 'the most advanced system for neuroradiological examinations', and is signed by Godfrey Hounsfield.

The CT scanner has led to the modern paradigm shift in medical investigation and treatment. Traditional radiological investigation was often invasive and the resulting treatment was also invasive. The modern paradigm is that of non-invasive diagnosis and minimally invasive

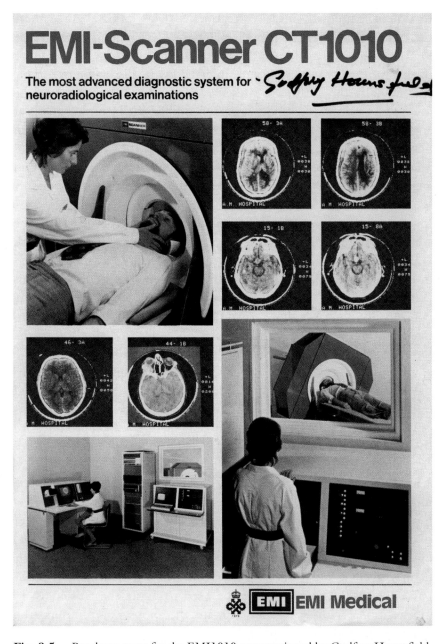

Fig. 8.5.   Brochure cover for the EMI1010 scanner signed by Godfrey Hounsfield.

treatment. Minimally invasive treatment has as its basis an accurate pre-treatment diagnosis. The CT scanner also changes the way radiological images were interpreted. In traditional radiology the presence of an abnormality was commonly inferred by the distortion of normal anatomy. In the head the presence of a brain tumour could be inferred by a displaced blood vessel when filled with contrast media at angiography or from a distorted cerebral ventricle which had been filled with air at pneumoencephalography. Both angiography and pneumoencephalography required the patient to be an inpatient and anaesthesia needed to be used since both techniques were physically unpleasant for the patient. In contrast, the CT scan could be performed as an outpatient and the patient only had to keep still in the scanner gantry. Unlike angiography or pneumoencephalography the CT scanner showed the abnormality directly without any inference as in the case of the lady with the left-sided frontal lobe tumour. This ability to see the abnormality directly has had several effects. The abnormality is shown more clearly and a likely diagnosis is easier to make and the extent of the abnormality is easier to define and so the radiological–pathological correlation is enhanced. Because the CT scan is non-invasive it can be repeated easily, unlike invasive techniques, and so the response of the disease to treatment can be assessed quite easily. This has greatly facilitated the monitoring of the effects of medical treatments in clinical trials. As the CT scan is non-invasive the threshold for performing a radiological examination is reduced, since doctors are understandably reluctant to perform potentially hazardous examinations without a very strong clinical indication. The introduction of the CT scanner has lowered the threshold for performing radiological investigations, and whilst this has had the effect of considerably increasing the work of X-ray departments it has also meant that abnormalities may be diagnosed at an earlier stage in their natural history, and earlier diagnosis means that treatment is facilitated. The CT scanner can also be used to guide the radiologist in interventional radiology and facilitate the biopsy of tumours, the drainage of fluid collections and radiofrequency ablation.

When the team at EMI were developing the whole body scanner it became apparent that a cross-section of the body would have significant utility in planning radiotherapy treatment. Prior to the introduction of CT scanning radiotherapy treatment planning was imprecise and time consuming. There was an imbalance between the accuracy of the treatment that could be delivered by the linear accelerator and the then available treatment plans. The CT scan allowed computer programs to guide the treatment beam in a process requiring only a few minutes. The radiotherapy planning system is linked to the CT diagnostic display console and the radiation isodose distribution curves can be overlaid onto the CT image. The CT density numbers could be used to calculate the effect of inhomogeneities in the tissues in the path of the radiation beam. This was the very problem that Allan Cormack had been considering back in 1956. The areas to be irradiated at therapy could be marked as could sensitive areas to be avoided, which could be located precisely.

The impact of CT scanning on the X-ray equipment industry is interesting. The CT scanner or EMI scan developed by EMI Medical Inc was quite unexpected by the large X-ray equipment companies and it took them some time to catch up. The X-ray industry had been concentrating on increasingly sensitive X-ray film-intensifying screen combinations with ever finer resolution. The EMI/CT scanner was initially of lower resolution and used an entirely different physical principle. There are stories told of Hounsfield approaching several eminent radiologists with his early ideas and being greeted without any enthusiasm. It is interesting to consider how the research that led to the CT scanner did not come from the major X-ray companies in the same way that the research that led to our modern low osmolar non-ionic contrast media did not develop in one of the large contrast-media companies, but in a small Norwegian company.[22] In the same way that the first paper by Torsten Almén[23] on the idea of a non-ionic contrast agent had no immediate impact in the radiological community so the significance of the papers of Allan Cormack was not recognised. In the mid-1960s EMI had only a minor involvement in medicine by way of its subsidiary SE Labs. By the mid-1970s EMI was a world leader in advanced medical technology with a full order book and a significant market potential which at that time was valued at £100 million per year. The story of the rise and decline of EMI

Medical Inc is interesting and today EMI has no medical connection at all.

The CT scanner is in clinical use for all parts of the body and it has transformed the lives of countless people. Godfrey Hounsfield was told by many patients and relatives how very grateful they were for the CT scanner and he felt humbled and pleased by this.

CT scanning has continued to develop since the 1970s and the modern multislice CT scanner has a central role in current medical imaging. Spiral CT represents a significant advance in the technology of CT scanning and has increased the clinical value of CT. The first clinical cases and performance measurements were presented as work in progress by Willi Kalender, Peter Vock and Wolfgang Seissler at the 75th anniversary meeting of the Radiological Society of North America in 1989.[24,25] The technique was then fully described in a paper in *Radiology* in 1990.[26] The development of spiral CT and now multislice scanning was made possible by the advances in computing. Data no longer have to be taken away for analysis but can be reconstructed almost instantaneously. In spiral CT, the X-ray source rotation and the patient table translation are made simultaneously and so the time for acquisition of the raw data is significantly reduced. The principles of spiral CT have been well reviewed by Vannier and Wang.[27] Willi Kalender has reviewed its uses[28] and describes the amazing results that can be achieved by modern multislice scanners. We now have improved spatial resolution with virtual endoscopy and faster scanning enabling complex dynamic studies. The most dramatic advances resulted from the provision of higher continuous X-ray power and improvements in computers. CT scanning has had inestimable effects on medical care and we all have a debt to Godfrey Hounsfield and Allan Cormack for their pioneering work.

References

1. Bull J. History of Computed Tomography. In: *Radiology of the Skull and Brain: Technical Aspects of Computed Tomography*, Newton TH, Potts DG (eds). St Louis: Mosby; 1981: n.p.

2. Thomas AMK, Banerjee AK, Busch U. *Classic Papers in Modern Diagnostic Radiology.* Berlin: Springer-Verlag; 2004.

3. Vaughan CL. *Imaging the Elephant, A Biography of Allan MacLeod Cormack.* London: Imperial College Press; 2008.

4. Cormack AM. Representation of a function by its line integrals, with some radiological applications. *J Appl Phys* 1964; 34: 2722–2727.

5. Wells, PNT. Sir Godfrey Newbold Hounsfield KT CBE. *Biogr Mems Fell R Soc* 2005; 51; 221–235.

6. Friedland W, Thurber BD. The birth of CT. *Am J Radiol* 1996; 167: 1365–1370.

7. Webb S. *From the Watching of Shadows. The Origins of Radiological Tomography.* Bristol and New York: Adam Hilger; 1990.

8. Webb S. Historical experiments predating commercially available computed tomography. *Brit J Radiol* 1992; 65: 835–837.

9. Webb S. The Invention of Classical Tomography and Computed Tomography. In: *The Invisible Light. 100 Years of Medical Radiology,* Thomas, AMK (ed.). Oxford: Blackwell Science; 1995: 61–63.

10. Oldendorf WH. The quest for an image of the brain: a brief historical and technical review of brain imaging techniques. *Neurol* 1978; 28: 517–533.

11. Cormack AM. Sampling the radon transform with beams of finite width. *Phys Med Biol* 1978; 23: 1141–1148.

12. Hounsfield GN. Historical notes on computerised axial tomography. *J Can Assn Radiol* 1976; 27: 135–142.

13. Hounsfield GN. Computer reconstructed X-ray imaging. *Phil Trans R Soc Lond A* 1979; 292: 223–232.

14. Hounsfield GN. The EMI Scanner. *Proc R Soc Lond B* 1977; 195: 28–289.

15. Ambrose J. You never know what is just around the corner. *Rivista di Neuroradiologia* 1996; 9: 399–404.

16. Ambrose J, Hounsfield G. Computerised transverse axial tomography. *Brit J Radiol* 1973; 46: 148–149.

17. Hounsfield GN. Computerized transverse axial scanning (tomography). Part 1. Description of system. *Brit J Radiol* 1973; 46: 1016–1022.

18. Ambrose J. Computerized transverse axial scanning (tomography). Part 2. Clinical application. *Brit J Radiol* 1973; 46: 1023–1047.

19. Perry BJ, Bridges C. Computerized transverse axial scanning (tomography). Part 3. Radiation dose considerations. *Brit J Radiol* 1973; 46: 1048–1051.

20. Ambrose JAE, Lloyd GAS, Wright JE. A preliminary evaluation of fine matrix computerized axial tomography (Emiscan) in the diagnosis of orbital space-occupying lesions. *Brit J Radiol* 1974; 47: 747–751.

21. Bull JWD. Foreword. In: *Computerised Axial Tomography in Clinical Practice*, du Boulay GH, Moseley IF (eds). Berlin: Springer-Verlag; 1977: n.p.

22. Grainger RG, Thomas AMK. History of Intravascular Iodinated contrast Media. In: *Textbook of Contrast Media*, Dawson P, Cosgrove D, Allison DJ (eds). Isis Medical Media; 1999: 3–14.

23. Almén T. Development of non-ionic contrast media. *Investigative Radiology* 1985; 20: 2–9.

24. Vock P, Jung H, Kalender WA. Single-breathhold voluminetric CT of the hepatobiliary system. *Radiol* 1989; 173(P): 377.

25. Kalender WA, Seissler W, Vock P. Single-breath-hold spiral volumetric CT by continuous patient translation and scanner rotation. *Radiology* 1989; 173(P): 414.

26. Kalender WA, Seissler W, Klotz E, *et al.* Spiral volumetric CT with single-breathhold technique, continuous transport, and continuous scanner rotation. *Radiology* 1990; 176: 181–183.

27. Vannier MW, Wang G. Principles of spiral CT. In: *Spiral CT of the Chest*, Rémy-Jardin M, Rémy J (eds). Berlin, Heidelberg, New York: Springer; 1996: 1–32.

28. Kalender WA. Spiral CT in the year 2000. In: *Spiral CT of the Chest*, Rémy-Jardin M, Rémy J (eds). Berlin, Heidelberg, New York: Springer; 1996: 321–329.

Chapter 9

THE DISCOVERY OF PROSTAGLANDINS

Rod Flower

9.1 Introduction

In 1982, John Vane, Bengt Samuelsson and Sune Bergström were awarded the Nobel Prize in Physiology or Medicine 'for their discoveries concerning "prostaglandins" and related biologically active substances'. The citations specified (amongst other items) Bergström's work on the purification and structural determination of prostaglandins, the elucidation of arachidonic acid metabolism by Samuelsson and the discovery of the mechanism of action of aspirin by Vane.

The award not only celebrated a lifetime of highly significant achievements on the part of the three investigators but was also noteworthy for another reason; prostaglandins were the first family of lipid mediators to be closely characterised. The notion that a group of potent substances, with diverse biological effects, could be derived from such a simple precursor as a fatty acid, fundamentally altered thinking about the role of lipids in cell signalling.

Although the significance of the prostaglandin field today stands as a monument to the work of numerous researchers, many of the seminal discoveries arose through an intellectual cross-fertilisation between a group of scientists in Stockholm, drawing largely upon physico-chemical and biochemical expertise, and a group of London-based researchers using mainly the techniques of bioassay, over a period roughly spanning the 1960s–1970s. This chapter focuses mainly upon that period and how these interactions led to the discovery of the prostaglandin system and its intimate linkage to disease and anti-inflammatory drug action.

9.2 Lipids: Just Fats?

The story of our emerging understanding of the biosynthesis and action of lipid mediators, however, had its roots in the early decades of the last century. At that time, little significance was attached to non-nutritional functions of lipids. They were generally regarded as a heterologous collection of 'greasy' substances that could be extracted from animal and plant tissues with organic solvents. Lipids were, it was conceded, important structural components of cells: 'fat' in the diet was a convenient source of energy and in adipose tissue the neutral lipids represented a useful metabolic store. Few believed that lipids (with the possible exception of acetylcholine) were candidates for intracellular signalling factors or local hormonal regulation.

Things changed in the 1930s. The seminal discovery of the 'essential' fatty acids by George Burr and Mildred Burr[1,2] and a realisation of their importance in the diet was one defining event. The wholly unexpected observation by George Hevesey (and one of the first uses of a radioactive isotope in medical research) that phosphorus in cell membranes was metabolically very labile was another (discussed by Rex Dawson et al.[3]). But of more significance to this chapter were some odd observations dating from the 1930s concerning the biological properties of semen.

The potent pharmacological properties of seminal plasma had been noticed by several groups. In Columbia University, Raphael Kurzrok and Charles Lieb[4] had already reported a stimulant effect on uterine smooth muscle; in London, Martin Goldblatt[5] described the hypotensive actions not only of human seminal plasma itself, but also of alcohol or acetone extracts. In 1935 he reported that the 'turbid, alkaline' fluid had pronounced hypotensive effects in anaesthetised cats or rabbits, and stimulated the rabbit isolated small intestine and guinea pig isolated seminal vesicle.[6] After some careful comparative work, Goldblatt concluded that the 'seminal depressor' factor could be distinguished from all the vasodepressors hitherto described.

Whilst studying with Henry Dale and John Gaddum in London in the 1930s, a young medical graduate from Stockholm, Ulf von Euler, had discovered a mysterious contractile substance in intestinal extracts that he subsequently dubbed 'substance P'.[7] After his return to Sweden he continued to search for other biologically active factors in different organs. After testing a wide variety of tissue extracts, including some from accessory genital organs from various animals, Euler tested human seminal fluid on the blood pressure of the rabbit, noting a dramatic hypotensive action.[8] He also noted that seminal fluid extracts contracted the atropinised rabbit jejunum. In addition to its presence in human semen, this vasodepressor activity was also detectable in extracts of human, dog and rabbit prostate tissue, as well as the vesicular glands of (sexually mature) bulls. The biological activity could not be accounted for by any compound known at the time and Euler was initially convinced that it was due to the presence of substance P. In a subsequent publication however,[9] he clearly demonstrated that the bulk of the biological activity in the extracts behaved instead as a low molecular weight lipid-soluble acid that contracted gastro-intestinal and uterine smooth muscle of the rabbit or guinea pig, as well as being a vasodepressor agent. Other known depressor substances such as histamine, adenosine, kallikrein, substance P and acetylcholine were ruled out, leaving Euler to conclude that he was dealing with an entirely novel substance. Because it was abundantly present in extracts of the prostate he named it 'prostaglandin'. Euler also extracted a similar depressor substance from the vesicular gland of monkeys (*Macacus rhesus*) which, by analogy with 'prostaglandin', Euler named 'vesiglandin'.[9–11]

The outbreak of the Second World War halted research in the prostaglandin area and when it resumed after the war it was a fellow Swede, Sune Bergström, who continued this work. Meanwhile, Euler himself proceeded to achieve distinction in quite a different field; in 1970 he shared, with Julius Axelrod and Bernard Katz, the Nobel Prize in Physiology or Medicine for his work on catecholamine metabolism.

But there was an interesting postscript to Euler's discovery. Although his elegant experimental work was never called into question it transpired that the name 'prostaglandin' was a misnomer. In fact, it is the seminal vesicle and not the prostate from which prostaglandins (in the male reproductive tract) are chiefly derived. The reason for this confusion was undoubtedly differences in the descriptions of the comparative reproductive anatomy of the different species he had investigated. However, the name stuck and whether strictly correct or not, 'prostaglandin' was the term given to the pharmacologically active lipids produced by the vesicular glands and it has remained in currency ever since. Little further work was carried out with vesiglandin, and it was the prostaglandins that dominated the interest of the post-war biomedical community.

9.3 Bergström's Work on Prostaglandin Purification

Polyunsaturated fatty acids, particularly the 'essential fatty acids', are prone to oxidation. This occurs spontaneously in the presence of atmospheric oxygen or through a reaction catalysed by lipoxygenases. Bergström had begun his work by investigating the auto-oxidation of cholesterol. It was a happy choice of topic as these reactions were later to prove of great significance. By coincidence, the laboratory in which he had begun these studies in 1940 was in Columbia University, where a few years earlier Kurzrok and Lieb had conducted those experiments on the biological activity of seminal fluid. Although Bergström had met Kurzrok during his visit to Columbia University he was not aware of this work on prostaglandins and in fact he did not become involved in the field until after his return to Sweden in 1947. At a meeting of the Physiological Society in Stockholm, Bergström presented a paper on the autoxidation work he had begun at Columbia together with other data on lipoxygenase-catalysed oxidation of linoleic acid. By another coincidence, Euler was also present at the meeting and he encouraged Bergström to take a fresh look at the samples of 'prostaglandins' that had been stored in the deep freeze since the war years.[12]

Bergström had brought back from his American trip one of the newest analytical tools then available — the Craig Countercurrent Distribution machine — and it was largely through the use of this equipment that he was able to announce, some two years later, that the biologically active principle in extracts of sheep vesicular glands had been purified about 500,000 times and was associated with a nitrogen-free unsaturated hydroxyl fatty acid with a UV absorption at 280 nm.

A new appointment at Lund University and the associated respon-sibility of running a new academic department interrupted Bergström's work on the prostaglandins for several years although during this time his team built up a substantial expertise in lipid analy-sis, and the techniques that they evolved to do this — especially reversed-phase chromatography — proved to be of inestimable value when he resumed his interest in the prostaglandins in the mid-1950s. When he did so, Bergström soon recognised that a major obstacle to further work was the tiny amounts of material he had prepared. To scale up his preparations he organised the collection of large numbers of sheep vesicular glands from abattoirs around the world for use in his further work. This paid handsome dividends and by 1957 Bergström and his collaborator Jan Sjövall isolated one prostaglandin factor (called by them 'prostaglandin F') in a crystalline form,[13] sub-sequently noting that it produced a contraction of the rabbit isolated duodenum at a concentration of 5 ng/ml, and also that it was not the only active acidic factor present in the crude extracts.

These important findings were greatly extended when Bergström moved, together with Sjövall, to the Karolinska Institute in Stockholm. In two papers published in 1960[14,15] the two researchers reported the isolation from vacuum-dried sheep vesicu-lar glands of two factors, one named prostaglandin E (because it partitioned in ether) and the other, prostaglandin F (because it par-titioned into phosphate buffer; 'fosfat', in Swedish). Again, the countercurrent system was used to prepare prostaglandin F, whereas prostaglandin E was purified using reverse-phase chromatography. Elemental analysis, ultraviolet and infrared spectroscopy together

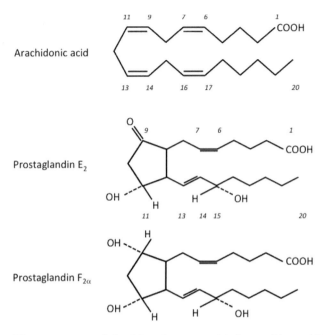

Fig. 9.1. The structures of the 20-carbon essential fatty acid, arachidonic acid (5, 8, 11, 14 eicosatetraenoic acid) and the first 2 prostaglandins to be identified and characterised by Bergström and Sjövall in 1960, prostaglandin E and prostaglandin F. The small italic numbers refer to the carbon numbering system, which is important in following the subsequent work on the reaction mechanism.

with, most significantly, data from what was probably the world's first functional gas chromatograph-mass spectrometer (GC-MS), suggested an empirical formula of $C_{20}H_{34}O_5$ for PGF and $C_{20}H_{36}O_5$ for the more lipid-soluble PGE. Prostaglandin E was also detected in ram semen by the Karolinska group. This was important since it linked the original observation of biological activity in seminal plasma to the presence of a prostaglandin.

The large amounts of pure crystalline material by then available greatly facilitated the subsequent analysis in which the prostaglandins were degraded by a variety of chemical treatments, and the structures of the resultant fragments deduced from the information provided by the new GC-MS. These structures were confirmed by chemical synthesis (see Fig. 9.1).

9.4 Bergström and Samuelsson's Work on Prostaglandin Biosynthesis

With the first prostaglandin structures elucidated, the interest of many scientists next turned to the question of their biosynthesis. Rune Eliasson[16] had already reported that the number of prostaglandins recovered from vesicular gland homogenates was substantially increased (some 20-fold) if they were incubated in a water bath at 37⁰C for an hour or more. This observation coupled with others (such as the fact that there was a definite pH optimum for the reaction) strongly suggested that some enzymatic process was at work.

The Karolinska group noticed that the structures of prostaglandins E and F bore a resemblance to the 20 carbon 'essential' fatty acids, particularly in the disposition of the *cis* double bonds. Indeed, the resemblance was sufficiently compelling to persuade the Karolinska group that these fatty acids could be the precursors from which prostaglandins were generated. How could this idea be tested? Curiously, Eliasson had already tested the effect of adding one of these fatty acids, arachidonic acid, to his minced vesicular glands but had observed no additional increase in prostaglandin formation. It seems likely now that the amount of arachidonic acid already present in the preparation was already maximal, but whatever the explanation the Karolinska group decided to try again using radioactive arachidonic acid, in the expectation that labelled prostaglandins would appear in the homogenates if the hypothesis was correct.

There was no commercial source of labelled arachidonic acid and the preferred synthetic route necessitated the catalytic reduction of an acetylenic derivative of arachidonic acid (5,6,11,14 eicosatetraynoic acid commonly known as TYA) with tritium gas. But the Karolinska group, now comprising Bengt Samuelsson and Henry Danielsson as well as Bergström, did not have access to this reagent so they contacted David van Dorp at the Unilever Research Laboratories in the Netherlands. Van Dorp's group had a long-standing interest in the essential fatty acids and, unknown to Bergström, had already considered the same idea. Bergström phoned van Dorp who, notwithstanding the fact that these two groups were nominally in 'competition', generously agreed to supply a sample of the labelled fatty acids that he was preparing for his own study of prostaglandin biosynthesis.

The crucial experiment was subsequently performed by both groups, and published simultaneously[17,18] in consecutive papers in *Biochim. Biophys. Acta*. Both the Dutch and Swedish groups reported that the radioactive arachidonic acid was indeed converted into labelled prostaglandin E_2. More extensive studies quickly followed in which it was demonstrated that the two other classes of prostaglandins (e.g. F_1, E_1 and E_3, F_3) were biosynthesised from fatty acid substrates with 3 (dihomo-γ-linolenic acid) or 5 (5,8,11,14,17 eicosapentaenoic acid) double bonds respectively, as opposed to the 4 double bonds in arachidonic acid. In all cases, the enzyme(s) responsible for the transformation were associated with the 'microsomal' ($100,000 \times g$) fraction of disrupted vesicular gland tissue. This enzyme system was at first called 'prostaglandin synthetase', but today it is generally known as fatty acid cyclo-oxygenase (often shortened to Cox).

9.5 Samuelsson's Work on the Role of Oxygen in the Biosynthetic Reaction

Comparing the structures of arachidonic acid and prostaglandins (see Fig. 9.1) it was clear that three atoms of oxygen had been introduced into the fatty acid substrate at C-9, C-11 and C-15. But did this oxygen originate from dissolved gaseous molecular oxygen, or from water, or from both these sources? The answer was provided by a series of ingenious experiments in which the GC-MS again proved crucial. When prostaglandins were extracted from preparations of the vesicular glands incubated with dihomo-γ-linolenic acid under an atmosphere of 'heavy' oxygen ($^{18}O_2$) fragments containing C-11 and C-15 were four mass units heavier than the native prostaglandins generated under $^{16}O_2$. At first it was not clear whether the oxygen at C-9 also originated from molecular oxygen or water but Samuelsson[19] was able to demonstrate not only that the ketone oxygen at C-9 originated from molecular oxygen, but that the ring oxygen atoms at C-9 and C-11 were both derived from the same molecule of oxygen gas. It was an entirely novel type of dioxygenase reaction and it had important mechanistic implications as it led Samuelsson to postulate the existence of a hypothetical intermediate in prostaglandin biosynthesis. It was a concept that was later to prove crucial to our understanding of prostaglandin biochemistry. In addition to this novel dioxygenase reaction that formed the ring of the prostaglandin molecule, there was also a mono-oxygenase reaction that inserted an atom of oxygen at C-15 in a manner extremely reminiscent of the activity of another enzyme, the plant lipoxygenase.

Sheep vesicular gland homogenates were invariably used as a source of enzyme and an interesting new product detected in these incubation mixtures was another species, prostaglandin D_2. It was clear that the existence of this product is entirely reasonable given the proposed mechanism of formation of prostaglandins E and F — that is, cleavage of the oxygen–oxygen bond of a hypothetical endoperoxide-like intermediate with or without reduction. Later, several other tissues were also found to generate prostaglandins from labelled arachidonic and other substrate acids, including the guinea pig lung that was to become significant later.[20]

9.6 Vane's Work with Prostaglandins

In John Vane's lab at the Royal College of Surgeons of England in London, the 'bioassay cascade' was one of his signature techniques[21] and in common use (see Fig. 9.2). In the experiments relevant here, a guinea pig isolated heart–lung preparation was suspended by a cannula in the trachea, through which the lung could be rhythmically inflated if required. Physiological Krebs' solution was pumped through a catheter inserted into the pulmonary artery through an incision in the right heart. The left heart was usually cut away to allow free drainage of the perfusing solution that was collected in a funnel and diverted to (or pumped over) a cascade over the bioassay tissues. Vane had observed that when arachidonic acid was infused into such a preparation (through the pulmonary artery catheter) it was converted to prostaglandins which in turn contracted the strips of isolated smooth muscle strips, such as the rat fundic strip or colon, that were selected for their sensitivity to prostaglandins.

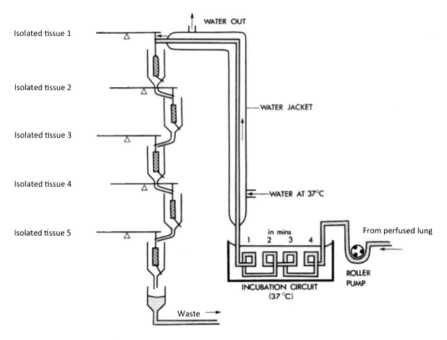

Fig. 9.2.   Vane's 'bioassay cascade'. In this type of experiment the outflow from guinea pig perfused isolated lung was pumped through a warming coil and over a 'cascade' of isolated smooth muscle strips that were chosen for their sensitivity to hormones under investigation. The effluent was either discarded or could be retained for further analysis. (From a slide in the author's personal collection.)

Significantly, it was not only the injection of fatty acid substrates that led to increased amounts of prostaglandin in the perfusate: many other substances including bradykinin, histamine and 'SRS-A' (Slow Reacting Substance of Anaphylaxis; a mysterious spasmogenic lipid generated during anaphylaxis) released prostaglandins from this preparation. The amounts of prostaglandins released by these stimuli were often in excess of the total mass of prostaglandins contained in the lung, the latter figure being obtained by estimating the concentration of prostaglandins extracted after homogenising the tissue in cold alcohol.[22,23]

The fact that prostaglandin release could be initiated directly by infusing arachidonic acid suggests that the rate-limiting step for prostaglandin formation was the availability of substrate. That one could release more prostaglandins than the tissue apparently contained was taken to indicate that prostaglandins are not stored within the tissue but were synthesised and released 'as required'. In other words, biosynthesis immediately preceded release. Finally, the observation that other substances could liberate prostaglandins without being substrates themselves suggested that they liberated arachidonic acid within the cell in such a way that it could be converted into prostaglandins and released.

9.7 The Discovery of 'RCS'

Another way of releasing prostaglandins from the perfused lung preparation was by inducing anaphylactic shock. A lung preparation was taken from a guinea pig that had been immunised to ovalbumin, and anaphylaxis was induced by injecting the antigen into the pulmonary arterial catheter. This procedure released several chemical mediators including histamine, prostaglandins and the mysterious SRS-A. It was whilst they were investigating this phenomenon that Vane and his colleague Priscilla Piper made a significant discovery. The experiment in question was designed to detect not only the release of substances generated during anaphylaxis, such as histamine and SRS-A, but also some others which the investigators thought at that time might be released, such as bradykinin, the prostaglandins and 5-HT. To do this a cascade of bioassay tissues had been carefully selected, including strips of guinea pig trachea (to detect SRS-A), cat terminal ileum (histamine), spirally-cut strips of rabbit aorta, rat stomach strip (prostaglandins and 5-HT), rat colon and chick rectum (prostaglandins).

Injection of the antigen released substances that contracted several tissues but analysis of the tracings indicated that no bradykinin or 5-HT was released but that histamine, SRS-A and prostaglandins were present. A curious observation was made in connection with the spirally cut strips of rabbit aorta used to detect 5HT. Normally, strips from female rabbits in oestrus were used, and these did not contract during anaphylaxis indicating that no 5HT release was occurring. But when strips of aorta from male rabbits were used instead a strong contraction was observed following antigen challenge (see Fig. 9.3). That

Anaphylaxis in isolated perfused lungs of Guinea-pig

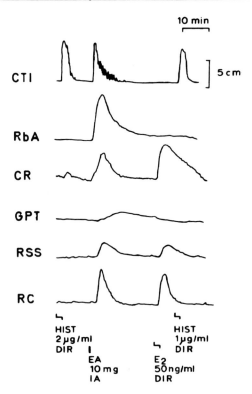

Fig. 9.3. The release of inflammatory mediators during anaphylactic shock of perfused isolated guinea pig lungs as analysed in a bioassay cascade of the type shown in Fig. 9.2. This illustrates an experiment in which strips of cat terminal ileum (CTI), rabbit aortic strip (RbA), chick rectum (CR), guinea pig trachea (GPT), rat stomach strip (RSS), and rat colon (RC) were used as the detecting tissues. 'Calibrating' infusions of histamine (Hist) and prostaglandin E_2 (E_2) were given directly over the isolated tissues, showing that histamine in a concentration of 1–2 ng/ml contracted the CTI and prostaglandin E_2 (50 ng/ml) contracted the CR, the RSS and RC. Egg albumin (EA; the sensitising antigen) was then injected through the perfused lung and this released biologically active substances that contracted the CTI, RbA, RSS, CR, GPT and RC. Histamine, prostaglandin E_2 and SRS-A was released during anaphylaxis but could not have been the only substances present as they did not contract the RbA. This alerted Vane's group to the presence of a further 'rabbit aorta contracting substance' (RCS), a finding that proved to be instrumental in the development of the discovery of the mechanism of action of aspirin and the discovery of thromboxane. (From a slide in the author's personal collection.)

this was not 5-HT was clear not only because the highly sensitive female aortas did not contract, but also because methysergide, a 5-HT antagonist, failed to reverse the contractions. In fact, subsequent experiments clearly demonstrated that the contraction of the male aortas could not be accounted for by any known mediators in the concentrations encountered in this type of experiment. Clearly a new substance had been identified and — tongue in cheek — it was immediately christened 'RCS', an acronym for Rabbit Aorta Contracting Substance and also for the Royal College of Surgeons.[22]

Several rather surprising properties of RCS soon came to light. Firstly, it was highly unstable — later estimates put its half-life at one to two minutes. Secondly, anaphylactic challenge was not the only method by which RCS could be released. Injections of bradykinin, partially purified SRS-A and to a lesser extent histamine, also released RCS. The most important finding of all, however, was that several anti-inflammatory drugs including aspirin prevented the release of RCS when the lung was challenged by the antigen or stimulated with bradykinin. It had been known for some time that aspirin could prevent bradykinin-induced bronchoconstriction in guinea pigs, and it was, in fact, in this context that they were being tested in this experimental model. Piper and Vane speculated that inhibition of RCS could be important in the action of aspirin.

The precise identity of RCS was to elude researchers for several years to come but meanwhile a vital clue came from some further biological experiments. A strong link was established with the prostaglandin system when it became evident that all stimuli which released prostaglandins, including arachidonic acid itself, invariably released RCS. Nor was the perfused lung the only organ that could release RCS. Pieces of chopped spleen released the substances when agitated and, most interesting of all, a crude microsomal preparation containing the cyclooxygenase enzyme when incubated with arachidonic acid in the fluid superfusing the bioassay tissues also generated a substantial amount of RCS.

Another significant observation was made in this experiment too: although very unstable, it was noted that as the RCS activity in a sample decreased so the prostaglandin content seemed to increase.

John Vane and Ryszard Gryglewski[24] speculated that the process of prostaglandin biosynthesis included RCS as an intermediate and that once formed, RCS spontaneously decayed to prostaglandins. The implication was that RCS was probably the 'endoperoxide' intermediate in prostaglandin biosynthesis postulated by the Karolinska and Unilever groups.

9.8 The Aspirin 'Enigma'

Aspirin, which had been synthesised in the 1890s, was a therapeutic enigma. By the early years of the 20th century its chief actions were known to be its antipyretic, anti-inflammatory and analgesic effects. With the passing of time several other drugs with a similar pharmacology were discovered: antipyrine, paracetamol, phenylbutazone, indomethacin and naproxen. These drugs were generally known collectively as the 'aspirin-like' drugs as they not only shared the therapeutic effects of aspirin but also its unwanted effects, such as gastric irritation, as well.

But despite widespread clinical use, little was known about the real mechanism of action of these drugs. They produced an anti-inflammatory effect that was qualitatively and qualitatively different from other anti-inflammatory drugs such as steroids. Their analgesic action, too, was of a different nature to that produced by the opioids. The biochemical effects of these drugs had been documented, and theories based upon these effects abounded. It was observed, for example, that most of the aspirin-like drugs uncoupled oxidative phosphorylation, that several salicylates inhibited dehydrogenase enzymes, especially those dependent upon pyridine nucleotides. Some amino-transferases and decarboxylases were also inhibited and so were several key enzymes involved in protein and RNA biosynthesis. All these inhibitory actions were at some time invoked to explain the therapeutic action of aspirin. A problem with most of these ideas was that the concentration of the drugs required for enzyme inhibition was (sometimes greatly) in excess of the concentrations typically found in the plasma after therapy, and there was invariably a lack of correlation between the ability of these drugs to inhibit a particular enzyme, and their activity as anti-inflammatory agents. Furthermore, there was no convincing reason why inhibition of any of these enzymes should produce the triple anti-inflammatory, analgesic and antipyretic effect of aspirin — let alone its characteristic unwanted effects.

Many pharmacologists were interested in this problem, including the British pharmacologist Harry Collier. Collier had termed aspirin an 'anti-defensive' drug[25] because of its ability to prevent the physiological defence mechanisms of pain, fever and inflammation from functioning normally. Together with his group he made the important finding that guinea pigs who had received aspirin were protected from the bronchoconstriction normally elicited in these animals by injection of bradykinin, ATP or SRS-A. Aspirin also prevented the contraction of the guinea pig isolated tracheo-bronchial muscle caused by SRS-A and bradykinin and also the nociceptive response to ATP in mice. Initially, Collier suggested that 'A-receptors' (which could be blocked by aspirin-like drugs) were involved in the spasmogenic response to these agents, but later he abandoned this concept, believing instead that these drugs inhibited some underlying cellular mechanism.

Stimuli which released prostaglandins from the guinea pig isolated lungs also released RCS and one of the mildest of these stimuli was ventilation of the lung. Using a modified version of his cascade superfusion assay, the 'blood-bathed organ' technique, whereby blood from an anaesthetised animal is passed over a bioassay cascade *ex vivo*, Vane knew that prostaglandins and RCS could also be released into the arterial circulation of an anaesthetised dog if it was mildly hyperventilated. When aspirin was given to the dog the release of these substances was greatly reduced. This experiment focused Vane's attention upon the whole question of prostaglandin release. While he was writing a review paper, it occurred to him that as the 'release' of prostaglandins actually equated with fresh synthesis, then stimuli that released prostaglandins were in fact 'turning on' the synthesis of these compounds. Vane's conclusion was that aspirin might be blocking the synthesis of prostaglandins.

As sheep seminal vesicles (by now the traditional source of Cox enzyme) were difficult to obtain in the UK, Vane resorted to the guinea pig lung homogenate preparation estimating prostaglandin $F_{2\alpha}$ generation by bioassay. Figure 9.4 shows the results of Vane's original experiment. There was a concentration-dependent inhibition of prostaglandin formation by aspirin, indomethacin and sodium salicylate whereas several other unrelated drugs such as morphine, hydrocortisone and mepyramine were without effect. Vane published the results of these experiments in *Nature* in 1971.[26] Three other papers from the RCS group that year added support to this finding and also extended it considerably. By coincidence one of these stemmed from an entirely independent line of investigation.

It had been known for a number of years that aspirin inhibited the aggregation of platelets in response to stimuli such as collagen or ADP and also prevented the release of a smooth muscle contractile substance presumed to be prostaglandin $F_{2\alpha}$. The hypothesis being investigated by Jim Smith and Bryan Willis was that this was brought

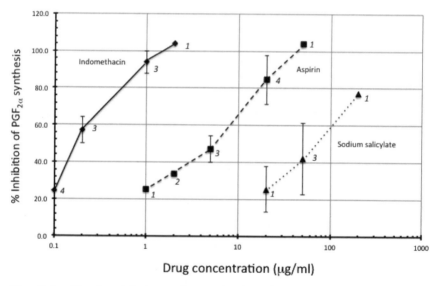

Fig. 9.4.   Vane's original experiment showing that aspirin, indomethacin and sodium salicylate inhibited the production of prostaglandin $F_{2\alpha}$ in homogenates of guinea pig lung. Inhibition (Y-axis) is presented as the mean and standard error of n observations. (Redrawn by the author from the data presented in Vane's paper of 1971.[26])

about indirectly by the release of phospholipase A_1 from platelets and that this enzyme was the target of the inhibitory action of aspirin.[27]

Once again the experimental protocol was simple: venous blood samples were obtained before and 1 hour after taking 600 mg aspirin orally. Platelets were isolated, washed, incubated with the potent aggregating agent thrombin and the supernatant tested for the presence of released nucleotides, phospholipase and various other enzymes, as well as prostaglandins. Only the prostaglandins were substantially inhibited.

In another human study,[28] Joe Collier and Rod Flower assessed the action of aspirin on the prostaglandins in human seminal plasma (which contains large amounts of prostaglandins, which are therefore easy to assay). Volunteers were given aspirin or a placebo for three days, and seminal fluid samples obtained, extracted, and the prostaglandin E and F content assessed by bioassay. Once again, the results were unequivocal with a substantial inhibition of both prostaglandins achieved after dosing with this drug.

In a further confirmatory study, Vane, together with Sergio Ferreira and Salvador Moncada,[29] demonstrated that the aspirin-like drugs blocked the prostaglandin release, elicited by electrical stimulation or catecholamine injection, from the perfused isolated dog spleen *in vitro*. It seemed that the aspirin effect was not restricted to tissue, species or route of administration.

The significance of all these findings was, of course, that they provided a major clue to the way in which the aspirin-like drugs exerted their therapeutic actions. At the time there was already accumulating evidence suggesting that prostaglandin E_1 was a potent pyretic agent and that F or E prostaglandins mimicked the inflammatory response when injected intradermally. Prostaglandins had also been detected in inflammatory exudates. Of course, only three aspirin-like drugs had been tested so far, but that situation soon changed when Vane's group published further data demonstrating that all the aspirin-like drugs blocked prostaglandin generation in concentrations within plasma levels found during therapy.[30] The discovery also had another implication — biologists now had a simple means of preventing prostaglandin synthesis and release and thereby assessing the functions of prostaglandins in biological systems.

9.9 The Detection and Isolation of an Intermediate in Prostaglandin Biosynthesis and RCS Characterised

Most investigators still thought of the prostaglandin family as comprising mainly E- and F-type compounds but this situation changed in 1973 when the Karolinska and Unilever groups succeeded in isolating two intermediates formed during prostaglandin biosynthesis. Not only did this add two further compounds to the prostaglandin family and clarify several outstanding questions concerning the biosynthetic mechanism, but it also led directly to the elucidation of the structure of RCS and to the discovery of additional prostaglandins and related compounds.

Further studies of prostaglandin biosynthesis strengthened Samuelsson's conviction that an endoperoxide intermediate really existed and the 'RCS' experiments of Piper and Vane provided circumstantial evidence for a labile prostaglandin related substance too. Mats Hamburg and Samuelsson had observed a discrepancy between the rate of oxygenation of the substrate arachidonic acid by sheep vesicular gland homogenates and the appearance of prostaglandin E_2, strongly suggesting that some intermediate was temporarily accumulating.[31] If Vane's RCS was this intermediate then clearly it could exist independently otherwise it could not have been detected using his superfusion bioassay techniques. So could this intermediate be extracted from the vesicular gland homogenates? This proved indeed to be the case and a hitherto undetected product was subsequently isolated from such incubation mixtures by thin layer chromatography. If the homogenate was first treated with a reducing agent then the compound disappeared and the amount of prostaglandin F increased. The unknown compound also gave a positive reaction with a reagent that detected peroxides. If extracted from the chromatography plate and re-analysed the mysterious compound changed completely to a mixture comprising mainly prostaglandin E_2 and prostaglandin D_2.

These results provided incontrovertible evidence for the endoperoxide intermediate whose existence Samuelsson had predicted almost ten years earlier, and showed furthermore that the material could be isolated from the reaction mixture as an independent substance. The notion of a stepwise synthesis of prostaglandins supplanted the idea that the entire pathway was the product of a single concerted enzyme reaction. Samuelsson and his colleagues went on to predict the existence of an *endoperoxide isomerase* enzyme that catalysed rearrangement of the intermediate into prostaglandin E compounds, and an *endoperoxide reductase* that transformed the endoperoxide into prostaglandin $F_{2\alpha}$ (see Fig. 9.5).

The subsequent publications from the Karolinska group were mirrored again by those of the Unilever group who reported not one, but two intermediates.[32] Convinced that they were Vane's RCS, these were originally dubbed 'prostaglandins R_1 and R_2' although they were later renamed G_2 and H_2 to maintain some consistency within the prostaglandin nomenclature scheme. Disappointingly, however, whilst preparations of prostaglandins G and H contracted the rabbit aortic strip in a manner reminiscent of RCS, there was a discrepancy between the stability of the two substances. RCS had a calculated half-life of some 30 sec in Krebs' solution but the half-life of the endoperoxides was approximately 5 min. Thus it seemed necessary to invoke the presence of yet another product to explain Vane's bioassay results.

Whilst inherently unstable, the endoperoxides could be maintained in cold dry acetone for several months, enabling reasonable estimations of their smooth muscle contractile activity to be made. But there was often a problem with interpretation of such experiments. It was often unclear what proportion of the observed response was caused by the endoperoxides themselves and what proportion caused by the breakdown, enzymatic or non-enzymatic, of the endoperoxides in the test system. Happily, there was another system that lent itself more readily to an analysis of endoperoxide synthesis and action — the platelet aggregation response.

It had already been ascertained[33] that incubation of arachidonic acid with sheep vesicular gland microsomes led to the rapid generation of an extremely potent but evanescent platelet aggregating substance. Given the acronym LASS (Labile Aggregation Stimulating Substance), the production of this material was blocked by aspirin, thus linking it strongly to the prostaglandin system. Willis suggested

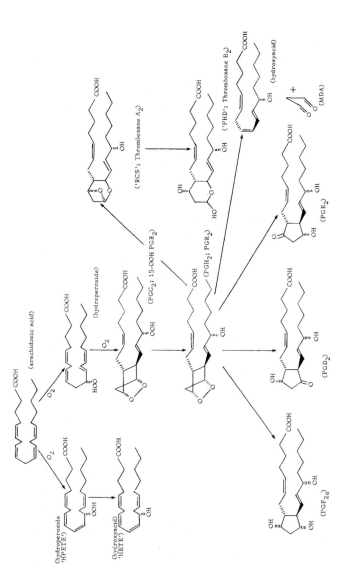

Fig. 9.5. The prostaglandin biosynthetic cascade as it was known after the seminal discoveries of Samuelsson's team in the mid-1970s. The only prostaglandins known at the beginning of the period covered by this chapter were prostaglandins E and F. In addition to prostaglandin D, which was discovered later, these prostaglandins can be formed by both enzymatic and non-enzymatic mechanisms although this was not clear to early workers. The fundamental discovery and isolation of the endoperoxides prostaglandin G₂ and H₂ provided the key to understanding the complex biosynthetic pathways. In some other tissues such as lung, a previously unidentified product originally termed 'PHD' was observed. This compound was later renamed thromboxane B₂ and the intermediate between prostaglandin H₂ and thromboxane B₂ was termed thromboxane A₂ and subsequently identified as Vane's RCS. (From a slide in the author's personal collection.)

that it was, in fact, the endoperoxide prostaglandin H_2. The Karolinska group had observed that addition of purified endoperoxides to platelet suspensions caused a dose dependent aggregation and, interestingly, a patient undergoing treatment for a bleeding disorder was found to have a Cox deficiency; platelets from this subject did not respond to arachidonic acid although prostaglandin G_2 produced aggregation as usual.[34] When the metabolism of arachidonic acid in aggregating platelets was carefully examined using a radioactive tracer technique a rather surprising finding was made. There was, in fact, little conversion to prostaglandins E, F or D at all. Instead, the major products were two totally novel compounds. They were identified by GC-MS as 12-hydroxy eicosatrienoic acid (12-HETE) and a more complex molecule dubbed 'PHD'.[35]

But it wasn't only platelets that synthesised PHD. When labelled arachidonic acid was incubated with guinea pig lung homogenates, or injected into perfused lung preparations, large amounts of both PHD and a hydroxyacid 12-HETE were formed. Even though it was now clear that the endoperoxides were not Vane's RCS, it was at least conceivable that PHD was somehow involved.[36]

There were several possible reaction mechanisms by which PHD could be formed, but Samuelsson and his colleagues proposed that a rearrangement of the endoperoxide prostaglandin G_2 with incorporation of one water molecule could account for the structure. Intriguingly, this conversion would require the generation of yet another transient intermediate. Could this be the elusive RCS?

An experiment which provided compelling evidence for the existence of such a short-lived intermediate in platelets was performed. A small amount of arachidonic acid was added to a suspension of platelets causing a partial aggregation. After 30 sec, a small aliquot of the partly aggregated suspension was added to a second cuvette containing fresh platelets that had been treated with indomethacin to block production of mediators by the platelets themselves. When this addition had been made it was observed that the platelets in the second cuvette aggregated. Clearly there was some substance present in the arachidonic acid-treated suspension that caused the second batch of platelets to aggregate. None of the known prostaglandins or indeed the endoperoxides G_2 or H_2 had an aggregating effect in the concentrations found in the sample and so it seemed that there must be a further biologically active substance present. But even more interestingly, when extracts containing this substance were tested on the rabbit isolated aortic strip it responded with a strong contraction that could not be explained by the presence of endoperoxides. The contractile substance was much more labile than the endoperoxides, with a half-life of only about 35 sec,[37] a figure almost identical to the half-life of RCS as estimated by Piper and Vane in the late 1960s.

It seemed as if the mystery of RCS was at last clarified. Evidently it was a labile intermediate generated during the transformation of the endoperoxides to PHD. A variety of putative intermediates were considered and eliminated by rigorous analysis until only one possibility remained. Because it was characterised first in platelets (thrombocytes) and contained an oxane ring it was called 'thromboxane'. The highly unstable intermediate (Vane's RCS) was termed thromboxane A_2 whilst the inactive breakdown product hitherto referred to as PHD was renamed thromboxane B_2 (see Fig. 9.5).

9.10 Impact of these Discoveries on Medical Science

Whilst an important chapter had come to an end, the prostaglandin story and its implications continued. As a result of Bergström's work, prostaglandins themselves (or their analogues) were introduced into clinical medicine for a variety of uses (e.g. as gastric anti-secretory and oxytocic drugs).

Samuelsson and the Karolinska group went on to elucidate the structures of further eicosanoid metabolites, including an entire new family of arachidonic acid metabolites, the leukotrienes.[38,39] The hitherto mysterious SRS-A was eventually revealed as a member of this family, thereby tying up another loose end in our story. Since SRS-A was implicated in allergic lung disease, the elucidation of the leukotriene biosynthetic pathway provided new targets for anti-asthma therapies, some of which are in clinical use.

Vane moved from his base at the Royal College of Surgeons to take up a post as Research and Development Director at the Wellcome

Foundation, at the time a prominent pharmaceutical company. He took his team with him and shortly after their arrival they discovered a further prostaglandin, prostacyclin — prostaglandin I_2 — synthesised from the endoperoxides by a new synthase enzyme.[40-43] The biological activity of prostacyclin was almost completely the opposite of thromboxane A_2, and its antiplatelet and vasodilator actions were shown to be crucial regulators of haemostatic mechanisms. An analogue is in clinical use for the treatment of pulmonary hypertension.

Vane's ideas about the mechanism of action of aspirin led to a revolution in non-steroidal anti-inflammatory drug (NSAID) therapies. New drugs were produced using Cox inhibition as a screening tool. When an isoform of Cox, Cox-2, was discovered, a new paradigm for NSAID action based upon this theory was born.[44-46] The result of this was the introduction of the selective Cox-2 inhibitors. Whilst these drugs initially attracted some controversy in the press because of the apparently increased incidence of cardiovascular disease amongst users, they are still regarded as powerful anti-inflammatories that have less gastric side effects than the 'older' NSAIDs and are in common clinical use, providing excellent analgesic and symptomatic improvement in arthritis and related conditions such as sports injuries and post-operative trauma.

References

1. Burr G, Burr M. A new deficiency disease produced by the rigid exclusion of fat from the diet. *J Biol Chem* 1929; 82: 345–367.
2. Burr G, Burr M. On the nature and role of the fatty acids essential in nutrition. *J Biol Chem* 1930; 86: 587–621.
3. Dawson R, Jungalwala F, Miller E *et al.* Synthesis and exchange of phopsholipids within the brain and liver cells. *Biochem Soc Symp* 1972; 35: 365–376.
4. Kuzrock R, Lieb C. Biochemical studies of human semen II. *Proc Soc Exp Biol Med* 1930; 26: 268–272.
5. Goldblatt MW. A depressor substance in seminal fluid. *J Soc Chem Ind (London)* 1933; 52: 1056.
6. Goldblatt MW. Properties of human seminal plasma. *J Physiol* 1935; 84: 208–218.

194   R. Flower

7. Euler USV, Gaddum J. An unidentified depressor substance in certain tissue extracts. *J Physiol* 1931; 72: 74–81.

8. Euler USV. *Prostaglandin Historical Remarks.* Oxford: Pergamon Press; 1982.

9. Euler USV. On the specific vaso-dilating and plain muscle stimulating substances from accesory genital glands in man and certain animals (prostaglandin and vesiglandin). *J Physiol* 1937; 88: 213–234.

10. Euler USV, Hammarstrom S. The occurence of prostgalandins in animal organs. *Skand Arch Physiol* 1937; 77: 96–99.

11. Euler USV. Further investigations into prostaglandin, the physiologically active substance of certain genital glands. *Skand Arch Physiol* 1939; 81: 65–80.

12. Bergström S. Prostaglandins — a group of hormonal compounds of widespread occurrence. *Biochem Pharmacol* 1963; 12: 413–414.

13. Bergström S, Sjövall J. The isolation of prostaglandin. *Acta Chem Scand* 1957; 11: 1086.

14. Bergström S, Sjövall J. The isolation of prostaglandin E from sheep prostate glands. *Acta Chem Scand* 1960;.14:.1693–700.

15. Bergström S, Sjövall J. The isolation of prostaglandin F from sheep prostate glands. *Acta Chem Scand* 1960;.14: 1693–700.

16. Eliasson R. Studies on prostaglandin; occurrence, formation and biological actions. *Acta Physiol Scand Suppl* 1959; 46: 1–73.

17. Bergström S, Danielsson H, Samuelsson B. The enzymatic formation of prostaglandin E2 from arachidonic acid: prostaglandins and related factors 32. *Biochem Biophys Acta* 1964; 90: 207–210.

18. Van Dorp D, Beerthuis RK, Nugteren DH *et al.* The Biosynthesis of Prostaglandins. *Biochim Biophys Acta* 1964; 90: 204–207.

19. Samuelsson B. On the Incorporation of Oxygen in the Conversion of 8, 11, 14-Eicosatrienoic Acid to Prostaglandin E1. *J Am Chem Soc* 1965; 87: 3011–3013.

20. Änggard E, Samuelsson B. Biosynthesis of prostaglandins from arachidonic acid in guinea pig lung. Prostaglandins and related factors. 38. *J Biol Chem* 1965; 240: 3518–3521.

21. Vane JR. The use of isolated organs for detecting active substances in the circulating blood. *Br J Pharmacol Chemother* 1964; 23: 360–373.

22. Piper PJ, Vane JR. Release of additional factors in anaphylaxis and its antagonism by anti-inflammatory drugs. *Nature* 1969; 223: 29–35.

23. Piper P, Vane J. The release of prostaglandins from lung and other tissues. *Ann N Y Acad Sci* 1971; 180: 363–385.

24. Gryglewski R, Vane JR. The generation from arachidonic acid of rabbit aorta contracting substance (RCS) by a microsomal enzyme preparation which also generates prostaglandins. *Br J Pharmacol* 1972; 46: 449–457.

25. Collier H, Shorley P. Analgesic antipyretic drugs asantagonists of bradykinin. *Br J Pharmacol Chemother* 1960; 15: 601–610.

26. Vane JR. Inhibition of prostaglandin synthesis as a mechanism of action for aspirin-like drugs. *Nat New Biol* 1971; 231: 232–235.

27. Smith JB, Willis AL. Aspirin selectively inhibits prostaglandin production in human platelets. *Nat New Biol* 1971; 231: 235–237.

28. Collier JG, Flower RJ. Effect of aspirin on human seminal prostaglandins. *Lancet* 1971; 2: 852–853.

29. Ferreira SH, Moncada S, Vane JR. Indomethacin and aspirin abolish prostaglandin release from the spleen. *Nat New Biol* 1971; 231: 237–239.

30. Flower R, Gryglewski R, Herbaczynska-Cedro K *et al.* Effects of anti-inflammatory drugs on prostaglandin biosynthesis. *Nat New Biol* 1972; 238: 104–106.

31. Hamberg M, Samuelsson B. Detection and isolation of an endoperoxide intermediate in prostaglandin biosynthesis. *Proc Natl Acad Sci USA* 1973; 70: 899–903.

32. Nugteren DH, Hazelhof E. Isolation and properties of intermediates in prostaglandin biosynthesis. *Biochim Biophys Acta* 1973; 326: 448–461.

33. Willis AL, Vane FM, Kuhn DC *et al.* An endoperoxide aggregator (Lass), formed in platelets in response to thrombotic stimuli: purification, identification and unique biological significance. *Prostaglandins* 1974; 8: 453–507.

34. Malmsten C, Hamberg M, Svensson J *et al.* Physiological role of an endoperoxide in human platelets: hemostatic defect due to platelet cyclo-oxygenase deficiency. *Proc Natl Acad Sci U S A* 1975; 72: 1446–1450.

35. Hamberg M, Samuelsson B. Prostaglandin endoperoxides. Novel transformations of arachidonic acid in human platelets. *Proc Natl Acad Sci USA* 1974; 71: 3400–3404.

36. Hamberg M, Samuelsson B. Prostaglandin endoperoxides. VII. Novel transformations of arachidonic acid in guinea pig lung. *Biochem Biophys Res Commun* 1974; 61: 942–949.

37. Hamberg M, Svensson J, Samuelsson B. Thromboxanes: a new group of biologically active compounds derived from prostaglandin endoperoxides. *Proc Natl Acad Sci USA* 1975; 72: 2994–2998.

38. Samuelsson B, Hammarstrom S, Murphy RC *et al.* Leukotrienes and slow reacting substance of anaphylaxis (SRS-A). *Allergy* 1980; 35: 375–381.

39. Samuelsson B, Borgeat P, Hammarstrom S *et al.* Leukotrienes: a new group of biologically active compounds. *Adv Prostaglandin Thromboxane Res* 1980; 6: 1–18.

40. Bunting S, Gryglewski R, Moncada S *et al.* Arterial walls generate from prostaglandin endoperoxides a substance (prostaglandin X) which relaxes strips of mesenteric and coeliac ateries and inhibits platelet aggregation. *Prostaglandins* 1976; 12: 897–913.

41. Moncada S, Gryglewski R, Bunting S *et al.* An enzyme isolated from arteries transforms prostaglandin endoperoxides to an unstable substance that inhibits platelet aggregation. *Nature* 1976; 263: 663–665.

42. Gryglewski RJ, Bunting S, Moncada S *et al.* Arterial walls are protected against deposition of platelet thrombi by a substance (prostaglandin X) which they make from prostaglandin endoperoxides. *Prostaglandins* 1976; 12: 685–713.

43. Whittaker N, Bunting S, Salmon J *et al.* The chemical structure of prostaglandin X (prostacyclin). *Prostaglandins* 1976; 12: 915–928.

44. DeWitt DL, Meade EA, Smith WL. PGH synthase isoenzyme selectivity: the potential for safer nonsteroidal anti-inflammatory drugs. *JAMA* 1993; 95: 40S–44S.

45. Meade EA, Smith WL, DeWitt DL. Differential inhibition of prostaglandin endoperoxide synthase (cyclooxygenase) isozymes by aspirin and other non-steroidal anti-inflammatory drugs. *J Biol Chem* 1993; 268: 6610–6614.

46. Mitchell JA, Akarasereenont P, Thiemermann C *et al.* Selectivity of non-steroidal anti-inflammatory drugs as inhibitors of constitutive and inducible cyclooxygenase. *Proc Natl Acad Sci USA* 1993; 90: 11693–11697.

Chapter 10

THE ANTIBODY PROBLEM AND THE GENERATION OF MONOCLONAL ANTIBODIES

Herman Waldmann and Celia P. Milstein

10.1 Introduction

In 1984 César Milstein, Niels Jerne, and Georges Köhler received the Nobel Prize 'for theories concerning the specificity in development and control of the immune system and the discovery of the principle for production of monoclonal antibodies'. All three scientists (Fig. 10.1) are connected through what we can call 'the antibody problem'. By this we mean the comprehensive explanation for how any individual can make so many different antibodies to any one antigen, so many antibodies to the universe of antigens, and how, with time, such antibodies can mature in their avidity.

In his presentation speech[1] Professor Hans Wigzell spoke of Niels Jerne as the great theoretician in modern immunology responsible for proposing that the immune system was pre-committed in its capacity to mount immune responses to foreign antigens, antigens selecting from amongst naturally produced antibodies (receptors) those with the appropriate specificity, so setting in train production of more of those antibodies.[2] This theory served as the basis of the clonal selection theory later propounded by Frank MacFarlane Burnet,[3] who extended Jerne's idea to explain that selection worked at the level of clonally distributed lymphocyte receptors. Wigzell also referred to two other theories of Jerne, one invoking the so-called transplantation antigens as a driving force in the thymus for generation of 'adaptive' cells of the immune system to develop in the thymus.[4] Although Wigzell

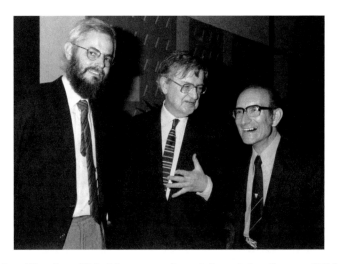

Fig. 10.1.   The three Nobel Laureates: from left to right, Georges Köhler, Niels Jerne and César Milstein.

praised the quality and impact of this theory, others have argued that much of what was proposed was incorrect.[5] Jerne's third theory,[6] the 'network theory', although seemingly influential in its time, has not, in retrospect, left a lasting legacy of insight into the immune system.[7]

With reference to Georges Köhler and César Milstein, Wigzell describes how the development of the hybridoma technique for production of monoclonal antibodies has revolutionised the use of antibodies in health care and research; how 'rare antibodies with a tailor-made-like fit for a given structure can now be made in large quantities';[1] and how the parent hybridoma cells can be stored in master-cell banks enabling worldwide use and offering a previously unmet precision in diagnosis and new possibilities for therapy. For both these scientists the discovery of monoclonal antibodies was a consequence of their relentless quest to explain the 'antibody problem'. It was never in their planning that they would generate new tools and drugs of such great use to humanity, but these arose simply as a by-product of asking an absolutely fundamental scientific question. All three scientists, all very different personalities, provide clear demonstrations that there is no one life-style recipe to the discovery of scientific truths.

10.2 Biographical Details of the Laureates

Recently, we have been provided with two 'official' biographies, giving us insights into the lives of Jerne and Köhler.[8, 9] A short biography of César Milstein written by David Secher can be found in the *Oxford Dictionary of National Biography* (ODNB).

10.2.1 *Niels Jerne*

Niels Jerne was born in London on 23 December 1911, the son of Hans Jensen and Elsie Marie Jerne of Danish extraction. The family soon moved to Holland where Niels grew up. He gained his baccalaureate in Rotterdam in 1928 and somewhat reluctantly 'studied' physics for two years at the University of Leiden. After working for three years with the banana company Elders and Fyffe, he moved to Copenhagen, got married and started a family with Tjek, a Dutch artist. There he transiently continued his education before entering a range of remunerative activities including employment in the meat industry under his father, and then into the standardisation section of the Serum Institute, dealing with antibody products, where he trained himself in biostatistics and serology and was first exposed to bench research. He never really experienced hardship as his father continued to support the family, but despite that support it seems that he took a long time to establish a career choice. Eventually he decided to complete his medical training, and completed a PhD thesis at the Danish Serum Institute where his interest in the antibody problem began.[10–12]

Thomas Söderqvist in his *Troubled Life of Niels Jerne*,[8] provides us with a picture of someone who did not seek to immerse himself in experimental science, but who was motivated to a theoretical approach to understanding the 'big' problems of immunology. Although able to influence and inspire many talented followers, he articulated a sense of feeling 'on the outside', perhaps a reflection of his lack of a firm home country. His somewhat complex personal life is seen as linking with some of his ideas on the immune system, perhaps explaining his passion for interconnecting networks, or analogies with language (as in his Nobel lecture).[13] His seeming lack of interest in the application of monoclonal antibodies, the complement system and AIDS as a disease of the immune system, and limited reference to the emerging principles of molecular biology (as if they offered no special intellectual avenues) is somewhat surprising given his obvious intellect.

With just one theory standing the test of time, one wonders whether Jerne would have been a choice for a Nobel Prize had not monoclonal antibodies been described when they were.[14] Jerne had charisma and was admired by the international research community, so that he was able to attract a range of remarkable scientists to the Basle Institute of Immunology, and he provided the intellectual environment from which major discoveries emerged. In the framework of the 'antibody problem' he brought in the molecular biologists Charles Steinberg and Sosumu Tonegawa, with the result that Tonegawa established that the genetic information encoding one chain of antibody in a B-cell was rearranged from two separate genetic elements in genomic DNA.[15] One of Jerne's earliest recruits was the Czech scientist Ivan Lefkovits, who, by limiting dilution analysis, established clearly that B-cells were pre-committed to respond to given antigens, and was able to measure the frequencies of such pre-committed cells.[16] Perhaps the boldness of Jerne's theories inspired many to perform ingenious experiments, and this alone might justify the award?

Another of Jerne's early recruits was Fritz Melchers, who much later took over the helm from Jerne. It was Melchers who recruited the young Georges Köhler as a graduate student. Köhler's PhD project was to investigate the diversity of antibodies that could be made to a particular part of the protein β-galactosidase and through this route Köhler found his entry into the antibody problem.[17] Recently the immunologist Klaus Eichmann has written an excellent biography of the scientific life of Georges Köhler which gives us a glimpse of the special qualities of this otherwise very private man.[9]

10.2.2 *Georges Köhler*

Georges Köhler was born on 17 April 1946 in Munich of a German father Karl, and a French mother Raymonde. When he was ten years old the family moved within Germany to the French border near Strasbourg. His high school record was remarkably undistinguished. On completing his baccalaureate in 1965 he went on to study biology at the Albert-Ludwigs University in nearby Freiburg. As part of his diploma work he studied mutations affecting DNA repair in *E.coli*, eventually completing his diploma in 1971, taking a little longer than most. On the recommendation of his then professor, Rainer Hertl, Köhler was introduced to Fritz Melchers as a potential graduate student, and so to the Basel Institute.

By all accounts Köhler's approach to the laboratory was somewhat relaxed, and not typical of the majority of the Institute's scientists. However, the intellectual ethos of the Institute was not lost on him, and the potential for using fluctuation analyses (so popular with phage scientists at the time) to isolate mutant antibody-producing cells was something that he and Melchers recognised. Unfortunately, the technology of the time was not up to the analysis of normal B-cells. It was then that Köhler's attention was drawn to the benefits of using malignant B-cell lines for such mutation studies, as was being practised in the laboratories of Matthew Scharff (Albert Einstein College, New York),[18] and of César Milstein (Cambridge, MRC Laboratory of Molecular Biology-LMB).[19, 20]

10.2.3 *César Milstein*

César Milstein was born on 8 October 1927 in Bahia Blanca, Argentina, the middle of three sons of Jewish parents, immigrants to Argentina. He worked towards a doctoral degree under the direction of Professor Stoppani,[21] Professor of Biochemistry at the Medical School, with no economic support other than that which his wife Celia and he could generate working part-time doing clinical biochemistry. His thesis was on enzyme kinetics. He was then granted a British Council Fellowship to work under the supervision of Malcolm Dixon, an enzymologist in the Department of Biochemistry, Cambridge. Working on the mechanism of metal activation of the enzyme phosphoglucomutase,[22] he was brought into a collaboration with Fred Sanger,[23] with whom he took a short-term appointment once his PhD was completed in 1960. He then returned to Argentina to run his own group. The political persecution of liberal intellectuals and scientists forced his resignation, and in 1963 he returned to work with Fred Sanger, by then the Head of the Division of Protein Chemistry in the newly-formed Laboratory of Molecular Biology of the Medical Research Council. Following Sanger's suggestion, Milstein shifted his interests from enzymes to antibodies — and specifically to the antibody problem.[24] Although also gifted as a theoretician, Milstein had a strong belief in experimentation to generate data, and with his strong background in biochemistry and protein sequencing he was well placed to make key discoveries. His attraction to the antibody problem is well displayed in the two influential reviews he wrote with Sydney Brenner[25] and Alan Munro[26] in 1966 and 1970 respectively. It was Milstein who, with David Secher in 1971, attacked the antibody problem by studying mutation in myeloma cells and who, with Richard Cotton[20] in 1973, introduced cell fusion technology in order to study expression of immunoglobulin genes in myeloma cell lines. It was also to Milstein's credit that he adapted his scientific repertoire to accommodate the rapidly evolving technologies of molecular biology, resulting in early papers on the isolation of RNA encoding immunoglobulin chains. Even in these forays into RNA came some seminal discoveries, such as the discovery of the leader sequence of secreted immunoglobulins, a discovery with broad implications for protein secretion.[27,28]

It is on this scientific background that the foundations of monoclonal antibodies were laid.

10.3 The Antibody Problem

What then was this 'antibody problem' that had attracted these three Laureates?

Put simply, immunologists have long known that mice, horses, sheep, and man can make vast numbers of different antibodies to a diverse array of foreign antigens. Karl Landsteiner taught us that such antibodies can have a very tight fit for the inciting antigen.[29] Others have taught us that this fit can become even greater as the immune response matures, or after it is boosted with a further antigen shot.[30] We have also long known that antibodies can switch in class from IgM, in primary responses, to IgG in subsequent responses (Fig. 10.2). Even prior to our understanding of the DNA basis of the genetic code, it was very difficult to imagine that there would be an unlimited set of genes encoding all possible antibodies that we might generate — be they poor fit or tight fit. This led many eminent scientists to advocate the 'instructive' theory for antibodies — one where the foreign antigen would form a template around which a nascent antibody molecule would define its shape, and then be committed to that shape in perpetuity[31,32] (see discussion by Lederberg[33]). Now, with our knowledge of complete animal genomes, we can recognise that to accommodate the antibody repertoire problem within the

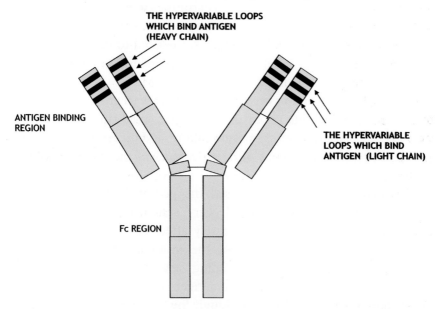

We generate antibodies such as this against a vast number of antigens. The antigen binding regions vary from antibody to antibody especially in the (black) hypervariable regions. The "antibody problem" related to how the immune system acquired the genetic information to make so many antibodies to the large universe of antigens. Were the genes all inherited in the genome, or were there somatic events which created the diversity, or was the answer a combination of both?

Fig. 10.2. A typical IgG molecule.

30,000 or so genes comprising the total human genome requires that we acknowledge this cannot be achieved by simply inheriting all necessary variable regions in the germ line, but that somatic events must shape that repertoire.

The desire to understand the somatic diversification of antibodies was able to build on previous Nobel Prize-winning work on the structure of antibodies and the recognition of variable and constant regions in antibody Heavy and Light chains.[34,35] This work benefited from the availability of monoclonal plasma cell tumours of mice[36] and men[37] (the myelomas), and the protein sequencing techniques developed by Sanger. The sequencing of many myelomas also identified the hypervariable regions of antibodies (three in each chain) as the sites which were more likely to vary from antibody to antibody. This raised the idea that there must be a somatic hypermutation mechanism selective to B-cells, and critical to driving diversity. The clonal selection theory predicted that genetic changes which committed to defined antibodies were changes that would not be present in the germ line but in cells committed to making antibodies.

The ability to commit certain myeloma lines to grow in tissue culture offered the exciting opportunity that one could study some of the somatic diversification events in tissue culture, and use natural or induced mutations to study functions of different parts of the immunoglobulin molecule.

Milstein and Scharff recognised the potential value of studying myeloma mutants. Milstein and Secher[38] systematically collected such mutants, only to find that they rarely affected the antigen binding sites, but rather other regions of the molecule. Scharff,[18] using a myeloma with a known antigen-binding capacity, adapted his screen to select mutants no longer binding to antigen, but again the frequency of informative mutants was disappointingly low. If there was a hypermutation mechanism it was not demonstrable with such approaches.

Cotton and Milstein[20] had the idea of fusing two myeloma cells together to ask questions about how two sets of genetic information for immunoglobulin Heavy and Light chains would function: would there be any allelic exclusion; would there be any gene scrambling so that gene bits for one immunoglobulin gene would assort with bits for another?

They observed that both sets of Heavy and Light chains could be expressed co-dominantly, and that there was no allelic exclusion or gene scrambling. This result would have predicted a successful outcome in rescue of a monoclonal antibody, were a normal B-cell to be fused to a myeloma cell line, but of course, that experiment took a while longer to achieve.

10.4 Cell Fusion

Cell fusion between two different tumour lines had been demonstrated some 50 years before as a rare event in tissue culture. Enhancing the frequency of the fusion event became possible by taking advantage of Sendai virus which was known for creation of syncitia *in vitro*.[39,40] Henry Harris and John Watkins[41] used this technology in 1965 to fuse normal cells with tumour cells, when they observed evidence that the normal cells could suppress the malignant phenotype. Part of the whole process of selecting the fused 'heterokaryons' was to find selective conditions where they would grow, whilst the unfused cells might be selected against. Previous work from the Waclaw Sybalski[42,43] and John Littlefield[44] laboratories had identified the potential of restoration by cell fusion of the enzyme hypoxanthine guanine phosphate ribosyltransferase (HGPRT) and use of selective culture conditions in the presence of hypoxanthine-aminopterin-thymidine (HAT) medium and other selection conditions to get around the problem. Richard Cotton, who had gained the necessary cell-fusion experience with Henry Harris in Oxford, was recruited by César Milstein to Cambridge where they applied these techniques to a selection of myeloma hybrids,[20] so setting the scene for the eventual fusion of normal B-cells to myelomas. In principle, normal B-cells would eventually die out in culture, and would need no selective agents to keep them from growing.

Milstein gave a seminar on his fusion work at the Basel Institute in 1973, and it was then that Köhler expressed his desire to come to Cambridge to work with him on the antibody problem.

After settling into Cambridge, and having immersed himself in some of the technology, Köhler and Milstein decided to try and fuse

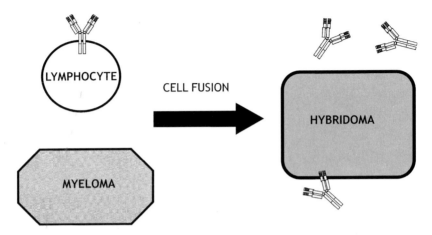

Tissue culture adapted myeloma cell lines have the capacity to secrete large amounts of immunoglobulin. If these are fused to B-cells which are immunised to defined antigens, then one can select from cultures of immortalised hybridomas making antibodies to those same antigens.

Fig. 10.3.   Hybridomas to make monoclonal antibodies.

normal antibody-producing cells to myeloma cells. The motive at that time was to isolate many antibody producing lines to a defined antigen, so that they could get further insights into the diversification process.

One of the authors (HW) was somewhat surprised when Georges Köhler rang him in Cambridge, and asked to be shown the Jerne plaque assay on sheep red blood cell monolayers,[45] as they would be selecting hybridomas towards this antigen (for ease of isolation). Although surprised that Jerne's method had not been learned by Köhler in Basel, HW happily led him through the steps.

As a consequence, HW was kindly invited to attend the famous 'Bull Session' when Milstein and Köhler presented their work-in-progress to members of the LMB. It was a somewhat low-key presentation with Köhler describing in some detail how they had obtained their monoclonal anti-SRBC hybridomas (Fig. 10.3). The mood of the meeting definitely changed when a muted question came from Sydney Brenner, asking, 'Can one make an antibody to anything? Could I make one to my mother-in-law?' It was at that point that many of us realised the importance of the discovery that had been made.

10.5 Why is the Discovery Important?

10.5.1 *The antibody problem*

In terms of the antibody problem, hybridomas making monoclonal antibodies did offer a way to follow maturation and diversification of responses driven by antigen. The direction taken by Milstein with his colleagues Claudia Berek, Matti Kaartinen and Gillian Griffiths[46–49] was to isolate many hybridomas during the course of an immune response to a defined haptenic determinant (oxazolone), and use RNA sequencing to identify evolving changes. This study gave clear evidence of somatic mutations and their impact on affinity maturation *in vivo*, and provided strong evidence for a hypermutation mechanism in B-cells. These findings, together with other seminal studies in the field, virtually eliminated the 'antibody problem' as a problem, leaving just the 'hypermutation' mechanism to be resolved. Recent work on cytosine deaminase by Tasuku Honjo[50] and Michael Neuberger[51] (a close collaborator of Milstein) suggests that it has a key role in the process, in addition to other editing mechanisms that probably operate.

10.5.2 *Impact of diagnostics and research tools*

There can be few areas of biomedical research and diagnosis that have not benefited from the availability of monoclonal antibodies (mAbs). In conjunction with sophisticated detection systems (such as fluorescent probes, enzymes and other amplification tags),[52,53] mAbs have revolutionised modern biomedical research. More than that, their ease of production has provided sufficient incentive for new and successful businesses to commercialise useful antibodies and make them readily available, 'à la carte' as Milstein used to say.

Not only have mAbs been useful in marking and purifying cells at different stages of differentiation, as well as interrogating the breadth of intracellular and membrane protein products, they have also, through their capacity to harness innate effector systems, such as complement or phagocyte Fc receptors, enabled ablative approaches to implicate defined cell types in function or pathology.[54]

It is hard to think of any advance in the past 50 years (aside from DNA sequencing) which has had such a huge impact on medical and biological research.

10.5.3 *Therapeutic antibodies*

The idea that antibodies might provide drugs with desirable specificities to hit cancers and microbial targets has been with us for over a century, as an inevitable by-product of recognising antibody diversity.[55] Polyclonal antibodies (aside from anti-toxins, anti-Rhesus, and anti-lymphocyte globulins) have never quite fulfilled that promise, as they carry logistic complexities that make them relatively unattractive commercial products. As Wigzell articulated in his Nobel presentation,[1] the mAb technology allows for standardisation (a word that should be dear to Jerne's background) and reproducible manufacturing processes for as long as is required. It is for that reason that major pharmaceutical companies and many start-up biotechnology companies have invested in antibody-based therapeutics.

This has taken a little time as the initial 'products' were, by their very nature, murine, and therefore potentially foreign to the patient.[56] The use of antibody engineering to convert murine antibodies to less immunogenic human forms was very much pioneered by Cambridge scientists close to Milstein[57–62] (Neuberger, Gregory Winter, Marianne Bruggemann, Waldmann) from which chimeric, then humanised, then 'fully' human antibody genes from bacteriophage and from appropriately 'engineered' mice emerged (Fig. 10.4). Although not fully solved,[63] the perception that immunogenicity is no longer a significant constraint on antibody utility has meant that therapeutic antibodies are now part of a major resurgence in drug discovery, generating multi-billion-dollar profits for those involved. Not only are they used for targeting cancer and microbes, but now for diverse targets even within the immune system itself.

Antibodies have proven useful drugs for many reasons. First, they lend themselves to bulk manufacturing and straightforward purification. Second, they provide a hitherto unrealised way of neutralising inflammatory molecules such as cytokines and chemokines, or blockading

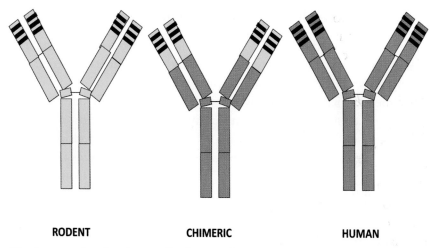

RODENT   CHIMERIC   HUMAN

The frameworks of rodent antibodies are shown in yellow, human frameworks in blue, and the antigen-binding loops in black. There are now many genetic engineering approaches to generating human monoclonal antibodies.

Fig. 10.4. The transition from monoclonal rodent antibodies to genetically engineered human antibodies.[57,60–62,67,68]

cell membrane-based growth receptors, particularly in cancer. Third, they can exploit natural amplification mechanisms such as complement and the phagocytic systems to kill unwanted cells. Fourth, they can deliver agonist signals through cell surface receptors which can be exploited to boost immunity or to encourage cells to commit suicide. As yet not properly realised is their potential to deliver a toxic chemical payload to cancers, but this is certain to evolve. As with all drugs, antibodies are not without their unwanted side effects, which are generally related to the molecules and cells to which they are targeted, and as these become better understood, then so too can they be better managed.

Perhaps one of the surprising outcomes of the use of antibodies as immunosuppressants has been the discovery that certain antibodies can deliver long-term benefit from short-term treatment by being able to harness mechanisms of immunological tolerance.[64–66] Such treatments could, in principle, enable cure of diseases such as multiple sclerosis and Type 1 diabetes.

10.6 Commercialisation of Monoclonal Antibodies

At the time of the discovery, Milstein had tried hard to ensure that the mAb technology was patented. However, the infrastructure for transferring technology from academia was very inadequate in the UK at that time (1975), and this is why, perhaps in those early days, the US was able to exploit the opportunities more effectively. However, with the advent of various 'humanisation' technologies, developed with Medical Research Council support, monoclonal antibodies did eventually bring to the UK the deserved commercial success from an ever developing billion dollar drug industry.

10.7 Translational Research

The 'antibody problem' as a fundamental question in biology was the driver for the three Nobel Laureates discussed here. None of them could have anticipated the huge research and commercial applications that would emerge from the journey they took. The lesson for those who fund science is to be extremely careful not to prescribe 'strategic areas' for investment in research. More often than not, targeted research may prove less cost-effective than allowing scientists to focus on outstanding fundamental questions in science, without pressure for a translational 'product'. This is not to say that scientists should not be made aware of the unmet needs that their research could answer, but where talent is obvious they should be left, and indeed encouraged, to do it their way.

References

1. Wigzell H. The Nobel Prize for phsyiology or medicine. In: *Nobel Lectures, Physiology or Medicine 1981–1990*, Lindsten J (ed.). Singapore: World Scientific Publishing Co.; 1993: 203–208.
2. Jerne NK. The natural-selection theory of antibody formation. *Proc Natl Acad Sci U S A* 1955; 41: 849–857.
3. Burnet FMS. The clonal selection theory of acquired immunity. *The Abraham Flexner Lectures of Vanderbilt University, 1958*. Cambridge: Cambridge University Press; 1959: ix, 209.

4. Jerne NK. The somatic generation of immune recognition. *Eur J Immunol* 1971; 1: 1–9.

5. Huseby E, Kappler J, Marrack P. TCR-MHC/peptide interactions: kissing-cousins or a shotgun wedding? *Eur J Immunol* 2004; 34: 1243–1250.

6. Jerne NK. Idiotypic networks and other preconceived ideas. *Immunol Rev* 1984; 79: 5–24.

7. Eichmann K. *The Network Collective: Rise and Fall of a Scientific Paradigm*. Basel and Boston: Birkhäuser; 2008.

8. Soderqvist T, Jerne NK. *Science as Autobiography: The Troubled Life of Niels Jerne*. New Haven, CT and London: Yale University Press; 2003.

9. Eichmann K. *Köhler's Invention*. Basel and Boston: Birkhäuser; 2005.

10. Jerne NK. A study of avidity based on rabbit skin responses to diphtheria toxin-antitoxin mixtures. *Acta Pathol Microbiol Scand Suppl* 1951; 87: 1–183.

11. Jerne NK. Bacteriophage inactivation by antiphage serum diluted in distilled water. *Nature* 1952; 169: 117–118.

12. Jerne NK. The unit in preference to the titre as a measure of agglutinating activity. *Bull World Health Organ* 1954; 10: 937–940.

13. Jerne NK. The generative grammar of the immune system. *EMBO J* 1985; 4: 847–852.

14. Köhler G, Milstein C. Continuous cultures of fused cells secreting antibody of predefined specificity. *Nature* 1975; 256: 495–497.

15. Tonegawa S, Steinberg C, Dube S et al. Evidence for somatic generation of antibody diversity. *Proc Natl Acad Sci U S A* 1974; 71: 4027–4031.

16. Lefkovits I. Precommitment in the immune system. *Curr Top Microbiol Immunol* 1974; 65: 21–58.

17. Köhler G. Frequency of precursor cells against the enzyme beta-galactosidase: an estimate of the BALB/c strain antibody repertoire. *Eur J Immunol* 1976; 6: 340–347.

18. Baumal R, Birshtein BK, Coffino P et al. Mutations in immunoglobulin-producing mouse myeloma cells. *Science* 1973; 182: 164–166.

19. Secher DS, Cotton RG, Milstein C. Spontaneous mutation in tissue culture-chemical nature of variant immunoglobulin from mutant clones of MOPC 21. *FEBS Lett* 1973; 37: 311–316.

20. Cotton RG, Milstein C. Letter: fusion of two immunoglobulin-producing myeloma cells. *Nature* 1973; 244: 42–43.

21. Stoppani AO, Milstein C. Essential role of thiol groups in aldehyde dehydrogenases. *Biochem J* 1957; 67: 406–416.

22. Milstein C. The mechanism of activation of phosphoglucomutase by chelating agents. *Biochem J* 1961; 79: 584–590.

23. Milstein C, Sanger F. The amino acid sequence around the serine phosphate in phosphoglucomutase. *Biochim Biophys Acta* 1960; 42: 173–174.

24. Milstein C. The amino acid sequence around the reactive serine residue in alkaline phosphatase from Escherichia coli. *Biochem J* 1964; 92: 410–421.

25. Brenner S, Milstein C. Origin of antibody variation. *Nature* 1966; 211: 242–243.

26. Milstein C, Munro AJ. The genetic basis of antibody specificity. *Annu Rev Microbiol* 1970; 24: 335–358.

27. Brownlee GG, Cartwright EM, Cowan NJ *et al.* Purification and sequence of messenger RNA for immunoglobulin light chains. *Nat New Biol* 1973; 244: 236–240.

28. Milstein C, Brownlee GG, Harrison TM *et al.* A possible precursor of immunoglobulin light chains. *Nat New Biol* 1972; 239: 117–120.

29. Landsteiner K, van der Scheer J. On cross reactions of immune sera to azoproteins. *J Exp Med* 1936; 63: 325–339.

30. Eisen HN, Siskind GW. Variations in affinities of antibodies during the immune response. *Biochemistry* 1964; 3: 996–1008.

31. Breinl F, Haurowitz F. Chemische untersuchung des prazipitates aus hamoglobin and anti-hamoglobin-serum and bemerkungen ber die natur der antikorper. *Z Phyisiol Chem* 1930; 192: 45–55.

32. Pauling L. A theory of the structure and process of formation of antibodies. *J Am Chem Soc* 1940; 62: 2643–2657.

33. Lederberg J. Genes and antibodies. Do antigens bear instructions for antibody specificity or do they select cell lines that arise by mutation? *Science* 1959; 129: 1659–1743.

34. Porter RR. Separation and isolation of fractions of rabbit gamma-globulin containing the antibody and antigenic combining sites. *Nature* 1958; 182: 670–671.

35. Edelman GM, Gally JA. A Model for the 7s Antibody Molecule. *Proc Natl Acad Sci U S A* 1964; 51: 846–853.

36. Potter M. Immunoglobulin-producing tumors and myeloma proteins of mice. *Physiol Rev* 1972; 52: 631–719.

37. Kunkel HG. Myeloma proteins and antibodies. *Am J Med* 1965; 39: 1–3.
38. Secher DS, Milstein C, Adetugbo K. Somatic mutants and antibody diversity. *Immunol Rev* 1977; 36: 51–72.
39. Okada Y. Analysis of giant polynuclear cell formation caused by HVJ virus from Ehrlich's ascites tumor cells. I. Microscopic observation of giant polynuclear cell formation. *Exp Cell Res* 1962; 26: 98–107.
40. Roizman B. Polykaryocytosis induced by viruses. *Proc Natl Acad Sci U S A* 1962; 48: 228–234.
41. Harris H, Watkins JF. Hybrid cells derived from mouse and man: artificial heterokaryons of mammalian cells from different species. *Nature* 1965; 205: 640–646.
42. Szybalski W, Smith MJ. Genetics of human cell lines. I. 8-Azaguanine resistance, a selective 'single-step' marker. *Proc Soc Exp Biol Med* 1959; 101: 662–666.
43. Szybalski W. Use of the HPRT gene and the HAT selection technique in DNA-mediated transformation of mammalian cells: first steps toward developing hybridoma techniques and gene therapy. *Bioessays* 1992; 14: 495–500.
44. Littlefield JW. Selection of hybrids from matings of fibroblasts *in vitro* and their presumed recombinants. *Science* 1964; 145: 709–710.
45. Jerne NK, Henry C, Nordin AA *et al.* Plaque forming cells: methodology and theory. *Transplant Rev* 1974; 18: 130–191.
46. Griffiths GM, Berek C, Kaartinen M *et al.* Somatic mutation and the maturation of immune response to 2-phenyl oxazolone. *Nature* 1984; 312: 271–275.
47. Berek C, Griffiths GM, Milstein C. Molecular events during maturation of the immune response to oxazolone. *Nature* 1985; 316: 412–418.
48. Berek C, Milstein C. The dynamic nature of the antibody repertoire. *Immunol Rev* 1988; 105: 5–26.
49. Milstein C, Even J, Berek C. Molecular events during the onset and maturation of the antibody response. *Biochem Soc Symp* 1986; 51: 173–182.
50. Honjo T, Muramatsu M, Fagarasan S. AID: how does it aid antibody diversity? *Immunity* 2004; 20: 659–668.
51. Neuberger MS, Rada C. Somatic hypermutation: activation-induced deaminase for C/G followed by polymerase eta for A/T. *J Exp Med* 2007; 204: 7–10.

52. Cuello AC, Galfre G, Milstein C. Development of a monoclonal antibody against a neuroactive peptide: immunocytochemical applications. *Adv Biochem Psychopharmacol* 1980; 21: 349–363.

53. Herzenberg LA, De Rosa SC. Monoclonal antibodies and the FACS: complementary tools for immunobiology and medicine. *Immunol Today* 2000; 21: 383–390.

54. Milstein C. The Nobel Lectures in Immunology. Lecture for the Nobel Prize in Physiology or Medicine, 1984. From the structure of antibodies to the diversification of the immune response. *Scand J Immunol* 1993; 37: 385–398.

55. Milstein C, Waldmann H. Optimism after much pessimism: What next? *Curr Opin Immunol* 1999; 11: 589–591.

56. Bruggemann M, Winter G, Waldmann H *et al.* The immunogenicity of chimeric antibodies. *J Exp Med* 1989; 170: 2153–157.

57. Neuberger MS, Williams GT, Fox RO. Recombinant antibodies possessing novel effector functions. *Nature* 1984; 312: 604–608.

58. Bruggemann M, Williams GT, Bindon CI *et al.* Comparison of the effector functions of human immunoglobulins using a matched set of chimeric antibodies. *J Exp Med* 1987; 166: 1351–1361.

59. Jones PT, Dear PH, Foote J *et al.* Replacing the complementarity-determining regions in a human antibody with those from a mouse. *Nature* 1986; 321: 522–525.

60. Riechmann L, Clark M, Waldmann H *et al.* Reshaping human antibodies for therapy. *Nature* 1988; 332: 323–327.

61. Bruggemann M, Caskey HM, Teale C *et al.* A repertoire of monoclonal antibodies with human heavy chains from transgenic mice. *Proc Natl Acad Sci U S A* 1989; 86: 6709–6713.

62. Winter G, Griffiths AD, Hawkins RE *et al.* Making antibodies by phage display technology. *Annu Rev Immunol* 1994; 12: 433–455.

63. Somerfield J, Hill-Cawthorne GA, Lin A *et al.* A novel strategy to reduce the immunogenicity of biological therapies. *J Immunol* 2010; 185: 763–768.

64. Benjamin RJ, Waldmann H. Induction of tolerance by monoclonal antibody therapy. *Nature* 1986; 320: 449–451.

65. Keymeulen B, Walter M, Mathieu C *et al.* Four-year metabolic outcome of a randomised controlled CD3-antibody trial in recent-onset

type 1 diabetic patients depends on their age and baseline residual beta cell mass. *Diabetologia* 2010; 53: 614–623.

66. Coles AJ, Cox A, Le Page E *et al.* The window of therapeutic opportunity in multiple   sclerosis: evidence from monoclonal antibody therapy. *J Neurol* 2006; 253: 98–108.

67. Winter GP. Antibody engineering. *Philos Trans R Soc Lond B Biol Sci* 1989; 324: 537–546; discussion 547.

68. Winter G, Milstein C. Man-made antibodies. *Nature* 1991; 349: 293–299.

Chapter 11

THE DISCOVERY OF THE LDL RECEPTOR AND ITS ROLE IN CHOLESTEROL METABOLISM

Gilbert Thompson

11.1 Introduction

In 1985 The Nobel Prize in Physiology or Medicine was awarded to Michael Brown and Joseph Goldstein, aged 44 and 45 respectively, 'for their discoveries concerning the regulation of cholesterol metabolism'. In his presentation speech, Professor Viktor Mutt of the Karolinska Institute commented that they had discovered, 'a physiological mechanism of great importance: the way in which mammalian cells strive to establish an equilibrium between their own synthesis and the cholesterol they obtain from circulating blood'. He went on to say that they had also elucidated 'important genetically-determined alterations from this mechanism' and that 'this knowledge forms a rational basis for development of methods for the treatment and prevention of the widespread disabling diseases known to be a consequence of derangement in plasma cholesterol concentrations', namely the various clinical manifestations of atherosclerosis. He concluded by noting how effectively Goldstein and Brown had collaborated together and suggested that partnerships like theirs should be emulated more often, both in science and other fields of human endeavour.[1]

11.2 Biographical Background of the Laureates

11.2.1 Joseph Goldstein

Joseph L. Goldstein was born in 1940 and grew up in South Carolina, US. He attended the local schools in his home town and then went to Washington and Lee University in Virginia, where he graduated *summa cum laude* in Chemistry in 1962. Having decided to do Medicine he sought and gained entry to the University of Texas Southwestern Medical School in Dallas. His talents were soon spotted by Donald Seldin, legendary head of the Department of Medicine, who ear-marked him as the future head of a division of Medical Genetics. When Goldstein obtained his MD in 1966 he was acknowledged as the outstanding graduate of his year. He spent the next two years as an intern and resident at the Massachusetts General Hospital in Boston, where the author happened to be working as a research fellow at the time. He struck one as a serious and intense yet open and friendly person, who spoke in rapid bursts with a pronounced Southern accent. After completing his residency he spent the next two years as a clinical associate at the National Institutes of Health (NIH) in Bethesda, where he looked after Don Fredrickson's patients, including some with homozygous familial hypercholesterolaemia (FH). While at the NIH he also worked on the biochemistry of protein synthesis in the laboratory of Marshall Nirenberg, winner of the 1968 Nobel Prize in Physiology or Medicine (see Chapter 6).

Following Seldin's advice he went to Seattle in 1970 to do a fellowship in Medical Genetics with Arno Motulsky at the University of Washington. During his two years there he undertook a major study of the genetic causes of hyperlipidaemia in myocardial infarction survivors [2-4] and also learned how to perform tissue culture. He returned to Dallas in 1972 and was appointed Assistant Professor in charge of the division of Medical Genetics, as Seldin had planned. He was promoted to Associate Professor in 1974 and Professor in 1976. The following year he became Chairman of the Department of Molecular Genetics and has remained so ever since.

11.2.2 *Michael Brown*

Michael S. Brown was born in 1941 in Brooklyn, New York, and moved to Pennsylvania with his family when he was 11. He went to high school in a small town near Philadelphia and thence to the University of Pennsylvania, where he graduated with a degree in Chemistry in 1962. His mother worked at the Smith Kline laboratories nearby, which may have stimulated his interest in medical research. He went to the University of Pennsylvania School of Medicine and got his MD in 1966, coming top of the class like Joe Goldstein did in Dallas. The two met for the first time later that year when they were interns at the Massachusetts General Hospital and quickly became friends. In 1968 Brown went to the NIH as a Clinical Associate in gastroenterology and spent some time in Earl Stadtman's laboratory, where he acquired skills in enzymology. In 1971 he embarked upon a fellowship in gastroenterology at the University of Texas Southwestern Medical School, having been persuaded to go there by Joe Goldstein. In addition to undertaking clinical duties such as endoscopy, Brown worked in John Dietschy's laboratory where the two of them, together with Marvin Siperstein, succeeded in solubilising and partially purifying from rat liver the enzyme hydroxyl methyl glutaryl co-enzyme A (HMG CoA) reductase, the rate limiting step on the cholesterol synthesis pathway.[5] He became Associate Professor in Internal Medicine in 1974, Professor in 1976 and Professor of Medical Genetics and Director of the Center for Genetic Diseases the following year.

Scientific collaboration between Brown and Goldstein started in 1972, after the latter had returned to Dallas from Seattle, and was precipitated by a phone call from the surgeon Tom Starzl, informing Siperstein that he was about to perform a portocaval shunt on a 12-year-old girl with homozygous FH in an attempt to lower her cholesterol. Siperstein was away so Brown flew to Denver to collect a skin biopsy from the patient;[6] the research that ensued is described below and formed the scientific basis for their Nobel Prize. At a personal level Brown seems less restless than Goldstein and has a more measured approach to life. He enjoys sailing and fishing whereas Goldstein is passionately fond of art.

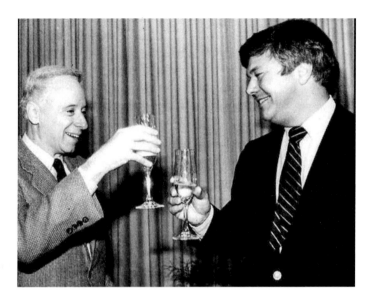

Fig. 11.1. Goldstein (left) and Brown celebrating the announcement in October 1985 that they had won the Nobel Prize. (Reproduced with permission of Drs JL Goldstein and MS Brown).

At the risk of oversimplification, Brown is the doer and Goldstein the thinker, although they often swap roles. Both are superb communicators and have been the joint recipients of numerous honours and prizes, including the Lasker Award for Basic Medical Research, which they received in the same year as their Nobel Prize (Fig. 11.1).

11.3 The Problem: Familial Hypercholesterolaemia 40 Years Ago

Goldstein and Brown were doing their internships in Boston in 1967 when Fredrickson, Robert Levy and Robert Lees published a five-part article in the *New England Journal of Medicine* introducing a novel classification of disorders of lipoprotein metabolism.[7] This article aroused enormous interest among clinicians regarding the role of lipids in atherosclerosis and cardiovascular disease. It also underlined the unique status of the NIH, where Fredrickson directed the Laboratory of Molecular Diseases in the National Heart Institute, as a referral centre for inherited forms of dyslipidaemia. Prominent among the latter were patients with familial hypercholesterolaemia, a disorder which fascinated Joe Goldstein when he went to work there two years later.

Familial hypercholesterolaemia is characterised by hypercholesterolaemia from birth and the subsequent development of tendon xanthomas and premature onset of atherosclerosis, as first described by Carl Muller in 1938.[8] Nick Myant noted that the dominantly-inherited increase in plasma cholesterol was largely confined to LDL cholesterol,[9] which can reach > 20 mmol/l in homozygotes and up to12 mmol/l in heterozygotes. The frequency of FH in the populations of Europe and North America averages about 1:500 for heterozygotes and 1:1000,000 for homozygotes but in some parts of the world is much higher. Regions with an increased prevalence include the Lebanon, South Africa and the French Canadian province of Quebec. In South Africa and Quebec the increased prevalence of FH represents a founder effect traceable to immigrant settlers from Europe, whereas in Muslim communities it reflects the frequency of first-cousin marriages.

In homozygotes the severe hypercholesterolaemia usually results in atheromatous involvement of the aortic root before puberty. Sudden death from myocardial infarction or acute coronary insufficiency before the age of 30 was the rule until plasmapheresis was introduced in 1975.[10] Post-mortem examination of homozygotes reveals that the aortic valve, sinuses of Valsalva and ascending arch of the aorta are grossly infiltrated with atheroma, with the coronary ostia often narrowed to pinhole size.

Now as then, heterozygous FH often remains undiagnosed until the onset of cardiovascular symptoms in adult life. In addition to hypercholesterolaemia there may be signs of cholesterol deposition, such as corneal arcus and tendon xanthomas. The increased frequency and premature onset of coronary heart disease is well documented, and in untreated subjects occurs about 20 years earlier than in the rest of the population. On coronary angiography triple vessel disease is common, often accompanied by disease of the left main stem. Post-mortem examination reveals severe atherosclerosis of the aorta, especially the abdominal portion. The aortic root is affected to a much lesser extent than in homozygotes but the coronary arteries show extensive involvement.

This, then, was the disorder which so intrigued Goldstein and Brown in 1972. Because hypercholesterolaemia was present in heterozygotes as well as in homozygotes they speculated that FH was probably not caused by an enzyme deficiency, as is common in recessively inherited disorders, but was more likely to be due to a defect in a protein involved in the feedback regulation of cholesterol synthesis.[11] They set about testing this hypothesis in a series of ingenious experiments using fibroblasts cultured from the skin of FH patients and normal subjects.

11.4 The Solution: Discovery of the LDL Receptor and its Partial or Complete Absence in FH

Working together in Dallas, combining Goldstein's cell culture skills and Brown's knowledge of enzymology, the pair set out to measure the activity of HMG CoA reductase in fibroblasts cultured from the skin of an FH homozygote whose serum cholesterol had reached 26 mmol/l.[12] They discovered that the activity of HMG CoA reductase was 60–80 times greater in the fibroblasts when incubated with lipoprotein-deficient plasma than in control fibroblasts. And unlike the latter, HMG CoA reductase activity in the homozygote's fibroblasts, determined by measuring the conversion of ^{14}C-HMG CoA to ^{14}C- mevalonate, was not suppressed by adding LDL to the culture medium (Fig. 11.2). Fibroblasts from FH heterozygotes exhibited a partial defect in regulation of HMG CoA reductase but Goldstein and Brown considered it unlikely that a defect in the gene encoding this enzyme could be the cause of FH.

They pursued their investigations further and demonstrated that ^{125}I-labelled LDL was bound to normal fibroblasts by a high affinity, saturable process which mediated the uptake and subsequent proteolytic degradation of LDL and resulted in suppression of HMG CoA reductase activity and therefore of cholesterol synthesis.[13] They showed that fibroblasts from FH homozygotes lacked these high

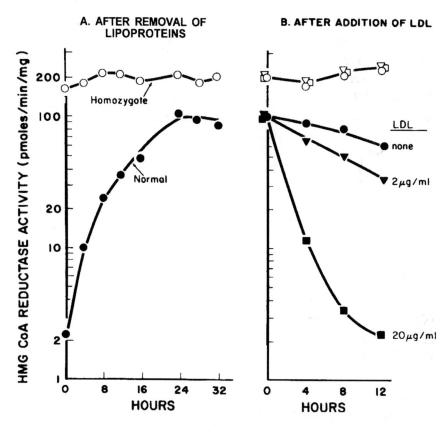

Fig. 11.2. HMG CoA reductase activity in cultured fibroblasts from a normal subject and patient with homozygous FH in (A) the absence and (B) the presence of LDL. (Reproduced with permission from ref. 12).

affinity binding sites, failed to degrade LDL and failed to suppress their HMG CoA reductase activity when exposed to LDL. Fibroblasts from FH heterozygotes showed intermediate levels of high affinity binding of LDL.

Goldstein and Brown concluded that high affinity binding of LDL results in endocytosis (internalisation) and lysosomal degradation of LDL, the ensuing hydrolysis of cholesterol esters leading to release of free cholesterol and inhibition of HMG CoA reductase. They proposed that FH was due to an abnormality of a dominantly

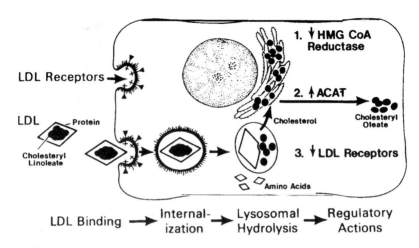

Fig. 11.3. Schematic diagram of the LDL receptor pathway, showing binding of LDL to receptors in coated pits followed by endocytosis and hydrolysis in lysosomes. The ensuing release of free cholesterol results in downregulation of HMG CoA reductase and LDL receptors and upregulation of ACAT. (Reproduced with permission from MS Brown and JL Goldstein. Receptor-mediated endocytosis: Insights from the lipoprotein receptor system. *Proc. Natl. Acad. Sci. USA* 1979; 76: 3330–3337).

inherited gene whose product is the LDL receptor (Fig. 11.3), defects of which result in reduced catabolism of LDL and increased cholesterol synthesis. The severity of the ensuing hypercholesterolaemia depends upon whether the receptor defect is partial, as in heterozygotes, or total, as in homozygotes.

At the time not everyone accepted Goldstein and Brown's explanation of the cause of FH. This became evident at a meeting they attended at Hammersmith Hospital in September 1975, organised by Nick Myant and the author. During the meeting Avedis Khachadurian described a number of families with a variant form of FH, characterised by the appearance of the features of homozygous FH in children whose parents were normocholesterolaemic. Cholesterol synthesis was greater than normal in cultured fibroblasts from these variant homozygotes but lower than in fibroblasts from homozygotes with classical FH. With the benefit of hindsight it is clear that Khachadurian was describing the condition now known as

Autosomal Recessive Hypercholesterolaemia (ARH) which, as the term implies, is aetiologically distinct from the commoner autosomal dominant i.e. classical form of FH. Later in the meeting, Alan Fogelman and George Popjak, with whom Myant had worked when Popjak was at Hammersmith Hospital during the 1950s, postulated that the greater than normal induction of HMG CoA reductase they observed in FH leucocytes incubated in lipid-free serum was secondary to excessive leakage of endogenously-synthesised cholesterol from these cells, not to a failure of down regulation of the enzyme consequent on defective LDL catabolism as Brown and Goldstein claimed.

However, *in vivo* evidence that LDL catabolism was indeed defective in FH came from several sources. Turnover studies at the NIH had previously shown that the fractional catabolic rate (FCR) of ^{125}I-labelled LDL in FH heterozygotes was only half that of normal subjects.[14] Non-steady state studies of LDL turnover in FH patients showed that the FCR of LDL remained subnormal even after a marked reduction in pool size following plasma exchange, suggesting that the catabolic defect was intrinsic and not secondary to the expanded pool.[15] Subsequent studies by James Shepherd *et al.* in Glasgow involved simultaneous administration of native LDL labelled with ^{125}I and ^{131}I-labelled LDL coupled with 1,2 cyclohexanedione, a chemical modification known to inhibit binding of LDL to fibroblasts.[16] Their results showed that the FCR of ^{125}I-labelled LDL but not that of ^{131}I-LDL-cyclohexanedione was reduced in FH heterozygotes compared with normal subjects, implying decreased receptor-mediated catabolism of LDL in FH.[17] Using the same technique the author and his colleagues in London demonstrated an analogous but more severe defect in two homozygotes.[18]

The likelihood that the abnormalities of receptor-mediated catabolism revealed by these turnover studies reflected impaired uptake of LDL by hepatic receptors was supported by *in vitro* binding studies, using cell membranes prepared from liver biopsies obtained during routine abdominal surgery from control subjects and FH patients.[19] The results showed that saturable binding of ^{125}I-LDL was reduced by approximately 50% in FH heterozygotes compared with normal subjects; when the data were pooled they showed an inverse correlation between the saturable binding of LDL by liver membranes and the concentration of cholesterol in plasma. This finding drew attention to the importance of LDL receptors in the liver in regulating plasma cholesterol, a premise which was later confirmed by the Dallas workers after Starzl performed a liver transplant in an FH homozygote and thereby restored her plasma cholesterol level to normal.[20]

The discovery of the LDL receptor gave a unique insight into the pathophysiology of cholesterol metabolism and was the main scientific advance for which Goldstein and Brown were subsequently awarded the Nobel Prize. However, this discovery was buttressed by several others they made during the intervening ten years, as described below.

11.5 The Scavenger Receptor and Atherosclerosis

The observation that cholesterol ester-filled macrophages or foam cells occurred in the atherosclerotic lesions of FH homozygotes intrigued Goldstein and Brown, since it implied that macrophages took up LDL cholesterol via an LDL receptor-independent pathway. They investigated this phenomenon using mouse peritoneal macrophages and showed that the latter took up and degraded acetyl LDL much faster than native LDL and continued to do so despite accumulating large amounts of cholesterol.[21] They demonstrated that this process reflected the presence of a high affinity binding site which recognised acetylated but not native LDL. They also showed that uptake and degradation of acetylated LDL markedly stimulated cholesterol esterification in mouse peritoneal macrophages and greatly increased their cholesterol ester content.[22] This reflected the activity of acylcholesterol acyltransferase (ACAT) within macrophages, which re-esterified cholesterol linoleate, the form in which cholesterol occurs in LDL, to cholesterol oleate, the form in which it accumulates in foam cells.

Human monocyte macrophages behaved in a similar manner and Goldstein and Brown suggested that some chemical or physical modification of LDL occurred in plasma or tissue fluid which made it a suitable ligand for what they termed a scavenger pathway for LDL in

FH. Subsequently it became clear that this pathway plays a key role in atherogenesis in general, not just in FH, and that oxidised LDL is probably its main substrate. Oxidised LDL can be produced *in vitro* by incubating LDL with endothelial cells, smooth muscle cells or macrophages. Lipid peroxidation leads to conversion of lecithin to lysolecithin and of oxidised fatty acids to aldehydes; the latter reacting with lysine groups on apoB to give it a negative charge and thus making it a suitable substrate for the scavenger receptor.

The discovery of the scavenger receptor was a crucial step in the development of the inflammatory-response-to-injury theory of atherosclerosis, which was originally proposed by Rudolf Virchow and has been elaborated more recently by Peter Libby[23] and others. Although definitive proof of a causal role for oxidised LDL is lacking there is ample evidence that it is present in atherosclerotic lesions where it stimulates the release of pro-inflammatory cytokines, inducing the formation of vascular cell adhesion molecules and promoting the attachment to the endothelium of blood-borne monocytes. After migrating into the arterial intima, monocytes take on the characteristics of macrophages and express scavenger receptors. The ensuing uptake of modified LDL results in the formation of cholesterol ester-engorged foam cells and leads to the formation of atheromatous plaques. The presence of severe hypercholesterolaemia from birth, as seen in FH homozygotes, accelerates this process and promotes the premature onset of aortic stenosis and myocardial infarction, both of which occurred in the 12-year-old who provided the skin fibroblasts for Goldstein and Brown's earlier studies.

11.6 Stimulation of Receptor-mediated Catabolism of LDL by Statins

In 1971, the Japanese microbiologist Akira Endo began searching for microbial metabolites which would inhibit HMG CoA reductase. His belief that this would provide a novel means of lowering plasma cholesterol was vindicated when, after testing more than 6,000 microbial strains, he and his colleagues isolated a potent inhibitor of cholesterol synthesis from *Penicillium citrinum*.[24] Initially known as ML-236B, this compound was later called compactin and became the first HMG CoA reductase inhibitor or statin to be used in humans.

Using the culture system for human fibroblasts devised by Goldstein and Brown, they and Endo showed that compactin was a potent inhibitor of cholesterol synthesis *in vitro* in cells both from normal subjects and patients with homozygous FH.[25] Another finding was that incubating cells with compactin resulted in a compensatory overproduction of HMG CoA reductase. This explained its lack of effect on the serum cholesterol of rats *in vivo* although in later studies Endo showed that the compound lowered cholesterol in dogs and monkeys. The first clinical studies were carried out in FH homozygotes by Akira Yamamoto *et al.* in 1980[26] and subsequently Hiroshi Mabuchi *et al.* showed that co-administration of compactin and a bile acid sequestrant to heterozygotes lowered their LDL cholesterol to an unprecedented extent.[27]

The mechanism of the LDL-lowering effect of statins and bile acid sequestrants was explored by Goldstein and Brown and their colleagues in Dallas. They administered [131]I- labelled LDL to FH heterozygotes before and during treatment with mevinolin (later re-named lovastatin) and showed that it caused a 27% decrease in LDL cholesterol and a 37% increase in the fractional catabolic rate of [131]I- LDL.[28] These effects were enhanced by concomitantly reducing bile acid absorption, either by administering a sequestrant or bypassing the terminal ileum, and were attributed to increased expression of LDL receptors on hepatocytes leading to greater uptake of LDL by the liver.[29] The much smaller cholesterol-lowering effect of statins in homozygotes is explained by the total or near total lack of LDL receptors in such individuals, any effect exerted by these drugs on the latter being attributable to decreased production of LDL secondary to reduced cholesterol synthesis.

During the 1990s, a series of clinical trials established unequivocally that lowering LDL cholesterol with statins resulted in significant decreases in cardiovascular and total mortality, with few serious side effects.[30] As a result these drugs are now used routinely to treat and prevent cardiovascular disease throughout the world. Endo received the Lasker–DeBakey Clinical Medical Research Award in 2008 for discovering statins (Fig. 11.4) and in his acceptance speech he acknowledged

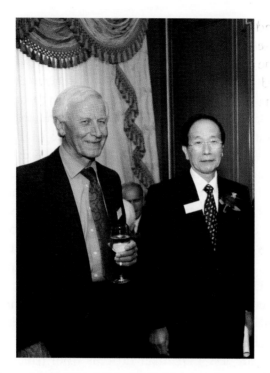

Fig. 11.4. The author (left) and Akira Endo (right) at the reception in New York following the presentation to the latter of the Lasker–DeBakey Clinical Medical Research Award in 2008.

the inspiration and support he had received from Goldstein and Brown over the years. It is largely due to their work that the mechanism of action of these remarkable compounds is so well understood.

11.7 Analysis of the LDL Receptor Gene and Mutations Causing FH

In 1982, Goldstein and Brown and their colleagues succeeded in purifying the LDL receptor from bovine adrenal cortex, yielding a glycoprotein with a molecular weight of 164,000.[31] The purified receptor had LDL binding properties which were identical to those of receptors expressed on intact cells. Two years later they cloned and sequenced the cDNA of the human LDL receptor.[32] The latter consisted of a protein containing 839 amino acids grouped into 5 domains: an amino terminal domain containing the binding site for LDL; a domain homologous with the precursor of the mouse epidermal growth factor receptor; a domain adjacent to the plasma membrane which is the site of O-linked glycosylation; a membrane spanning domain that anchors the receptor to the cell surface; and a cytoplasmic carboxy terminal. They isolated the LDL receptor gene the following year and showed that it contained 18 exons.[33]

These advances paved the way for analysis of the various different mutations of the LDL receptor gene which cause FH and well over a thousand of these have been described to date. The nature of the underlying mutation can exert a marked influence on the severity of the clinical phenotype. For example, FH heterozygotes with a mutation in exon 4, which encodes a critical part of the receptor's LDL-binding domain, have higher LDL cholesterol levels than those with mutations in other parts of the gene which do not affect this domain.[34] Anne Soutar and colleagues explained these findings by showing that lymphoblastoid cells cultured from FH patients with 'severe' mutations that cause receptor deficiency degrade less LDL than do cells from patients with 'mild' mutations, which are often single amino acid substitutions that enable LDL receptors to be expressed but impair their ability to bind LDL.[35]

Several years earlier Brown and Goldstein[36] had investigated a homozygote with a most unusual mutation and the results of their studies provided an important insight into the process whereby LDL undergoes endocytosis. Fibroblasts from this patient (JD) were able to bind ^{125}I-LDL, unlike the fibroblasts from other homozygotes, but differed from normal fibroblasts in their inability to transport LDL into the cell and inhibit HMG CoA reductase. Subsequent studies revealed that the failure of JD's receptors to internalise LDL was due to their inability to cluster in clathrin-coated pits on the cell surface[37] whereas in normal fibroblasts LDL binds to receptors within these pits, which then invaginate to form endocytic vesicles and deliver LDL to lysosomes. More recent studies revealed that the mutation responsible causes a single amino acid substitution, of cysteine for tyrosine, in the cytoplasmic domain of the LDL receptor[38] and that this prevents receptors from clustering in coated pits. The unravelling of this defect gave important insights into normal LDL metabolism and provides a classic example of the meticulous scientific detective work which has emanated from the Goldstein and Brown laboratory in Dallas non-stop for the past 38 years.

11.8 Impact of these Discoveries on Medical Science

The announcement of Goldstein and Brown's Nobel Prize helped boost the morale of those working in the field of lipids and atherosclerosis at a time when there were serious doubts in some quarters regarding the relevance of cholesterol to coronary disease. Their discovery of the LDL receptor provided a novel mechanism for the physiological uptake by cells of cholesterol transported in LDL and for the latter's catabolism by the liver. Equally important, it not only established the nature of the genetic defect in familial hypercholesterolaemia, and thus led to DNA analysis becoming an important screening test for the disease, but it re-emphasised the causal nature of the link between LDL cholesterol and atherosclerosis. Furthermore, Goldstein and Brown's subsequent discovery of the scavenger receptor resulted in increased understanding of the pathogenesis of atherosclerosis and the key role played by chemically-modified LDL in this process. Lastly, together with Endo, they helped define the mechanism of action of compactin, which was never marketed but was the prototypic statin, thereby making a fundamental contribution to the development of its successors. The introduction of these compounds into clinical practice in 1987 resulted in a dramatic improvement in the prognosis of patients with FH[39, 40] and has revolutionised the management and prevention of cardiovascular disease throughout the world.[41]

References

1. *Nobel Lectures, Physiology or Medicine 1981–1990*, Lindsten J (ed.). Singapore: World Scientific Publishing Co.; 1993: 273–274.
2. Goldstein JL, Hazzard WR, Schrott HG *et al.* Hyperlipidemia in coronary heart disease. I. Lipid levels in 500 survivors of myocardial infarction. *J Clin Invest* 1973; 52: 1533–1543.

3. Goldstein JL, Schrott HG, Hazzard WR *et al.* Hyperlipidaemia in coronary heart disease. II. Genetic analysis of lipid levels in 176 families and delineation of a new inherited disorder, combined hyperlipidemia. *J Clin Invest* 1973; 52: 1544–1568.

4. Hazzard WR, Goldstein JL, Schrott HG *et al.* Hyperlipidaemia in coronary heart disease. III. Evaluation of lipoprotein phenotypes of 156 genetically defined survivors of myocardial infarction. *J Clin Invest* 1973; 52: 1569–1577.

5. Brown MS, Dana SE, Dietschy JM *et al.* 3-hydroxy-3-methylglutaryl coenzyme A reductase. Solubilization and purification of a cold-sensitive microsomal enzyme. *J Biol Chem* 1972; 248: 4731–4738.

6. Foster DW, Wilson JD. Presentation of the Kober Medal to Joseph L. Goldstein and Michael S. Brown. *J Clin Invest* 2002; 110: S5–9.

7. Fredrickson DS, Levy RI, Lees RS. Fat transport in lipoproteins — an integrated approach to mechanisms and disorders. *N Engl J Med* 1967; 276: 34–42, 94–103, 148–156, 215–225, 273–281.

8. Muller C. Angina pectoris in hereditary xanthomatosis. *Arch Intern Med* 1939; 64: 675–700.

9. Myant NB. The metabolic lesion in familial hypercholesterolaemia. In: *Cholesterol Metabolism and Lipolytic Enzymes*, Polonovski J (ed.). New York: Masson Publishing; 1977: 39–52.

10. Thompson GR, Lowenthal R, Myant NB. Plasma exchange in the management of homozygous familial hypercholesterolaemia. *Lancet* 1975; 1: 1208–1211.

11. Goldstein JL, Brown MS. The LDL receptor. *Arterioscler Thromb Vasc Biol* 2009; 29: 431–438.

12. Goldstein JL, Brown MS. Familial hypercholesterolemia: Identification of a defect in the regulation of 3-hydroxy-3-methylglutaryl coenzyme A reductase activity associated with overproduction of cholesterol. *Proc Natl Acad Sci USA* 1973; 70: 2804–2808.

13. Goldstein JL, Brown MS. Binding and degradation of low density lipoproteins by cultured human fibroblasts. *J Biol Chem* 1974; 249: 5153–5162.

14. Langer T, Strober W, Levy RI. The metabolism of low density lipoprotein in familial type II hyperlipioproteinemia. *J Clin Invest* 1972; 51: 1528–1536.

15. Thompson GR, Spinks T, Ranicar A *et al.* Non-steady-state studies of low density lipoprotein turnover in familial hypercholesterolaemia. *Clin Sci Mol Med* 1977; 52: 361–369.

16. Mahley RW, Innerarity TL, Pitas RE *et al.* Inhibition of lipoprotein binding to cell surface receptors of fibroblasts following selective modification of arginyl residues in arginine-rich and B apoproteins. *J Biol Chem* 1977; 252: 7279–7287.

17. Shepherd J, Bicker S, Lorimer AR *et al.* Receptor-mediated low density lipoprotein catabolism in man. *J Lipid Res* 1979; 20: 999–1006.

18. Thompson GR, Soutar AK, Spengel FA *et al.* Defects of receptor-mediated low density lipoprotein catabolism in homozygous familial hypercholesterolemia and hypothyroidism *in vivo. Proc Natl Acad Sci USA* 1981; 78: 2591–2595.

19. Harders-Spengel K, Wood CB, Thompson GR *et al.* Difference in saturable binding of low density lipoprotein to liver membranes from normocholesterolemic subjects and patients with heterozygous familial hypercholesterolemia. *Proc Natl Acad Sci USA* 1982; 79: 6355–6359.

20. Bilheimer DW, Goldstein JL, Grundy SM *et al.* Liver transplantation to provide low-density-lipoprotein receptors and lower plasma cholesterol in a child with homozygous familial hypercholesterolemia. *N Eng J Med* 1984; 311: 1658–1664.

21. Goldstein JL, Ho YK, Basu SK *et al.* Binding site on macrophages that mediates uptake and degradation of acetylated low density lipoprotein, producing massive cholesterol deposition. *Proc Natl Acad Sci USA* 1979; 76: 333–337.

22. Brown MS, Goldstein JL, Krieger M *et al.* Reversible accumulation of cholesteryl esters in macrophages incubated with acetylated lipoproteins. *J Cell Biol* 1979; 82: 597–613.

23. Libby P. Inflammation in atherosclerosis. *Nature* 2002; 420: 868–874.

24. Endo A, Kuroda M, Tsujita Y. ML-236A, ML-236B, and ML-236C, new inhibitors of cholesterologenesis produced by Penicillium Citrinum. *J Antibiot (Tokyo)* 1976; 29: 1346–1348.

25. Brown MS, Faust JR, Goldstein JL *et al.* Induction of 3-hydroxy-3-methylglutaryl coenzyme A reductase activity in human fibroblasts incubated with compactin (ML-236B), a competitive inhibitor of the reductase. *J Biol Chem* 1978; 253: 1121–1128.

26. Yamamoto A, Sudo H, Endo A. Therapeutic effects of ML-236B in primary hypercholesterolemia. *Atherosclerosis* 1980; 35: 259–266.

27. Mabuchi H, Sakai T, Sakai Y *et al*. Reduction of serum cholesterol in heterozygous patients with familial hypercholesterolemia. Additive effects of compactin and cholestyramine. *N Eng J Med* 1983; 308: 609–613.

28. Bilheimer DW, Grundy SM, Brown MS *et al*. Mevinolin and colestipol stimulate receptor-mediated clearance of low density lipoprotein from plasma in familial hypercholesterolemia heterozygotes. *Proc Natl Acad Sci USA* 1983; 80: 4124–4128.

29. Kovanen PT, Bilheimer DW, Goldstein JL *et al*. Regulatory role for hepatic low density lipoprotein receptors *in vivo* in the dog. *Proc Natl Acad Sci USA* 1981; 78: 1194–1198.

30. Baigent C, Keech A, Kearney PM *et al*. Cholesterol treatment Trialists' (CTT) Collaborators. Efficacy and safety of cholesterol-lowering treatment: prospective meta-analysis of data from 90,056 participants in 14 randomised trials of statins. *Lancet* 2005; 366: 1267–1278.

31. Schneider WJ, Beisiegel U, Goldstein JL *et al*. Purification of the low density lipoprotein receptor, an acidic glycoprotein of 164,000 molecular weight. *J Biol Chem* 1982; 257: 2664–2673.

32. Yamamoto T, Davis CG, Brown MS *et al*. The human LDL receptor: a cysteine-rich protein with multiple Alu sequences in its mRNA. *Cell* 1984; 39: 27–38.

33. Sudhof TC, Goldstein JL, Brown MS *et al*. The LDL receptor gene: a mosaic of exons shared with different proteins. *Science* 1985; 228: 815–822.

34. Gudnason V, Day IN, Humphries SE. Effect on plasma lipid levels of different classes of mutations in the low-density lipoprotein receptor gene in patients with familial hypercholesterolemia. *Arterioscler Thromb* 1994; 14: 1717–1722.

35. Xi-Ming Sun, Patel DP, Knight BL *et al*. Comparison of the genetic defect with LDL-receptor activity in cultured cells from patients with a clinical diagnosis of heterozygous familial hypercholesterolemia. *Arterioscler Thromb Vasc Biol* 1997; 17: 3092–3101.

36. Brown MS, Goldstein JL. Analysis of a mutant strain of human fibroblasts with a defect in the internalization of receptor-bound low density lipoprotein. *Cell* 1976; 9: 663–674.

37. Anderson RG, Goldstein JL, Brown MS. A mutation that impairs the ability of lipoprotein receptors to localise in coated pits on the cell surface of human fibroblasts. *Nature* 1977; 270: 695–699.
38. Davis CG, Lehrman MA, Russell DW *et al.* The JD mutation in familial hypercholesterolemia. Amino acid substitution in cytoplasmic domain impedes internalization of LDL receptors. *Cell* 1986; 45: 15–24.
39. Neil A, Cooper J, Betteridge J *et al.* Reductions in all-cause, cancer, and coronary mortality in statin-treated patients with heterozygous familial hypercholesterolaemia: a prospective registry study. *Eur Heart J* 2008; 29: 2625–2633.
40. Versmissen J, Oosterveer DM, Yazdanpanah M *et al.* Efficacy of statins in familial hypercholesterolaemia: a long term cohort study. *BMJ* 2008; 337: a2423.
41. Lasker Foundation. *Lasker~DeBakey Clinical Medical Research Award: Akira Endo.* Available at: http://www.laskerfoundation.org/awards/2008_c_description.htm [Accessed 7 June 2011].

Chapter 12

THE INVENTION OF THE POLYMERASE CHAIN REACTION AND USE OF SITE-DIRECTED MUTAGENESIS

Anne K. Soutar

12.1 Introduction

In 1993 Michael Smith and Kary Mullis (Fig. 12.1) shared the Nobel Prize in Chemistry for their 'contributions to the development of methods within DNA-based chemistry'. Half the prize was awarded to Smith 'for his fundamental contributions to the establishment of oligonucleotide-based site-directed mutagenesis and its development for protein studies' and half to Mullis 'for his invention of the polymerase chain reaction (PCR) method'.[1] Both trained as organic chemists and became pioneers in the synthesis of short nucleic acids of defined sequence known as oligonucleotides, but it appears from all that has been written that they could hardly be more different in character or in their approaches to science. What they do have in common is that their research was largely curiosity-driven and certainly neither set out to tackle a clinical problem or change the face of medicine. Nonetheless, their research into the ways in which oligonucleotides could be used to analyse and manipulate DNA sequences was complementary and fundamentally changed the means available to investigate how genes function. Indeed, building on the work of other molecular biologists, Nobel Prize winners or otherwise, they provided the basis that made possible the explosion of knowledge about the human genome in health and disease during the last decade that has raised such expectations of a brave new world.

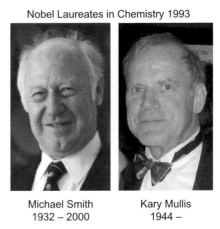

Nobel Laureates in Chemistry 1993

Michael Smith
1932 – 2000

Kary Mullis
1944 –

Fig. 12.1.   Nobel Laureates in Chemistry, 1993.

12.2 Michael Smith (1932–2000)

12.2.1 *Biographical sketch: early life and education**

Michael Smith was born in 1932 to a family of modest means living in Marton Moss on the northwest coast of England, sandwiched between Blackpool, a then popular seaside town, and the more up-market resort of Lytham St Anne's.[2,3] His father worked in the family market garden business growing vegetables (despite a penchant for chrysanthemums, according to his son) and his mother worked as a bookkeeper for a local tobacconist's shop. Michael was a grammar-school boy, benefiting from the newly instated 11+ examination which gave scholarships to bright children of less well-off parents to enable them to attend schools that provided a highly academic education. Although a less than perfect system, and blatantly unfair to many who did not 'pass' for whatever reason, many of England's brightest and best at this time depended on it for a leg-up onto the professional ladder.

---

* Biographical details of Michael Smith are from references 1–3.

From his brief autobiography at the time of the Nobel Prize[3] and a later and more detailed biography,[4] Smith seems to have needed both persistence and determination in the face of adversity to continue his academic education, often giving the impression that he believed he never quite reached the highest educational standards; indeed, a faint Lancashire gloom pervades much of his description of the earlier part of his life. Yet later photographs show him to be a smiling and genial person with whom one would be happy to share a pint down at the local. All these characteristics probably stood him in good stead for his career in research and, together with what appears to be his genuine modesty, made him a much respected and well-liked person through-out his adult life.[4] Despite these feelings of being second best, he graduated with a good upper second in chemistry from the University of Manchester in 1953, sufficient to enable him to obtain a State Scholarship to support him there as a graduate student. He worked on the stereochemistry of cyclohexane diols under the supervision of HB Henbest, and although the route was not entirely smooth his PhD was awarded in 1956 and the work resulted in several publications. No mean achievement for the son of a northern small-time market gardener, but nonetheless Smith clearly felt that his lack of social skills and the class system in the UK would prevent him from pursuing an academic career. He apparently planned to spend a year abroad after obtaining his PhD to gain research experience before joining industry.

12.2.2 *From postdoctoral fellow to independent scientist*

This plan of joining industry was not to be. Having 'failed in numerous applications' to obtain a fellowship to work on the west coast of the US[3] he was taken on at short notice by Gorind Khorana, then working at the University of British Colombia (UBC) in Vancouver, and arrived there in early autumn 1956. This was a stroke of good fortune indeed, although this may not have immediately been apparent to Smith. Nowadays Vancouver can hold its own compared with American west coast cities, but was then in its infancy, being neither a fashionable city nor having a strong academic community. However, it did have the advantage of nearby mountains that provided unlimited scope for Smith's love of outdoor activities, and excellent research opportunities with an enthusiastic and inspirational young supervisor. Khorana himself was to share the 1968 Nobel Prize in Physiology or Medicine with Robert Holley and Marshall Nirenberg 'for their interpretation of the genetic code and its function in protein synthesis', and no doubt Smith's work[5] made a contribution to this.

Research with Khorana was a change of direction from cyclohexane diols for Smith, as his first project was to standardise a method for chemical synthesis of nucleoside-5' triphosphates, based on Khorana's synthesis of ATP in 1954. This led to a general procedure for the preparation of nucleoside-3',5' cyclic phosphates, compounds such as cyclic AMP and cyclic GMP, whose importance was just emerging.[6] Michael Smith has written that, 'One particular pleasure of that period was the development of the methoxyl-trityl family of protecting groups for nucleoside-5'-hydroxyl groups (one synthesis of trimethoxytritanol erupted and left a large orange stain on the laboratory ceiling); this class of protecting group is still in use in modern automated syntheses of DNA and RNA fragments.'[2] Smith remained a postdoctoral fellow in Vancouver with Khorana for the next four years, developing in confidence and enjoying life to the full. There, through mutual friends, he met and eventually married Helen Wood Christie. Helen, who worked as a technician in a nearby lab, was the daughter of a Professor and Head of Forestry at UBC. She and Smith shared an interest in music and a love of outdoor pursuits.

In 1960, funding for Khorana in Vancouver became less secure and he moved to the University of Wisconsin where he was offered a tenured position. Smith went too, as part of the group, but in 1961 fulfilled his desire both to become independent and to return to Vancouver by accepting a position as Head of Chemistry at the Laboratory of the Fisheries Research Board of Canada. He remained there until 1966, ostensibly working on fisheries-related topics, but managing meanwhile to retain some research interest in nucleic acids despite understandable resistance from his employers. He financed his nucleic acid research with competitive funding from the National Institutes of Health (NIH) in the

US. In 1966, he was relieved to be offered a position as a Medical Research Associate of the recently formed Medical Research Council of Canada, supported by Dr Marvin Darrach, then Head of the Department of Biochemistry at UBC, as this salary enabled him to devote himself to full-time academic research and to participate freely in university activities in the Department of Biochemistry. During his time there he developed long-standing collaborations and friendships with colleagues, postdocs and students and continued his research into the synthesis and use of specific oligonucleotides.

12.2.3 *Work that led to the Nobel Prize*

One of the ideas behind Smith's earlier research was the question of whether oligonucleotides could be used to isolate genes — these days we are used to predicting the amino acid sequence of a protein from the DNA sequence of its gene, but at that time DNA sequencing was in its infancy, while the amino acid sequence of several proteins had been determined. One could predict the possible gene sequence for a protein, but it would be an inexact science because most amino acids can be encoded by up to four codons or triplets of nucleotides. Would this enable one to design an oligonucleotide that would bind specifically to a DNA fragment containing the gene of interest? Could one bind the oligo to a column and use it to isolate a gene?

To test these ideas, Smith's graduate student, Caroline Astell, synthesised specific pairs of oligonucleotides that complemented each other, and then determined their ability to bind — 'hybridise' — to form a stable double-stranded DNA fragment. At that time, chemical synthesis of oligonucleotides was painfully slow and each step so inefficient that large amounts of starting material were needed and the desired product had to be purified at each step. Once armed with sufficient oligonucleotides, they were able to show that there was a defined temperature, the melting temperature or Tm, at which two complementary oligonucleotides formed a stable duplex, and that this was dependent on their length and their composition, as DNA duplexes rich in guanine-cytosine pairs (G-C) melted at higher temperatures than adenosine-thymine (A-T)-rich pairs. Crucially, they found that the presence of a single mismatch in the pair did not prevent hybridisation, but did decrease the stability and therefore the Tm of the duplex, although the importance of this finding was not immediately obvious and Smith was concerned about how it could be taken further. Indeed, he considered the possibility of switching his research to a study of membrane proteins, but after a brief sabbatical with Ed Reich at the Rockefeller Institute in 1971, he returned to Vancouver determined to continue with nucleic acids. An enzymologist called Shirley Gillam joined his group and developed an enzymic method for synthesising oligonucleotides with polynucleotide phosphorylase. The first requirement was to purify the enzyme,[7] as there were no companies supplying all these materials in the kit form to which we have ready access today. Gillam eventually succeeded in extending a short chemically-synthesised oligonucleotide of just 4 bases to one containing 11 or 12 bases, and the whole process became quicker and much less tedious.[8] The ability of Smith's lab to synthesise oligonucleotides attracted the attention of other molecular biologists, one of whom was Fred Sanger at the MRC Laboratory for Molecular Biology (LMB) in Cambridge, who was developing new enzymatic methods for sequencing DNA and wanted Smith to produce short defined oligonucleotides to prime the reaction at specific sites on the DNA template.

This resulted in an important step in Smith's research career, as in 1975 he took the opportunity of sabbatical leave to spend a year with Fred Sanger's group in order to learn the developing techniques for DNA sequencing. Smith struggled at times in Cambridge to make the experiments work, but while there he participated in the determination of the entire sequence of bacteriophage φ X 174[9] that led to Sanger's second Nobel Prize in Chemistry. This was awarded in 1980, half to Paul Berg, 'for his fundamental studies of the biochemistry of nucleic acids, with particular regard to recombinant-DNA', the other half jointly to Walter Gilbert and Sanger, 'for their contributions concerning the determination of base sequences in nucleic acids'.[10] Smith also took full advantage of his time at LMB to interact with the many other young researchers who were attracted to this hothouse of molecular biology research. In particular, he had discussions with Clyde Hutchinson III, a visiting scientist from North Carolina with expertise in the biology of bacteriophage φ X 174 (whose DNA Sanger's group were sequencing) about the potential of using oligonucleotides for inserting specific mutations into DNA — the process that became known as site-directed mutagenesis and would win Smith the Nobel Prize.

On his return to Vancouver, he pursued and developed these ideas, often in collaboration with others, meanwhile gaining increasing recognition for his work from other molecular biologists worldwide. He also became increasingly involved in departmental politics; his devotion to his work also took its toll on his marriage, but although he and Helen separated, they remained on sufficiently good terms for Smith to invite his estranged wife to the Nobel ceremony in Stockholm. In 1978, Smith's group published two key papers: one was the first description of site-directed mutagenesis, resulting from the collaboration with Clyde Hutchinson in Chapel Hill[11] and the second, in collaboration with Ben Hall in Seattle, was on the use of a specific oligonucleotide to isolate the gene for yeast cytochrome c.[12] These two pioneering techniques are described in Figs 12.2 and 12.3. It is difficult to pin-point any 'Eureka' moment in Smith's research; like much excellent science, it was more a case of painstaking stepwise progress towards goals, punctuated by many small day-to-day successes and achievements.

Having shown that it was possible to introduce a specific mutation into a gene, Smith continued developing his method for site-directed mutagenesis, improving the yield of mutants and now using it to produce cDNA that would express a variant protein with a specific amino acid substituted so that its effect on function could be determined, an early example being cytochrome c.[13] As more DNA sequences became known, mutagenesis became an important tool to investigate the relationship between structure and function in a protein, and opened the way to 'improving' the activity of an enzyme, even to the concept of designer enzymes. Smith developed more collaborations to study different proteins and continued to

244   *A. K. Soutar*

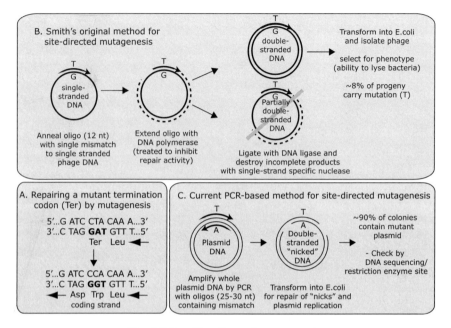

Fig. 12.2. Site-directed mutagenesis.

A: Smith proved his method for site-directed mutagenesis worked by repairing a defect in a phage enzyme needed to lyse bacteria, replacing a termination codon (TAG) with that encoding the amino acid tryptophan (TTG) (note the coding strand is the lower strand in the figure). B: In Smith's original method,[11] an oligonucleotide 12 nucleotides (nt) in length, that matched the sequence of a single-stranded phage but contained a single mismatch (G To T), was annealed to single-stranded DNA from the phage. He then extended the oligonucleotide by addition of single nucleotides, catalysed by the enzyme DNA polymerase that had first been treated to inactivate the enzyme's inherent DNA repair activity (now known as the Klenow fragment). The new strand was then circularised by ligation with DNA ligase and the mixture treated with a nuclease specific for single-stranded DNA to remove any partial products. The treated DNA was transfected into bacteria and the phage progeny screened for those that were able to lyse the bacterial cells i.e. in which the defect had been repaired. He then checked by restriction enzyme digestion and DNA sequencing, but the yield of mutants was low. C: With the advent of PCR with an accurate polymerase, site-directed mutagenesis based on Smith's principle has become a simple, rapid and effective procedure, whereby two much longer nucleotides, both containing the mismatch, are annealed to double-stranded DNA, extended by PCR and transformed directly into bacteria that ligate and replicate the plasmid of which almost 100% carry the mutation.

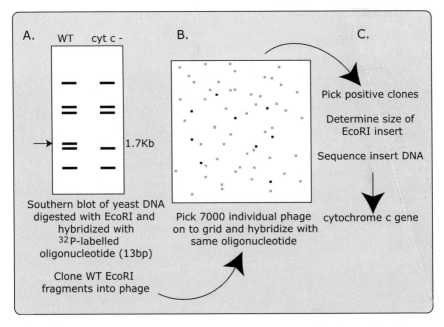

Fig. 12.3. Identification of a cloned gene with a specific oligonucleotide.

Smith used his knowledge of the denaturation and hybridisation properties of oligonucleotides to utilise one to isolate a fragment of yeast genomic DNA containing the gene for cytochrome c. Genomic DNA from yeast was digested with the restriction enzyme *Eco*RI, and the separated fragments transferred to a membrane that was hybridised with a ^{32}P-labelled oligonucleotide probe 13 bases in length that Smith and Gillam had synthesised to match the sequence encoding part of the cytochrome c protein[8] A: The short probe hybridised to too many fragments because it was difficult to control the conditions sufficiently well for such a short probe, but one fragment of 1.7Kb present in wild type (WT) was absent from a mutant lacking cytochrome c (cyt c-). Smith cloned the *Eco*RI fragments from wild type yeast into a bacteriophage and picked 7,000 single phage plaques onto a grid and transferred them to a membrane (each phage would contain a single *Eco*RI fragment). When hybridised with the same oligonucleotide probe, the background noise was considerable (grey spots) and there were a large number of positive phage (black spots). B: He then isolated and determined the size of the cloned inserts at C; one of about 1.7 Kb contained the yeast gene for cytochrome c[12].

participate in research, even though he was by now involved in the establishment and running of a new Biotechnology Laboratory at UBC.

Around this time, Smith, with Ben Hall and Earl Davie from the University of Washington at Seattle, co-founded Zymos, a Biotech company that focused on producing recombinant proteins as pharmaceuticals. Smith insisted that UBC was given shares in Zymos in recompense for his time. Within two years the company was renamed ZymoGenetics and had joined up with a Danish pharmaceutical company called Novo Nordisk to produce their first commercial product, insulin, launched in 1988. At this point Novo Nordisk acquired ZymoGenetics, and Smith became less involved, acting as an occasional consultant. He had enjoyed the rewards the company provided, particularly his company car — a white Mazda R X 7 sports car with 'Zymos' number plates that no doubt helped to ease any potential male mid-life crisis. Selling his shares in ZymoGenetics eventually made him a wealthy man, but he was by all accounts generous to his family, friends, colleagues and UBC.

Smith was awarded the Nobel Prize in 1993; the story goes that he missed the vital phone call from Sweden because he had gone to bed without his hearing aid — he had always suffered from poor hearing — and first heard about the prize on the morning news on the radio. Smith was, by all accounts, delighted, but not altogether surprised. He realised that it was important for Canadian science, and was willing to attend the numerous functions to which he was invited. He was the one asked to make the speech at the Nobel dinner, probably because he was considered a more reliable option than Mullis, of whom more below. Smith donated half his Nobel Prize money to support postdoctoral fellowships for research into schizophrenia and the other half to The Vancouver Foundation to fund public science education and the Society for Canadian Women in Science and Technology. He was also assiduous in ensuring that the people in his lab who had contributed so much to the experimental work received due recognition.[4] Apart from the celebrity naturally associated with the Nobel Prize, Smith apparently did not change his lifestyle, and continued to build up biomedical research at UBC, working right up until his untimely death in October 2000.

12.3 Kary Mullis (1944–)

12.3.1 *Biographical sketch: early life and education*

Kary Mullis was born in Lenoir, in rural North Carolina, in December 1944. We learn little about his family and early life from his brief Nobel autobiography[14] or his autobiographical book entitled *Dancing Naked in the Mind Field*,[15] except that he spent the first five years of his life on his maternal grandparents' farm and probably returned there most summers. He paints a picture of a rural idyll in which he and his cousins experienced a joyous freedom that seems barely possible today — but he does say that he remembers mostly the summers; perhaps the farm was less appealing in the depths of winter. At some point his family must have moved to the city of Colombia, because he attended school there at Drexel High, before going to study chemistry at Georgia Tech. What we do learn of these years suggests that Mullis was lucky to survive them. Having acquired a basic chemistry set as a Christmas present at the age of nine, which he augmented with products obtained without any restrictions from local chemist and hardware shops, he apparently set about experimenting with explosives and combustibles. He must have been a precocious and highly intelligent child; his parents are shadowy figures mentioned rarely in his writings, but his mother seems to have shown great forbearance.

Despite the lucrative and compelling distractions offered by vacation work in a local chemical company, Mullis successfully obtained his degree at Georgia Tech and was awarded public funding to study for a PhD, apparently choosing biochemistry over astrophysics: 'With Mars and Mercury in conjunction in Sagittarius, I was not going to specialise in something well-defined or manageable. I didn't think of myself as a worker or specialist.'[15] Presumably his future biochemistry supervisor, JB Neilands at the University of California in Berkeley, was unaware of this before accepting Mullis as a graduate student, unless everyone in Berkeley at that time was guided by the stars and did not consider hard work essential for a career in research. Certainly Neilands, whose research was focused on iron transport in bacteria, must have been fairly laid back himself, because Mullis's enthusiasm for experimenting in organic chemistry did not stop when he arrived in Berkeley. By the early 1960s he had moved on to the synthesis of mind-altering chemicals that he tested on himself and friends with gusto, while always remaining one small step inside the law. This was also apparently with the encouragement of his first wife Richards, who he had married while at Georgia Tech. How much effort was spent on his PhD project in the lab is not clear, because he attended many courses unrelated to biochemistry, even successfully submitting a letter to *Nature* in 1968 entitled, 'Cosmological Significance of Time Reversal'.[16] *Nature* letters from that time do not appear in publication database searches, so it is not possible to assess the impact of this paper on the scientific community. However, it did apparently persuade the examination committee that he could obtain his PhD without having taken all the required courses.[15]

When he eventually obtained his PhD in 1973, Mullis moved to Kansas where his new wife Cynthia was going to attend medical school. According to Mullis's Nobel lecture,[17] at this stage he planned to become a writer, but soon realised he needed to work as a scientist, and obtained a position with Richard Zakheim and Leone Mattioli in Pediatric Cardiology at the University of Kansas Medical School. It was his first introduction to human biology. His research project, which lasted two years, involved the role of angiotensin in pulmonary vascular physiology, and resulted in three published papers, although none with Mullis as first author. After this, another marriage apparently over, he returned to Berkeley, again with no job. According to Nicholas Wade, who interviewed Mullis for the *New York Times* in 1998,[18] Thomas White, a friend of Mullis, persuaded and assisted him to go back to science, first to a postdoctoral position in Pharmaceutical Chemistry at the University of California in San Francisco, working with Wolfgang Sadee on endorphins in rat brain.

12.3.2 *Joining the Cetus Corporation: work that led to the Nobel Prize*

White then encouraged Mullis to join him at Cetus, formed in 1971 as one of the first biotech companies. Mullis was taken on by Cetus Corporation in 1979, and his job was to synthesise oligonucleotides for use by other members of the company. He was soon put in charge of the DNA synthesis lab, and began to introduce automated methods, leaving himself free time: as he states in an interview with authors writing about PCR as a business venture,[19] 'We nucleotide chemists found ourselves successfully underemployed. Laboratory machines, which we loaded and watched, were making almost more oligonucleotides than we had room for in the freezer.... In my laboratory at Cetus, there was a fair amount of time available to think and to putter.'

Like Smith, Mullis became interested in denaturation of double-stranded DNA, but he used computer models to investigate the effects of time and temperature on the interaction between two strands of DNA. He apparently made use of re-iterative loops in these analyses, a process in which the result of each calculation becomes the input for the next calculation, providing powerful exponential growth. Thinking about these two ideas led to his concept that a particular region of highly complex DNA could be amplified by annealing a pair of oligonucleotide primers to double-stranded DNA that define a specific region and extending them in a re-iterative process: the polymerase chain reaction (Fig. 12.4).

Unlike Smith, Mullis does profess to a single 'Eureka' moment when the idea of PCR crystallised. It occurred while he was driving late one night in April 1983, as Mullis himself has described on more than one occasion. It was a brilliant concept; an idea so simple and obvious in retrospect that one cannot imagine, as Mullis himself at first thought, that no one had come up with it before. Mullis apparently also believed that same night that he would be awarded a Nobel Prize for this discovery.[15] However, it took some considerable time to develop the concept into a procedure that would work routinely, and this achievement required hard, and probably rather tedious work in

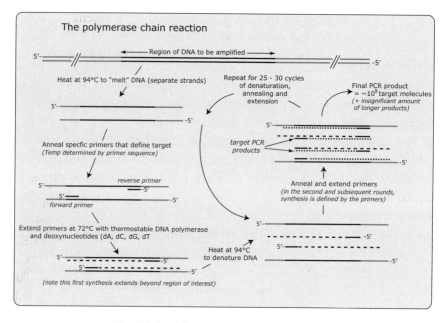

Fig. 12.4.   The polymerase chain reaction.

In the polymerase chain reaction as conceived by Mullis and developed by his colleagues at Cetus,[20-22] double-stranded DNA is denatured by heating and then annealed to two oligonucleotides, the forward and reverse primers, that between them define a region to be amplified. The oligonucleotides are then extended by the stepwise addition of single nucleotides catalysed by the enzyme Taq polymerase. In a series of cycles of denaturation, annealing and extension, more than 10[6] copies of the DNA fragment are produced. Taq polymerase is isolated from *Thermus aquaticus*, a thermophilic bacterium that grows in hot springs, and the isolated enzyme is able to withstand the repeated cycles of high temperature without loss of activity.

Mullis's view, by other colleagues at Cetus. In any event, Mullis was either too busy with other work or distracted by domestic issues even to test his idea experimentally until six months later. His early attempts were not successful: in the first, he mixed human DNA, two primers that were predicted to amplify a region of human nerve growth factor gene, the four deoxynucleotide substrates and some DNA polymerase, and left the mixture at 37°C for the reaction to proceed. With the benefit of hindsight, not surprisingly he failed to detect any product. A month later he tried again, this time trying a few cycles of denaturation and extension, adding fresh enzyme, but again to no avail.[19]

Eventually, with the help of a young technician called Fred Faloona and by switching to a simpler target, Mullis managed to amplify a small fragment of a DNA plasmid. The product was only weakly detectable by autoradiography (a radiolabelled nucleotide was included in the reaction), but it was enough to persuade the lawyers at Cetus to start preparing a patent, although Robert Fildes, President of Cetus, was less impressed. By June 1984, Mullis had succeeded in amplifying a short region of the beta-globin gene and was convinced the technique would work, but still felt that senior colleagues at Cetus did not show sufficient interest when he presented it at a Cetus in-house meeting. Despite this, Mullis was given a one-year trial period to develop PCR, focusing on the procedure as an aid to diagnosis of inherited diseases such as sickle cell anaemia, where the company believed there would be huge commercial profit. A PCR group at the company was formed to bring together sufficient technical and intellectual expertise to move the project forward, and comprised Henry Erlich, Norman Arnheim, Randy Saiki, Glenn Horn, and Steven Scharf, as well as Mullis and Faloona.[19]

Cetus appeared to be more concerned about protecting its patents for PCR as a diagnostic tool than publishing or developing it as a basic science method, and the first paper describing the use of PCR did not appear in print until December 1985, with Mullis as the middle of seven authors. The plan was to publish two papers: a theoretical paper with Mullis as first author, and a paper from Erlich's group demonstrating the practical use of the technique.[19] However, the practical paper was ready for publication well before the theory one,[20] and Mullis was only able to publish a paper on PCR with himself as first author two years later, and then not in a high impact research journal:[21] this can only have added to his ill feelings towards Cetus. As far as the development of PCR was concerned, the next major advance was Mullis's suggestion to use a thermostable DNA polymerase. With considerable effort, other scientists at Cetus were finally able to purify the enzyme from *Thermus aquaticus*, a bacterium that survives in burning springs. This greatly simplified the process, as it was no longer necessary to add fresh enzyme after each denaturation cycle and the reactions were much faster,[22] and Cetus immediately obtained a patent on the process.

The potential of PCR, especially for genetic diagnosis, was quickly recognised by molecular biologists worldwide when Mullis presented at the Cold Spring Harbour symposium in 1986, and Cetus at last began to realise that they had a very commercial product. Meanwhile, relationships had become strained in the Cetus PCR group about who should receive credit for its invention and development, and this reached such a state that Mullis, in discussion with White, agreed to leave the company in late 1986, with five months' salary and having earlier received a $10,000 bonus.[19] Cetus continued to develop and expand PCR as a major business enterprise, eventually selling the rights to Roche for $300 million. First Cetus's, and then Roche's prices made it expensive for research labs to utilise the reagents and the PCR machine developed in collaboration with PerkinElmer. This only encouraged other companies to find inventive ways of circumventing their licensing procedures, eventually bringing PCR within the reach of any lab.

Mullis essentially gave up experimental scientific research in 1986, from then on making his living by lecturing and as a consultant to other companies,[23] the continuation of which was no doubt made possible by his Nobel Prize. His lectures now focus less on PCR and more on other increasingly controversial issues that he appears to relish, such as his perception that there is no evidence that HIV causes AIDS, or that climate change is a myth. Views on Mullis are polarised: John Martin was sufficiently incensed to write to *Nature* after he had invited Mullis to talk at an international meeting in Toledo on PCR: 'Just before the lecture, he told me he would not speak on PCR, but would tell his ideas about AIDS.... His talk was in style rambling and ... inappropriate for young scientists. His only slides (on what he called "his art") were photographs ... of naked women with coloured lights projected on their bodies. The Council of the European Society of Clinical Investigation will not be inviting Dr Mullis to speak at further meetings.'[24] Mullis, of course, was not slow to respond to this letter with apparent glee, suggesting that others were only too pleased to invite him and to remunerate him well for his efforts.[15] Nonetheless, numerous anecdotes, such as his stated pride in addressing the Empress of Japan as 'sweetie' or his belief in astrology and supernatural phenomena, or indeed his 'joke' that women beyond 10,000 days of age are of no interest to him reveal him as a difficult person to warm to;[15] no doubt others find Mullis's approach to life to be more appealing and entertaining, but it has to be said that these probably do not include many active research scientists.

12.4 How these Nobel Prize-winning Discoveries Changed Medicine

12.4.1 *The impact of PCR and site-directed mutagenesis on medical practice*

The influence of PCR and site-directed mutagenesis on research has been far reaching and revolutionary, and its implications for medical practice are numerous (Fig. 12.5). Its most obvious benefit is the relative ease with which the precise genetic defect underlying an inherited disease can be defined. Before PCR, mapping of genetic variation or a defective gene relied on identification of restriction fragment length polymorphisms, that is, single nucleotide polymorphisms (SNPs) that changed a restriction enzyme site, and following their inheritance in families by Southern blotting. With the advent of PCR and high throughput genome sequencing, the number of known SNPs multiplied exponentially. This made fine mapping both quicker and more accurate, and permitted identification of the causal defect in numerous single gene disorders.[25] The clinical benefits of finding the cause of a single gene defect are clear: first, identification of the causal gene and pathway involved may lead to novel therapeutic approaches; second, carriers who may not yet have developed the phenotype can readily be identified and given preventative advice and treatment where feasible; and third, for serious early life-threatening disorders, prenatal or pre-implantation diagnosis is possible.[26] Gene replacement therapy becomes possible once the defect is known, but in most cases this remains beset by difficulties that have yet to be overcome.[27] Of course these genetic advances have raised new and serious ethical issues, but these are more than outweighed by the benefits.

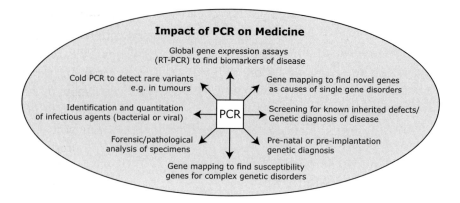

Fig. 12.5.   Diagram showing the impact of PCR on medicine.

Rapid analysis of genetic variation by PCR has also allowed genetic association studies to investigate the inheritance patterns of more complex genetic disorders such as coronary heart disease, diabetes, schizophrenia and obesity, where variation in several genes, each of which has a small effect, is believed to combine to contribute to an individual's risk. Association is sought between a particular phenotypic trait and a region of the genome, defined by the presence or absence of an SNP, either in candidate genes or in the currently fashionable genome-wide association studies (GWAS). Several such studies have now identified linkage of the phenotype to specific regions of the genome and in some cases to actual gene variants, although any clinical benefits are yet to be realised.[28] Nonetheless, the potential remains high for identifying new metabolic pathways as targets for therapy or that might trigger the onset of a chronic disease. Personalised medicine, where an individual's genotype could be used to predict whether or not they will benefit from a drug, or, perhaps more importantly, exhibit an adverse side effect to a drug that might be highly efficacious for others in the population with a different genotype remains high on the agenda for the pharmaceutical industry.[29]

PCR has made possible the rapid and accurate detection of a specific gene or organism in minute amounts of biological material, whether it be human tissue or fluid, a single cell from a developing embryo, a histological specimen preserved in wax or forensic samples. Quantitative RT-PCR, where mRNA is first copied with reverse transcriptase to produce cDNA that can be amplified by PCR, allows measurement of the expression of genes in such material. In purely practical terms, this has brought about unprecedented changes in the ability to analyse biological specimens, for example for the presence of infectious organisms. The need to grow the infectious agent and carry out detailed and time-consuming analysis of its biological properties has been replaced with a simple assay that can provide an accurate 'near-patient' result within hours or even minutes.[30] With the high sensitivity of PCR came the need for careful control of possible contamination and evaluation of the significance of detecting small amounts of the infectious agent, but the methods have been refined over the years to deal with these issues.[31] DNA fingerprinting,[32] where highly variable regions of the genome that are specific for a single individual are analysed, is dependent on PCR and has made possible dramatic advances in forensic medicine.

Another expanding clinical use of RT-PCR is the identification of biomarkers of human disease by gene expression profiling, although this is still in its infancy; a recent *Nature* editorial points out that the rapidly growing numbers of reported biomarkers all need careful evaluation before they can be applied in a clinical setting.[33] Nonetheless, some biomarkers have already been proven useful, for example two commercially available kits that measure expression of several genes in breast tumours can help to predict the likelihood of recurrence or whether the cancer is likely to respond to a particular treatment.[34, 35]

Site-directed mutagenesis has had less obvious practical impact on medicine, but the knowledge gained about the function of proteins from its use has been invaluable in unravelling the intricacies of metabolic and other signalling pathways during cell division, differentiation and development. Genetic variation can either affect the expression of a gene or the function of the protein that it encodes. Convincing evidence that a mutation affects function can only be obtained by site-directed mutagenesis to introduce the variant into the cloned gene, so that it can be expressed *in vitro* and the properties of the expressed variant protein determined.

12.4.2 *An example of how PCR and site-directed mutagenesis changed research into inherited disease*

Perhaps the best way to illustrate the impact of PCR and site-directed mutagenesis on research into inherited disease is with my own personal experience. My research focused on familial hypercholesterolaemia (FH), an inherited disorder of lipoprotein metabolism caused by defects in the function of the low density lipoprotein receptor, first identified by Joseph Goldstein and Michael Brown, themselves Nobel Prize winners.[36] In 1986 I was trying to identify the genetic defect in a homozygous FH patient whose cells in culture made an abnormal LDL receptor protein that had interesting properties and we were keen to know why (as were the editors of the journal in which we were trying to publish our findings). The only way forward was to make a cDNA library from the patient's mRNA and identify clones carrying fragments of the LDL receptor that could then be sequenced to identify the mutation: a lengthy and tedious procedure that did not guarantee success. In the nick of time, a young clinical colleague from another department (Tim Cox, now Professor of Medicine at Cambridge) reported at a work-in-progress meeting that he had just used 'PCR' to identify a mutation and I thought, if he can do that, then so can I.

Deciding it should be possible to amplify cDNA made by copying the patient's mRNA with reverse transcriptase, I unknowingly carried out one of the first RT-PCR reactions. I chose pairs of primers to amplify convenient overlapping 500 base pair fragments of the coding region, giving no thought to primer composition or secondary structure, nor to possible primer-dimer formation. It was an expensive venture, as both the primers and the enzyme were then very costly for a small lab. Heath Robinson would have admired the equipment we had available. It had, I believe, started life in the histology department as an automated means of fixing and staining histological slides, and comprised a series of three water baths, with a long mechanical arm that transferred between them, with much clunking, a rack of slides (or tubes). The excellent workshop at what was then the Royal Postgraduate Medical School had converted this into a PCR machine (and shortly thereafter designed and produced a beautiful custom-made machine). The original took up half a lab's worth of floor space and required almost 24 hours to complete a reaction. Its proud owners were reluctant to allow access to it, as it was already oversubscribed for their own work, but somehow I managed to persuade them to allow me to have a go, and my very first PCR reaction worked like a dream. Five bright bands were visible on the agarose gel: now all I had to do was to sequence them.

DNA sequencing then depended on producing single-stranded DNA as a template, and this could be achieved with phage M13. It had not occurred to me to put restriction enzyme sites in the primers, assuming they needed to be perfectly matched to the template, and thus planned to clone the products into M13 as blunt-ended fragments. Unaware then that Taq polymerase always added a few extra dAs (deoxyadenine nucleotides) at the end of each synthesis, leaving an overhang on the 3′ end, I was confounded by the inexplicable problems that M13 cloning posed. Eventually I obtained a few colonies from each fragment and sequenced them, manually of course, with radiolabelled dideoxy NTPs (nucleotide triphosphates) and on long ultrathin polyacrylamide gels that were a technical nightmare from start to finish. If you were lucky, you could read about 200 base pairs of sequence per gel, and with a short and a long run for each reaction, could extend the read to 300–350 per reaction. When I sequenced my few precious M13 clones, they all had at least one base pair change from the published sequence, but these variants were unique to each clone: clearly artefacts. This was caused by what became well known as the error rate of Taq polymerase. However, in one fragment, each of five clones had a single base pair substitution that was predicted to change an amino acid residue from proline to leucine: this was my 'Eureka' moment. The icing on the cake was that the base substitution introduced a new restriction enzyme site, making it possible to confirm the presence of the mutation in amplified genomic DNA from the patient and to screen other members of the patient's large family.[37] DNA-based diagnosis of FH was possible!

In this case it had not been difficult to deduce that the amino acid change — the only one detected in this patient, and a non-conservative substitution — was the cause of the disorder, but this was not always to be the case, at which point site-directed mutagenesis came into play. For the next point mutation we identified, we used an oligonucleotide containing the single base substitution to introduce a mutation into the cDNA for the LDL receptor and then expressed it or the normal cDNA in cultured cells that lacked normal LDL receptors. Assaying the expressed LDL receptor protein and its function enabled us to show without doubt that the mutation in the patient's DNA resulted in defective LDL receptor function.[38]

Today, with the constant improvements in PCR and sequencing, it is possible to find a new variant in the LDL receptor gene of a patient within just a few days. Proving it is definitely the cause of the disorder can still take time and is crucial for DNA-based diagnosis to be of clinical value, and with the projected expansion of high throughput sequencing of human genomes, determining the significance of genetic variation will become increasingly important. I have never met either Mullis or Smith, but am indebted and grateful to them both, as should be many others, for their contributions to molecular biology.

References

1. Nobelprize.org. The Nobel Prize in Chemistry 1993. Available at: http://nobelprize.org/nobel_prizes/chemistry/laureates/1993/index. html [Accessed 8 June 2011].
2. Nobelprize.org. Michael Smith — Nobel Lecture. Available at: http://nobelprize.org/nobel_prizes/chemistry/laureates/1993/smith-lecture.html [Accessed 8 June 2011].
3. Nobelprize.org. Michael Smith-Autobiography. Available at: http://nobelprize.org/nobel_prizes/chemistry/laureates/1993/smith. html [Accessed 8 June 2011].
4. Astell C. *No Ordinary Mike: Michael Smith, Nobel Laureate*. Vancouver: Ronsdale Press; 2004.
5. Smith M, Rammler DH, Goldberg IH *et al*. Studies on Polynucleotides. XIV.1 Specific Synthesis of the C3″-C5″ Interribonucleotide Linkage. Syntheses of Uridylyl-(3″→5″)-Uridine and Uridylyl-(3″→5″)-Adenosine. *J Am Chem Soc* 1962; 84: 430–440.

6. Nobelprize.org. Earl W. Sutherland, Jr. — Nobel Lecture. Available at: http://nobelprize.org/nobel_prizes/medicine/laureates/1971/suth erland-lecture.html [Accessed 8 June 2011].

7. Gillam S, Smith M. Enzymatic synthesis of deoxyribo-oligonucleotides of defined sequence. Properties of the enzyme. *Nucleic Acids Res* 1974; 1:1631–1647.

8. Gillam S, Rottman F, Jahnke P *et al.* Enzymatic synthesis of oligonu- cleotides of defined sequence: synthesis of a segment of yeast iso-1-cytochrome c gene. *Proc Natl Acad Sci USA* 1977; 74: 96–100.

9. Sanger F, Coulson AR, Friedmann T *et al.* The nucleotide sequence of bacteriophage phiX174. *J Mol Biol* 1978; 125: 225–246.

10. Nobelprize.org. The Nobel Prize in Chemistry 1980. Available at: http://nobelprize.org/nobel_prizes/chemistry/laureates/1980/index. html [Accessed 8 June 2011].

11. Hutchison CA 3rd, Phillips S, Edgell MH *et al.* Mutagenesis at a spe- cific position in a DNA sequence. *J Biol Chem* 1978; 253: 6551–6560.

12. Montgomery DL, Hall BD, Gillam S *et al.* Identification and isolation of the yeast cytochrome c gene. *Cell* 1978; 14: 673–680.

13. Pielak GJ, Mauk AG, Smith M. Site-directed mutagenesis of cytochrome c shows that an invariant Phe is not essential for function. *Nature* 1985; 313: 152–154.

14. Nobelprize.org. Kary B. Mullis — Autobiography. Available at: http://nobelprize.org/nobel_prizes/chemistry/laureates/1993/mullis .html [Accessed 8 June 2011].

15. Mullis KB. *Dancing Naked in the Mind Field*. New York: Pantheon Books; 1998.

16 Mullis KB. Cosmological Significance of Time Reversal. *Nature* 1968; 218: 663–664.

17. Nobelprize.org. Kary B. Mullis — Nobel Lecture. Available at: http://nobelprize.org/nobel_prizes/chemistry/laureates/1993/mullis- lecture.html [Accessed 8 June 2011].

18. Wade N. Scientist at Work/Kary Mullis; After the 'Eureka,' a Nobelist Drops Out. Available at: http://www.nytimes.com/1998/09/15/ science/scientist-at-work-kary-mullis-after-the-eureka-a-nobelist- drops-out.html?scp=2&sq=mullis&st=nyt [Accessed 8 June 2011].

19. Fore J Jr., Wiechers IR, Cook-Deegan R. The effects of business practices, licensing, and intellectual property on development and dissemination of the polymerase chain reaction: case study. *J Biomed Discov Collab* 2006; 1: 7.

20. Saiki RK, Scharf S, Faloona F *et al*. Enzymatic amplification of beta-globin genomic sequences and restriction site analysis for diagnosis of sickle cell anemia. *Science* 1985; 230: 1350–1354.

21. Mullis KB, Faloona FA. Recombinant DNA Part F: Specific Synthesis of DNA *in vitro* via a Polymerase-Catalyzed Chain Reaction. In: *Methods in Enzymology*, Vol. 155, Wu R (ed.). New York: Academic Press Inc.; 1987: 335–350.

22. Saiki RK, Gelfand DH, Stoffel S *et al*. Primer-directed enzymatic amplification of DNA with a thermostable DNA polymerase. *Science* 1988; 239: 487–491.

23. Dr Kary Banks Mullis: personal website. Available at: http://www.karymullis.com/ [Accessed 8 June 2011].

24. Martin JF. Bad Example. *Nature* 1994; 371: 97.

25. Peltonen L, McKusick VA. Genomics and medicine. Dissecting human disease in the postgenomic era. *Science* 2001; 291: 1224–1229.

26. Handyside AH. Preimplantation genetic diagnosis after 20 years. *Reprod Biomed Online* 2010; 21: 280–282.

27. Human genome Project Information: Gene Therapy. Available at: http://www.ornl.gov/sci/techresources/Human_Genome/medicine/genetherapy.shtml#status [Accessed 8 June 2011].

28. Ku CS, Loy EY, Pawitan Y *et al*. The pursuit of genome-wide association studies: where are we now? *J Hum Genet* 2010; 55: 195–206.

29. Hamburg MA, Collins FS. The path to personalized medicine. *N Engl J Med* 2010; 363: 301–304.

30. Belgrader P, Benett W, Hadley D *et al*. PCR detection of bacteria in seven minutes. *Science* 1999; 284: 449–450.

31. Mothershed EA, Whitney AM. Nucleic acid-based methods for the detection of bacterial pathogens: present and future considerations for the clinical laboratory. *Clin Chim Acta* 2006; 363: 206–220.

32. Jeffreys AJ. Genetic fingerprinting. *Nat Med* 2005; 11: 1035–1039.

33. Editorial. Valid concerns. *Nature* 2010; 463: 401–402.

34. Buyse M, Loi S, van't Veer L *et al.* Validation and clinical utility of a 70-gene prognostic signature for women with node-negative breast cancer. *J Natl Cancer Inst* 2006; 8: 1183–1192.

35. Cobleigh MA, Tabesh B, Bitterman P *et al.* Tumor gene expression and prognosis in breast cancer patients with 10 or more positive lymph nodes. *Clin Cancer Res* 2005; 11: 8623–8631.

36. Nobelprize.org. The Nobel Prize in Physiology or Medicine 1985. Available at: http://nobelprize.org/nobel_prizes/medicine/laureates/1985/ [Accessed 8 June 2011].

37. Soutar AK, Knight BL, Patel DD. Identification of a point mutation in growth factor repeat C of the low density lipoprotein-receptor gene in a patient with homozygous familial hypercholesterolemia that affects ligand binding and intracellular movement of receptors. *Proc Natl Acad Sci USA* 1989; 86: 4166–4170.

38. Webb JC, Sun XM, Patel DD *et al.* Characterization of two new point mutations in the low density lipoprotein receptor genes of an English patient with homozygous familial hypercholesterolemia. *J Lipid Res* 1992; 33: 689–698.

Chapter 13

THE DISCOVERY OF THE PATHOPHYSIOLOGICAL ROLE OF NITRIC OXIDE IN BLOOD VESSELS

Keith M. Channon

13.1 Introduction

The Nobel Prize in Physiology or Medicine was awarded in 1998 to Robert F. Furchgott, Louis J. Iganarro and Ferid Murad, 'for their discoveries concerning nitric oxide as a signalling molecule in the cardiovascular system'. In his presentation speech at the Karolinska Institute, on 10 December 1998, Professor Sten Lindahl of the Nobel Committee described the discovery of 'a short-lived gas, nitric oxide, NO, that was endogenously produced and acted as a signalling molecule between cells' as 'unexpected and unique. It initiated a new chapter in biomedical research.' The award of the Nobel Prize recognised the independent work by each of the prize winners over the preceding 30 years. Each part was a necessary component of the discovery that finally crystallised in the mid-1980s: Furchgott's identification of the obligate role of a factor derived from the endothelium in the relaxation of blood vessels; Murad's characterisation of guanylate cyclase and the second messenger cGMP (cyclic guanosine monophosphate); and Ignarro's linking of the chemistry of guanylate cyclase activation to nitric oxide. The discovery of nitric oxide as a signalling molecule has fundamentally altered our understanding of pathophysiology not only in cardiovascular disease, but in areas as diverse as neuroscience, reproductive medicine, infection and inflammation.

13.2 Biographical Backgrounds of the Laureates

13.2.1 *Robert Furchgott*

Robert F. Furchgott was born in 1916 in Charleston, South Carolina, and grew up during the years of the Depression. After high school he went initially to the University of South Carolina, but after the family moved he was able to transfer to the University of North Carolina at Chapel Hill, where he graduated in chemistry. He moved to Northwestern University in Chicago as a graduate student in 1937, where he gained his PhD in 1940 for work on serum albumin and the chemistry of erythrocyte membranes. He secured a postdoctoral position with Dr Ephraim Shorr, Associate Professor of Medicine at Cornell University Medical School in New York City, and during the early years of the Second World War worked on putative circulating factors relating to haemorrhagic shock. He published his first papers in 1943 and then in 1945 described the characteristics of 'vasoexcitatory' and 'vasodepressor' factors that were released in response to ischaemia.[1] These experiments were portentous of Furchgott's future work, and led to him developing *in vitro* bioassays for vasoactive factors using strips of smooth muscle, such as helically-cut rabbit aorta, that would assume iconic importance more than 30 years later.

In 1949 Furchgott moved from New York to take up an Assistant Professorship in Pharmacology at Washington University in St Louis. Here, he built on his work with isolated rabbit aortic strip preparations with his technician Marilyn (Wales) McCaman, who later became his first graduate student. In 1953, Furchgott published a paper entitled 'Reactions of strips of rabbit aorta to epinephrine, isoproterenol, sodium nitrite and other drugs', which reported the observation that acetylcholine produced only contractions, whereas acetylcholine was known to be a very potent vasodilator *in vivo*.[2] As Furchgott later admitted, 'Little did I suspect then what I was able to show many years later — namely, that relaxation of arteries by acetylcholine is strictly endothelium-dependent, and that my method of preparing the strips inadvertently resulted in the mechanical removal of all the endothelial cells.' Furchgott moved again in 1956 to become Chairman of the new Department of Pharmacology at the

State University of New York (SUNY) College of Medicine in Brooklyn. There, he built an expanding department and pursued research in quite broad areas, for example in photorelaxation of blood vessels, receptor theory and adrenergic receptor mechanisms. In 1978, Furchgott began testing the relative effects of adrenergic Beta$_1$ vs. Beta$_2$ adrenergic responses in the isolated rabbit aorta preparation that he had used for over 30 years. In an accidental finding due to a technician's error, the muscarinic agents acetylcholine and carbachol induced relaxation rather than the expected contraction, following their inadvertent administration without washing out a previous nora-drenaline constriction. Why this effect had been previously missed for many years turned out to be related to the newer method of using aortic rings rather than strips — which results in preservation rather than loss of the endothelial cell layer. Work in Furchgott's lab using rubbed or collagenase-treated rings or strips quickly established that the endothelial cells were an obligate requirement for the relaxation response to acetylcholine, observations that were published in *Nature* in 1980[3] (Fig. 13.1). There followed more sophisticated 'sandwich'

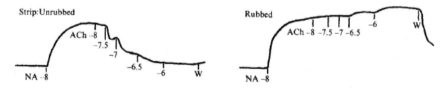

Fig. 13.1. The first demonstration of endothelium-dependent relaxation of vascular smooth muscle.

Tension recordings were made from strips of rabbit aorta which were suspended in organ chambers in physiological buffer, and constricted with noradrenaline (NA, 10^{-8} M). After approximately five minutes of stable constriction, exposure to increasing concentrations of acetylcholine (ACh, 10^{-8} M to 10^{-6} M) resulted in progressive relaxation of the constricted ring, but this response was abolished in parallel rings in which the endothelium had been gently rubbed off, although relaxation still occurred rapidly after washing with fresh buffer (W). Similar results were obtained in experiments where endothelium was removed by collagenase digestion. The presence or absence of endothelium was evaluated by silver staining on *en face* vessel preparations. From Furchgott and Zawadzki (ref. 3). (Reprinted with permission from Macmillan Publishers Ltd: *Nature* 288: 373–376, © 1980).

experiments that combined aortic strips or rings with or without endothelium, and characterisation of responses to other agonists, such as bradykinin, led to the concept of the 'endothelium-derived relaxing factor', a term coined in 1982.[4] Whilst Furchgott acknowledged that others had previously reported that intact vessel preparations could relax in response to muscarinic stimulation[5] none had made the key connection with the obligate role of the endothelium. It was Furchgott's critical contribution to identifying and characterising the fundamental phenomenon of endothelium-dependent relaxation that led him and others to focus on the underlying mechanisms — both upstream to identify the mediator derived from endothelial cells, and downstream to identify the pathways mediating relaxation in vascular smooth muscle cells.

13.2.2 *Ferid Murad*

Ferid Murad was born in 1936, the son of an Albanian immigrant. He grew up in Indiana, working long hours as a child in the family's restaurant business, but his intellectual ability also enabled him to excel at grade school and high school. He was awarded a Rector Scholarship at DePauw University in Greencastle, Indiana, where he was a pre-med and chemistry major. He went on to enter the newly-established MD-PhD program at Western Reserve University in 1958. Murad immersed himself in the pharmacology research programme under the supervision of Earl Sutherland and Theodore Rall, investigating how multiple hormones including catecholamines, cholinergics, ACTH, vasopressin, etc. could increase or decrease adenylyl cyclase activity and cyclic AMP formation. In doing so, Murad developed a focus on the second messenger cGMP, facilitated by his move to the University of Virginia in Charlottesville in 1970, where he isolated and characterised the soluble and particulate forms of the cGMP synthetic enzyme, guanylate cyclase. Whereas much of Murad's work was focused on how other receptor-mediated agonists led to increased cGMP levels, the potential link with nitric oxide came through his observations on the association between 'nitrovasodilators' and cGMP. In particular, he showed how both inorganic nitrates (such as sodium azide) and organic nitrates (such as glyceryl trinitrate) led to parallel changes in cGMP and smooth muscle relaxation. He hypothesised that the chemical activator of cGMP synthesis by guanylate cyclase might be nitric oxide. In December 1976, postdocs Shuji Katsuki and William Arnold chemically generated nitric oxide gas and bubbled it through a guanylate cyclase preparation, observing an immediate and striking increase in cGMP formation. These experiments led to the key paper from Murad's laboratory, published in 1977[6] describing how 'nitric oxide activates guanylate cyclase and increases cGMP levels in various tissue preparations', thus providing one of the key links between endothelium, nitric oxide and vasorelaxation.

13.2.3 *Louis Ignarro*

Louis J. Ignarro was born in 1941, the first of two sons to parents who had emigrated from Italy in the 1920s. Ignarro grew up and went through high school in Long Island, New York, before going to Columbia University, graduating in chemistry and pharmacy in 1962. From New York he moved to a graduate programme in pharmacology at the University of Minnesota, where he developed an interest in cardiovascular pharmacology and enzymology, being taught by Paul Boyer who went on to win the Nobel Prize in Chemistry in 1997. He worked hard to achieve his PhD, and published the data from his thesis in four back-to-back papers in the *Journal of Pharmacology and Experimental Therapeutics* — a feat that Ignarro admits to not coming close to achieving again. From Minnesota, he moved to a postdoctoral position at the National Heart, Lung and Blood Institute (NIH) in the laboratory of Elwood Titus, where he studied beta adrenoceptor chemistry. Progress was slower and more difficult than during his PhD studies. Although the NIH provided a stimulating academic environment, in 1968 Ignarro took up an offer from Geigy Pharamceuticals to head a research group that contributed to the development of the non-steroidal anti-inflammatory drug, diclofenac. During his time at Geigy, his continued work in chemistry and pharmacology led to an interest in the newly described nucleotide cGMP. When Geigy merged with Ciba Pharmaceuticals, Ignarro decided to move back to academic research, taking a position as Assistant Professor of Pharmacology at Tulane University School of Medicine in New Orleans in 1973. It was here that his interest in cGMP flourished, initially in the heart and inflammatory cells, but later in blood vessels. Influenced by Murad's work on cGMP,[6] Ignarro set out to test whether nitric oxide might be the factor that induced vasorelaxation by increasing cGMP in vascular smooth muscle cells. In analogous experiments to those conducted by Murad's group testing the direct effects of nitric oxide gas on cGMP formation, Ignarro bubbled nitric oxide gas through an organ chamber preparation of constricted bovine coronary artery and observed striking vasorelaxation. The effect was inhibited by free haemoglobin (a known scavenger of nitric oxide), and by methylene blue (an inhibitor of guanylate cyclase). Published in 1979, these observations provided another key link that implicated nitric oxide as the vasorelaxant activator of guanylate cyclase.[7] Further work by Ignarro's group tested the role of nitric oxide in platelet aggregation, an effect also found to involve cGMP, but then turned to address in more detail how nitrovasodilators generate nitric oxide, and how nitric oxide could activate guanylate cyclase and lead to vasorelaxation. These studies identified the importance of thiol groups, and nitrosothiol formation, in the biological actions of nitric oxide — an early indication of the pleitropic signalling actions of nitric oxide, beyond cGMP formation, that would be appreciated much more in future. Mike Wolin, a postdoctoral researcher in the laboratory, identified that heme iron, bound to guanylate cyclase, was the target for enzymatic activation by nitric oxide,[8] thus completing the links between nitric oxide, guanylate cyclase, cGMP and vasorelaxation that had been forged by the Murad and Ignarro groups.

13.3 Identification of Endothelium-Derived Relaxing Factor

By 1982, many of these mechanistic studies on the 'downstream' pharmacology of nitric oxide, explaining the mechanism of action of vasodilator drugs, had been completed and published. But the focus remained on pharmacology rather than physiology — the 'upstream' question of how nitric oxide could be relevant to physiological activation of guanylate cyclase remained uncertain, because the chemistry of nitric oxide, a reactive gas discovered by Joseph Priestly in 1772, was not imagined to have direct biological relevance. Indeed, the presumption that the effects of nitric oxide were an unexpected pharmacological action of a gas usually associated with toxic effects of pollutants seemed to fundamentally influence the interpretation of experimental data — as evidenced by Ignarro's paper on 'Coronary arterial relaxation by cigarette smoke, nitrosonornicotine and nitric oxide', published in 1980.[9] As a consequence, the focus was on how other nitric oxide-like mediators might be the physiological activators of gualylate cyclase. Indeed, more than seven years passed between the publications describing endothelium-dependent relaxation, the ability of nitric oxide to relax vascular smooth muscle and activate guanylate cyclase, and the papers finally ascribing the 'endothelium-derived relaxing factor' (EDRF) to release of endogenous nitric oxide. During this time, there continued a vigorous level of activity and debate. Furchgott, through successive studies published from 1980 to 1984 with Peter D. Cherry, John V. Zawadzki and Desingarao Jothianandan, rapidly characterised the various agonists and receptors that could elicit relaxation in arteries from different species and vascular territories, and established that the elusive EDRF was not an arachidonic acid metabolite, as they had originally hypothesised.[4] Furthermore, they established that EDRF action was mediated by cGMP, and inhibited by free haemoglobin and by methylene blue, 'suggesting...that EDRF is a labile free radical'.[10] In 1980–1981, Ignarro's focus remained on elucidating how nitrovasodilators released nitric oxide in tissues and led to vasodilatation. Nitroglycerine required cysteine to activate guanylate cyclase, whereas nitrite required thiols, leading to the identification of S-nitrosothiols as NO intermediates and NO donors. In the Murad lab there was a similar focus, with a presumption that nitric oxide, even if it might be an endogenous nitrovasodilator, would presumably have to be generated from some other intermediate nitro compound or compounds. A more direct potential link between Furchgott and Murad on endothelium-dependent relaxation and nitric oxide/cGMP, following a visit and seminar by Furchgott at the University of Virginia in 1980, did not progress because Murad's group moved to Stanford in 1981. However, Michael Peach visited in 1982, and with Robert Rapoport, a new research fellow in the Murad lab, there developed a more direct interest in EDRF. Rapoport published five papers during 1983, including one in *Nature*,[11] establishing that EDRF, and the various agonists responsible for its production, were inextricably linked with activation of smooth muscle cGMP formation. By 1983, work in the Ignarro lab had also turned to study endothelium-dependent relaxation, although, like Murad, the focus was more on the generation of cGMP as the mediator of vasorelaxation, rather than the possibility that EDRF might be nitric oxide. However, by 1984, Ignarro had observed that inhibition of guanylate cyclase with methylene blue also inhibited vasorelaxation elicited by acetylcholine, and noted the similarity with the vasorelaxation and cGMP formation elicted by nitric oxide gas.[12] From 1984 to 1986, the Ignarro lab turned in earnest to testing whether EDRF might be nitric oxide, using the direct approach of analyzing the 'effluent' from vessel rings stimulated with acetylcholine or bradykinin.[13] The activation of guanylate cyclase by these vascular rings was dependent upon exactly the same stimuli and characteristics as the EDRF response, and in particular the requirement for heme iron in guanylate cyclase, a characteristic of nitric oxide mediated activation of the enzyme.

During this period, others in the burgeoning field of EDRF made major contributions. In England, Salvador Moncada's group, working in the Wellcome Research Laboratories in Kent, had become interested in EDRF through their discovery of thromboxane synthase and prostacyclin, another potent vasodilator. In contrast to the experiments with vascular strips or rings pursued by Furchgott and Ignarro, Moncada developed the novel and innovative approach of cultured porcine endothelial cells on microbeads, and applied the effluent from the cells to 'reporter' rings of vascular tissue.[14] Richard Gryglewski, working in Moncada's group, used this system to make a number of key observations: that EDRF had a short half-life (seven seconds); that EDRF was rapidly inactivated by superoxide radicals (challenging and clarifying many of the prior presumptions about EDRF 'inhibitors');[15] and that EDRF shared many of the other pharmaco-logical properties of nitric oxide identified by Murad and Ignarro. Although Moncada's group were latecomers to the EDRF-cGMP field, only publishing their first papers in 1986, they made rapid progress. Richard Palmer used the Moncada group's endothelial cell system to recapitulate the effects of EDRF with authentic nitric oxide gas, just as Ignarro's and Murad's groups had done with guanylate cyclase. Furthermore, Palmer made the huge advance of establishing the first assay of nitric oxide that could be used to quantify nitric oxide in biological systems, by measurement of the chemilumines-cence generated by the reaction of nitric oxide with ozone,[16] a technique that remains in widespread use today, 25 years later.

In early 1986 the frenetic activity focused on solving the identity of EDRF came to a head. Ignarro, using the heme iron 'reporter' of guanylate cyclase, an absolute requirement for EDRF action, had shown that the spectral shift caused by formation of the nitrosyl-heme adduct was identical for nitric oxide as it was for EDRF,[17] and now felt sufficiently confident to propose, at a conference at the Mayo Clinic in June 1986 (the IV International Symposium on the Mechanisms of Vasodilatation), that EDRF was nitric oxide. At the same meeting, Furchgott independently reported his own identical conclusion. Whilst the Mayo conference was the first public statement of the new discovery, it was clear that several groups had reached the same conclusion at very much the same time. In the following months, a flurry of papers formally reported the key experiments. In these papers, it was Palmer and Moncada who, in June 1987, first titled their definitive *Nature* paper, 'Nitric oxide release accounts for the biological actions of EDRF',[16] and by December 1987 Ignarro's subsequent *PNAS* paper declared confidently that, 'Endothelium-derived relaxing factor produced and released from artery and vein is nitric oxide'.[18] The key finding that was to produce unprecedented cascades of new discoveries and a Nobel Prize within 12 years, had at last been made. The Mayo conference proceedings gave Furchgott and Ignarro the principal recognition for the final push that identified EDRF as nitric oxide, whereas Murad's work made a less overt contribution. Nevertheless, it was the sustained and systematic studies contributed by Furchgott, Murad and Ignarro over many years that were the justification for their particular recognition in the award of the Nobel Prize — even though the route, through detailed and at times distracting studies on cGMP biochemistry, was perhaps more circuitous than it might have been. Moncada's group was not recognised by the Nobel committee, despite publishing the first formal paper identifying EDRF as nitric oxide. Moncada's contributions might have been judged as too late in the long process of discovery — it is noteworthy that Moncada's first ever paper on EDRF was not published until April 1986, just two months before Furchgott and Ignarro proposed the identity of EDRF at the Mayo Clinic conference. Moncada's more long-standing and major contributions, since the early 1970s, had been in the field of prostaglandin research with Sir John Vane, himself a Nobel Prize winner in 1982; this had equipped Moncada with a strong portfolio of techniques and models to study vascular responses mediated by the endothelium. Moncada's first paper on EDRF described the endothelial cell bioassay system, but in the context of differentiating the EDRF response from that of prostacyclin.[14]

13.4 Physiological Significance of Nitric Oxide

The announcement of the identity of EDRF as nitric oxide by Furchgott, Ignarro and Moncada sparked a growing wave of new interest and activity that was driven ever larger and wider as new groups joined in to add to the initial discovery. The long-held presumption that nitric oxide could never be an endogenously-produced signalling molecule was rapidly replaced with a search for the cellular sources of nitric oxide. As early as 1982 Takeo Deguchi had reported that L-arginine activated guanylate cyclase in crude tissue lysates.[19] John B. Hibbs showed in 1987 that nitrite accumulation in macrophage conditioned medium was increased by L-arginine, but inhibited by L-arginine analogues such as N-methyl-L-arginine.[20] The synthesis of nitric oxide from L-arginine was confirmed rapidly in reports from Marletta's laboratory in 1987[21] and from Palmer & Moncada, published in *Nature* in 1988.[22] An avalanche of papers quickly identified and characterised the enzymes responsible for the generation of nitric oxide from L-arginine. By 1990 David Bredt and Solomon Snyder had characterised the first nitric oxide synthase enzyme, NOS1, from neuronal tissue.[23] This was followed by NOS2 from inflammatory cells and finally NOS3 from endothelial cells,[24] the latter by Murad's laboratory, who, having arguably missed out on the excitement generated by Furchgott and Ignarro in 1986, now once more made major contributions. The NOS enzymes turned out to be complex homodimeric oxidoreductases that oxidise the guanidine nitrogen of L-arginine, using molecular oxygen and NADPH, with novel enzymatic mechanisms, including activation by calcium-calmodulin, a heme-containing active site, a flavin domain with homology to the P450 oxidoreductases and a requirement for the cofactor tetrahydrobiopterin. Each of the three NOS enzymes were encoded by different genes that were cloned in the next few years. The NOS genes were early and notable genes to be knocked out in mouse models, beginning with NOS1 in 1993[25] and rapidly followed by NOS3 and NOS2, then double knockouts, mice with transgenic NOS overexpression and multiple disease models that placed nitric oxide at the centre of fundamental processes such as neurotransmission, memory and behaviour, neuronal injury and ischaemia, blood pressure regulation, vascular disease, inflammation and infection, host immunity and septic shock.

In 1992, the cover of *Science* proclaimed NO as the molecule of the year, perhaps reflecting the exuberance and confidence of the era, despite it being little more than five years since the discovery of nitric oxide. Nevertheless, the call made by *Science* in its accolade has stood the test of time, and not just in the award of the Nobel Prize, six years later. Few if any individual signalling molecules have achieved and maintained the profile, importance and continued scientific novelty of nitric oxide. Since the early papers published in *Nature*, new discoveries have continued unabated for 30 years, with new *Nature* papers reporting novel aspects of endothelial nitric oxide biology, right up to the present day. Within 5 years of the discovery of nitric oxide, more than 1,000 papers were being published per year, and this rose inexorably to around 6,000 publications per year by 1999, a rate that has been maintained since. The 'longitudinal' persistence of nitric oxide research with time has been accompanied by an unprecedented 'lateral' expansion, originating in the vascular endothelium that has permeated all branches of molecular and cellular biology, chemistry and biomedical sciences. During this period, the NO field has generated authors, publications and impact that rank in the very highest level in the medical sciences. Robert Furchgott's papers have been cited more than 25,000 times, with 8,700 citations of his classic *Nature* paper with John Zawadski. Louis Ignarro's publications have been cited 32,000 times (h-index 86); his 1987 *PNAS* paper identifying EDRF as NO has been cited more than 3,000 times. Ferid Murad's papers have attracted more than 28,000 citations, and other EDRF 'greats' have also made massive contributions to the literature. Although he was not one of the Nobel Laureates, Salvador Moncada's papers are amongst the most notable in the NO-EDRF field — his 1987 *Nature* paper identifying EDRF as NO has been cited more than 8,000 times, more than 20-fold more frequently than Ignarro's and his 1991 *Pharmacological Reviews* paper has been cited more than 12,000 times, making it one of the most highly cited scientific papers. Indeed, Moncada has 20 papers, each cited 1,000 times or more each, with an h-index of 155. The 'family tree' of scientists that has issued from the laboratories that pioneered EDRF research in the 1980s is now in its third generation, and includes within its prolific pedigree many leading names in the biomedical sciences that have gone on to populate every branch of science and medicine, across the globe.

13.5 Therapeutic Consequences of the Discovery of the Role of Nitric Oxide

How has the discovery of nitric oxide influenced biomedical sciences? In almost every way possible. Nitric oxide introduced an entirely new signalling paradigm, an endogenously-produced free radical gas that interacts with heme iron to alter the function of target enzymes. But even after this initial novelty had been appreciated, other more widely-applicable nitric oxide-mediated signalling modes were discovered, through S-nitrosylation, interaction with reactive oxygen species and nitration, in fundamental roles such as gene expression, post-translational regulation of numerous proteins and the function of the mitochondrial respiratory chain. The biology of the nitric oxide synthases has revealed new aspects of gene regulation, molecular and cellular biology and enzymology — both mechanism and regulation. For example, nitric oxide synthase regulation by serine and threonine phosphorylation, cofactor and substrate interactions, subcellular trafficking, protein–protein interactions, endogenous L-arginine inhibitors and the duality of nitric oxide vs. superoxide production ('nitric oxide synthase uncoupling'), mediated by tetrahydrobiopterin, that further widens the signalling repertoire, each have fundamental pathophysiological importance. The cellular physiological ramifications of the discovery of nitric oxide have been legion. In the circulation, nitric oxide has pivotal roles in oxygen delivery by haemoglobin, oxygen sensing and ischaemia, blood flow and angiogenesis and cardiac function. The solving of the identity of EDRF ushered in a new and vibrant era of research into the importance of the endothelium, rapidly promoted from a largely overlooked cellular lining of the blood vessel. Through studies on nitric oxide, we now understand the endothelium's critical roles in blood pressure and blood flow regulation, mechanotransduction, inflammation, thrombosis and vascular disease pathogenesis, leading to the concept of endothelial dysfunction and the validation of the endothelium itself as a primary therapeutic target. Indeed, the concept of endothelial dysfunction was key to the wider appreciation of the importance of cardiovascular risk factors as diverse as smoking, cholesterol, diabetes and hypertension.

Clinically, the potential of nitric oxide as a therapeutic target in human disease has yet to be fully realised. The massive impact of the discovery of nitric oxide has remained principally in the fields of physiology and pharmacology, rather than in clinical medicine. The discovery of nitric oxide has not yet yielded a therapeutic equivalent to monoclonal antibodies, or aspirin, or statins — although, characteristically, nitric oxide's ubiquitous roles permeate even these diverse fields. For example, the 'pleiotropic' effects of statins on the vascular wall are, in part, mediated by increased nitric oxide production. The role of nitric oxide as a signalling molecule in the vascular wall led to

understanding of the mechanism of action of nitrate-based vasodilator drugs, and later to tolerance to organic nitrates. These drugs, in
use since the 1870s as a treatment for angina, were notably used by
Alfred Nobel himself, and remain in widespread use today, but not
because of the Nobel status of nitric oxide.

The most significant therapeutic success from the discovery of nitric
oxide is the development of phosphodiesterase (PDE) inhibitors,
notably the PDE5 inhibitor sildenafil, launched as Viagra by Pfizer in
1998. Of the nitric oxide Nobel Laureates, it was Ignarro who, in the
late 1980s, worked on the relaxation of smooth muscle in the corpus
caversonum, responsible for penile erection. Using techniques borrowed
from the EDRF experiments of earlier years, Iganarro showed in strips
of corpus cavernosum smooth muscle that nitric oxide was released from
the non-adrenergic non-cholinergic (NANC) nerve fibres, leading to
cGMP formation and vasorelaxation.[26] The characteristics of the
response ultimately revealed a parallel pathway for nitric oxide released
from the NANC nerve fibres as that released from endothelial cells.
Ignarro had identified that phosphodiesterase inhibitors were effective in
augmenting cGMP in cavernosal smooth muscle, making it a promising
treatment for erectile dysfunction, findings published in the *New
England Journal of Medicine* in 1992.[27] The development of sildenafil, a
selective phosphodiesterase type 5 (PDE5) inhibitor, originally developed as a possible treatment for hypertension or angina, owed its
effectiveness as a treatment for erectile dysfunction to the fact that PDE5
was the abundant PDE in cavernosal smooth muscle. In the past 10
years Viagra has become a global blockbuster with annual sales of more
than $1 billion. The PDE5 isoform is also abundant in the pulmonary
vasculature, so sildenafil has also proved useful as a treatment for pulmonary arterial hypertension. Thus, the discovery of the nitric oxide
pathway, and perhaps Ignarro's work in particular, has led to major therapeutic advances. However, apart from sildenafil, the therapeutic
application of the vast knowledge arising from the discovery of nitric
oxide has been very limited. Attempts to target vascular nitric oxide production in the treatment of conditions such as septic shock, hypertension
and vascular disease have all been unsuccessful. In part, these failures
reflect the enthusiasm to test therapeutic potential using drugs with

limited specificity, such as non-specific nitric oxide synthase inhibitors or nitric oxide donors, in disease states where the pathophysiological role of nitric oxide remains poorly understood, even today. Has the recognition of the discovery of nitric oxide been a Nobel Prize that changed medicine? Undoubtedly yes, even thus far. But the continued new understanding of the protean mechanisms, whereby nitric oxide regulates cell signalling and metabolism, promises to deliver, in the future, many more 'new avenues for patient treatment and diagnoses of various diseases', as predicted by Lindahl in Stockholm in 1988.

References

1. Shorr E, Zweifach BW, Furchgott RF. On the occurrence, sites and modes of origin and destruction, of principles affecting the compensatory vascular mechanisms in experimental shock. *Science* 1945; 102: 489–498.

2. Furchgott RF, Bhadrakom S. Reactions of strips of rabbit aorta to epinephrine, isopropylarterenol, sodium nitrite and other drugs. *J Pharmacol Exp Ther* 1953; 108: 129–143.

3. Furchgott RF, Zawadzki JV. The obligatory role of endothelial cells in the relaxation of arterial smooth muscle by acetylcholine. *Nature* 1980; 288: 373–376.

4. Cherry PD, Furchgott RF, Zawadzki JV *et al.* Role of endothelial cells in relaxation of isolated arteries by bradykinin. *Proc Natl Acad Sci USA* 1982; 79: 2106–2110.

5. Jelliffe RW. Dilator and constrictor effects of acetylcholine on isolated rabbit aortic chains. *J Pharmacol Exp Ther* 1962; 135: 349–353.

6. Arnold WP, Mittal CK, Katsuki S *et al.* Nitric oxide activates guanylate cyclase and increases guanosine 3':5'-cyclic monophosphate levels in various tissue preparations. *Proc Natl Acad Sci USA* 1977; 74: 3203–3207.

7. Ohlstein EH, Barry BK, Gruetter DY *et al.* Methemoglobin blockade of coronary arterial soluble guanylate cyclase activation by nitroso compounds and its reversal with dithiothreitol. *FEBS Lett* 1979; 102: 316–320.

8. Wolin MS, Wood KS, Ignarro LJ. Guanylate cyclase from bovine lung. A kinetic analysis of the regulation of the purified soluble enzyme by

protoporphyrin IX, heme, and nitrosyl-heme. *J Biol Chem* 1982; 257: 13312–13320.

9. Gruetter CA, Barry BK, McNamara DB *et al*. Coronary arterial relaxation and guanylate cyclase activation by cigarette smoke, N'-nitrosonornicotine and nitric oxide. *J Pharmacol Exp Ther* 1980; 214: 9–15.

10. Furchgott RF, Cherry PD, Zawadzki JV *et al*. Endothelial cells as mediators of vasodilation of arteries. *J Cardiovasc Pharmacol* 1984; 6 Suppl 2: S336–343.

11. Rapoport RM, Draznin MB, Murad F. Endothelium-dependent relaxation in rat aorta may be mediated through cyclic GMP-dependent protein phosphorylation. *Nature* 1983; 306: 174–176.

12. Ignarro LJ, Burke TM, Wood KS *et al*. Association between cyclic GMP accumulation and acetylcholine-elicited relaxation of bovine intrapulmonary artery. *J Pharmacol Exp Ther* 1984; 228: 682–690.

13. Ignarro LJ, Harbison RG, Wood KS *et al*. Activation of purified soluble guanylate cyclase by endothelium-derived relaxing factor from intrapulmonary artery and vein: stimulation by acetylcholine, bradykinin and arachidonic acid. *J Pharmacol Exp Ther* 1986; 237: 893–900.

14. Gryglewski RJ, Moncada S, Palmer RM. Bioassay of prostacyclin and endothelium-derived relaxing factor (EDRF) from porcine aortic endothelial cells. *Br J Pharmacol* 1986; 87: 685–694.

15. Gryglewski RJ, Palmer RM, Moncada S. Superoxide anion is involved in the breakdown of endothelium-derived vascular relaxing factor. *Nature* 1986; 320: 454–456.

16. Palmer RM, Ferrige AG, Moncada S. Nitric oxide release accounts for the biological activity of endothelium-derived relaxing factor. *Nature* 1987; 327: 524–526.

17. Ignarro LJ, Byrns RE, Buga GM *et al*. Endothelium-derived relaxing factor from pulmonary artery and vein possesses pharmacologic and chemical properties identical to those of nitric oxide radical. *Circ Res* 1987; 61: 866–879.

18. Ignarro LJ, Buga GM, Wood KS *et al*. Endothelium-derived relaxing factor produced and released from artery and vein is nitric oxide. *Proc Natl Acad Sci USA* 1987; 84: 9265–9269.

19. Deguchi T, Yoshioka M. L-Arginine identified as an endogenous activator for soluble guanylate cyclase from neuroblastoma cells. *J Biol Chem* 1982; 257: 10147–10151.

20. Hibbs JB, Jr., Vavrin Z, Taintor RR. L-arginine is required for expression of the activated macrophage effector mechanism causing selective metabolic inhibition in target cells. *J Immunol* 1987; 138: 550–565.

21. Iyengar R, Stuehr DJ, Marletta MA. Macrophage synthesis of nitrite, nitrate, and N-nitrosamines: precursors and role of the respiratory burst. *Proc Natl Acad Sci USA* 1987; 84: 6369–6373.

22. Palmer RM, Ashton DS, Moncada S. Vascular endothelial cells synthesize nitric oxide from L-arginine. *Nature* 1988; 333: 664–666.

23. Bredt DS, Snyder SH. Isolation of nitric oxide synthetase, a calmodulin-requiring enzyme. *Proc Natl Acad Sci USA* 1990; 87: 682–685.

24. Pollock JS, Forstermann U, Mitchell JA *et al.* Purification and characterization of particulate endothelium-derived relaxing factor synthase from cultured and native bovine aortic endothelial cells. *Proc Natl Acad Sci USA* 1991; 88: 10480–10484.

25. Huang PL, Dawson TM, Bredt DS *et al.* Targeted disruption of the neuronal nitric oxide synthase gene. *Cell* 1993; 75: 1273–1286.

26. Ignarro LJ, Bush PA, Buga GM *et al.* Nitric oxide and cyclic GMP formation upon electrical field stimulation cause relaxation of corpus cavernosum smooth muscle. *Biochem Biophys Res Commun* 1990; 170: 843–850.

27. Rajfer J, Aronson WJ, Bush PA *et al.* Nitric oxide as a mediator of relaxation of the corpus cavernosum in response to nonadrenergic, noncholinergic neurotransmission. *N Engl J Med* 1992; 326: 90–94.

Chapter 14

THE DISCOVERY OF *HELICOBACTER PYLORI*

Chris Hawkey

14.1 Synopsis

The 2005 Nobel Prize in Medicine or Physiology was awarded to Barry Marshall and Robin Warren (Fig. 14.1) for their discovery of the bacterium, *Helicobacter pylori*, and the demonstration that it was the cause of active gastritis and peptic ulcer. Remarkably this was achieved through studies conducted in their spare time by two men who were not in formal academic posts. One of them was a medical registrar in training. Neither had published any research before their two letters to the *Lancet* in 1983,[1,2] which heralded a small series of pivotal papers that created one of the great paradigm shifts of the 20th century. Over the course of four years they showed that *H. pylori* was associated with gastritis and peptic ulcer,[3,4] that it could induce gastritis acutely[5] and that eradication prevented peptic ulcer relapse.[6] They used serology to show that the bacterium was widespread,[7] recognised that hydrolysis of urea to ammonia enabled it to survive gastric acid[8,9] and used this property to develop and commercialise highly specific and reliable gastric biopsy urease[10] and breath tests[11] for clinical use. By 1992 widespread initial disbelief had been replaced by enthusiasm for the new paradigm and a consensus statement from the National Institutes of Health (NIH) that placed *H. pylori* at the centre of peptic ulcer management.[12] Two years later the World Health Organisation[13] declared it a class 1 carcinogen, the cause of most cases of gastric cancer and mucosa-associated lymphoid tissue (MALT) lymphoma.

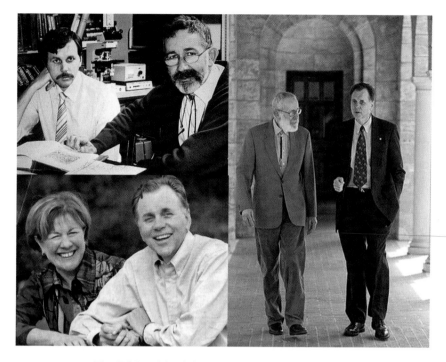

Fig. 14.1.   Top left: Marshall and Warren in 1984.
Bottom left: Contemporary photograph of Barry Marshall with his wife, Adrienne.
Right: The Nobel Prize winners.

14.2 Biographies

14.2.1 *Robin Warren*

14.2.1.1 *Family*

Born in Adelaide on 11 June 1937, Robin Warren was descended, on his father's side, from a family that had migrated from Aberdeen in 1840. His great grandfather was an entrepreneurial farmer, whose sons settled in vast areas of South and Western Australia and his father was one of Australia's leading winemakers. His mother's ancestors gave rise to a dynasty of Adelaide doctors although she, for financial reasons, instead trained as a nurse.

14.2.1.2 *Education*

Warren attended the Westbourne Park Primary School. Shy and poor at sport, he became interested in photography and cycling and absorbed in constructing a crystal radio set. His secondary education was at St Peter's College (also attended by the Nobel Prize winners Howard Florey and Lawrence Bragg). Shortly before matriculation he was diagnosed as suffering from grand mal epilepsy and his mother received patrician advice (echoing that offered to ulcer patients at the time) that he should be kept at home in a protected environment and not go to university or medical school. Fortunately this advice was not taken and he obtained a Commonwealth Scholarship to study medicine at Adelaide University in 1955.

14.2.1.3 *Professional and personal life*

After medical school he became an intern at Queen Elizabeth Hospital, Woodville, where he met his future wife, Winifred. He characterises himself at that time as an innocent with an uncomplicated enthusiasm for all that he did and learnt. After two years as Registrar in Haematology and Clinical Pathology in Adelaide he moved to Melbourne where he completed his training in 1968. He was trying to move to a position in Port Moresby in Papua New Guinea when, by his own account, he received a visit from an unidentified man who turned out to be Rolf ten Seldam, Professor of Pathology at the Royal Perth Hospital, who announced, 'you are working with me next year'. Warren worked as a pathologist in Perth for the rest of his career.

14.2.1.4 *Personality*

Warren was an individualistic and idiosyncratic man who, despite his shyness, sometimes wore a leather bootlace tie, drank large amounts of strong black coffee and smoked small cheroots. His appointment was a clinical one and his only publications were a few case reports prior to his ground-breaking letter to the *Lancet* in 1983.

14.2.2 Barry Marshall

14.2.2.1 Family

Like Robin Warren, there were times when Barry Marshall's life might have headed in a direction that would not have included the discovery of *H. pylori*. He was born (on 30 September 1951) and spent most of his first seven years in Kalgoorlie, a town which sprang up in the desert after the Irishman Paddy Hannan struck gold there in 1892. Local young men usually left school at 16 to go down the mines, earning high salaries that supported a wild drinking and partying social life, where barmaids are known as Skimpies. His father was 19 years old and in the final year of his apprenticeship as a fitter when Marshall was born. His mother quit nursing training at the age of 18 to have him. Marshall's parents left Kalgoorlie twice, the first time to drive to a new Uranium mine in Rum Jungle. They never made it because their Model A Ford broke down irretrievably in Carnarvon. They lived there for two years on an island a hundred yards from the beach, in a house with an outside toilet.

14.2.2.2 Education

The family returned to Kalgoorlie, where Marshall's grandparents owned a hotel, but later moved to Perth when he was seven, in part because his mother was anxious that the children should have aspirations beyond the Kalgoorlie lifestyle. Barry did well enough at school to be top of his class sporadically, but school work was not everything. Other achievements are said to have included winning a yo-yo competition to impress his then girlfriend and, like many Western Australians, he became an enthusiastic surfer. Like Warren, Marshall had natural curiosity and was inventive, interested in electricity and electronics (although a careless mis-wiring of an electric drill led to his father 'jumping rather high' when he used it). His interest in electronics led him to construct a home computer capable of word processing in 1981, which he feels gave him an edge when it came to doing literature surveys.

14.2.2.3 *Professional and personal life*

Marshall attended Newman College High School and then chose to do medicine rather than electrical engineering as he felt his maths was not strong enough. He went to the University of Western Australia from 1968 to 1974, where he met his wife Adrienne, a psychology student who was to be a strong continuing influence in his life. They married in 1972 and had four children.

In 1978 he trained as a registrar in general medicine, rotating through a wide range of disciplines. Doing gastroenterology in 1981 he needed a project and was sent by his boss, Tom Walters, to meet Warren and gather clinical information on the patients in whose gastric biopsy samples Warren had observed bacteria. Perhaps because he lacked the tunnel vision an established gastroenterologist might have brought to the issue, he showed immediate interest in the notion that an undescribed bacterium could be the cause of gastritis and peptic ulceration.

14.2.2.4 *Personality*

The two men, one shy and perfectionist, the other outgoing and apparently brash, were superficially different but had important similarities, particularly their inquisitiveness, and seem to have got on well from the start. Over four years they revolutionised the understanding of peptic ulcer. The more outgoing of the two, Barry Marshall, travelled the world after the discovery of *H. pylori* (Fig. 14.2) and for a time moved to the University of Virginia, but the pull of Western Australia (and possibly the push of his wife Adrienne) proved irresistible and he returned as Professor of Medicine in the University of Western Australia in 1997. Always the entrepreneur, he continued to try to commercialise applications arising from *H. pylori*, including its potential for drug and vaccine delivery

14.3 The Medical Problem that was Addressed

14.3.1 *Gastric ulcers*

A gastric ulcer (Fig. 14.3) is still sometimes called by the French *La Maladie Cruveilhier* after Jean Cruveilhier, who gave an early

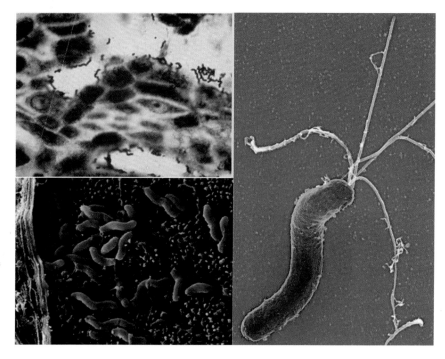

Fig. 14.2. Images of *Helicobacter pylori*.

Top left: Bacteria in gastric biopsy taken ten days after ingestion of *H. pylori* (courtesy of Barry Marshall).

Bottom left: Coloured scanning electron micrograph of *H. pylori* on mucosal surface (Science Photo Library).

Right: Coloured electron micrograph showing *H. pylori* with flagella (Science Photo Library).

(though not the first) description of gastric ulceration.[14–16] He did this as a pathological anatomist, despite initially finding autopsies so distasteful that he fled medical school to become a priest, only to be bullied back to medicine by his father. He noted that a gastric ulcer would develop as 'an erosion of the mucosa as a result of the morbid process...[of]...inflammation,...[which]...becomes an ulcer, which shows all the attributes of a syphilitic ulcer'. Cruveilhier also described duodenal ulcers, which were less common at the time but became extremely common 100 years later, early in the 20th century. His

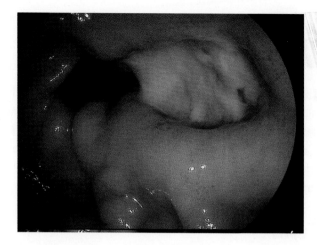

Fig. 14.3.   Chronic pre-pyloric gastric ulcer.

observation that 'idiopathic' ulcers were similar to syphilitic ulcers and his inference of a bacterial aetiology was prescient. Sporadically, spiral bacteria were reported in gastric specimens[16] but more than 150 years would pass before Warren and Marshall confirmed Cruveilhier's suggestion with their identification of *H. pylori*.

Cruveilhier recognised symptoms of indigestion, often occurring 'when there is no food in the stomach', with an epigastric distribution sometimes radiating to the spine. His treatments included leeches applied to the epigastrium and anus, mustard plasters to the calves and a diet of rice mixed with syrup of quince, emulsified with syrup of diacodium. Even by 1918, *Taylor's Practice of Medicine* recommended that patients with peptic ulcers be treated by extreme rest, food, 'given for a few days entirely by the rectum', to be followed with an ounce or two of milk every two to three hours, peptonised by the liquor pancreaticus of Benger.[17] Interestingly, Taylor mentions that 'bismuth is also of value'. Mustard plasters were still in vogue.

14.3.2 Duodenal ulcers

Gastric ulcers appeared to be more common than duodenal ulcers, at least based on post-mortem findings in the 19th century.[18] In the 20th century there was a sudden and dramatic increase in the number of patients with symptoms of duodenal ulcer and, where objective evidence was obtained, of duodenal ulcers themselves. This was often described as an epidemic without a specific infectious aetiology being implied. Instead, as is often the case when firm understanding is lacking, the stress of the 20th century and bad diet were blamed even though several pathologists reported ulcers to be associated with bacteria, as Cruveilhier had speculated. These included Stone Freeman, who found spirochaetes in 40% of gastric resections for ulcers or cancer and influenced Barry Marshall's thinking.[19]

14.3.3 *Aspirin*

The 20th century witnessed another epidemic of ulcers. This story (which some dispute) allegedly starts with Felix Hoffman, a synthetic chemist working with Bayer, whose father suffered with arthritis but got indigestion when he took salicylic acid for it.[20] In response his son tried to synthesise a better tolerated salicylic acid by acetylating it in 1897. Perhaps flushed with success he later applied the same chemical reaction to morphine and produced a cough linctus which the factory's employees said made them feel heroic. So Bayer called it heroin. Initially heroin was developed in preference to aspirin, which was suspected of weakening the heart. However, Hoffman, with a perseverance that echoes that of Warren and Marshall, conducted a secret trial of aspirin (against orders) to prove its tolerability. Aspirin was eventually launched in 1899. By 1937, however, the first evidence of gastric toxicity emerged in a paper published in the *Lancet* by Arthur Douthwaite and GAM Lintott, who gave aspirin to subjects, performed rigid endoscopy and made water colour paintings of the acute mucosal lesions they observed.[21]

14.3.4 *False theories and treatments*

Since the cause (apart from aspirin) of ulcers was entirely unknown it attracted capricious theories, the most prevalent of which was that they were due to psychological stress. This arose because of animal

experiments in which extreme physical stress resulted in gastroduodenal ulceration, which was interpreted as a paradigm for psychological stress rather than as the model for the stress ulcers seen in
patients with burns or on Intensive Care Units that it actually is. In
the early 1960s Tadataka (Tachi) Yamada, a young 16-year-old
immigrant from Japan to the US was diagnosed as suffering from an
ulcer. The stress of travel from Japan was felt to be the cause and
relaxation was recommended to help the ulcer to heal. The young
Tachi Yamada was therefore advised to take up smoking!
Interestingly, at about that time Susumo Ito[22] had performed a blind
suction gastric biopsy on himself and had shown a spiral bacteria
which proved to be ubiquitous amongst Japanese and was the cause
of Tachi Yamada's dyspepsia.

As well as stress reduction, many ulcer patients were treated with
variants of diets that had been in existence since Cruveilhier's time
(although the use of leeches and feeding per rectum had by then
been abandoned). The most famous diet was the Sippy diet which
consisted of milk and antacids and was named after its originator
Bertram Sippy. In part this was intended to neutralise excess production of hydrochloric acid, originally identified by William Prout.
Because ulcers and dyspepsia were so common they were an
attractive target for the pharmaceutical industry. The Nobel Prize-
winning pharmacologist Jim Black, who had already applied
receptor pharmacology to commercialise beta blockers, now developed the H2 receptor antagonists, along with Bill Duncan, Geoff
Durant, Robin Gannelin and Mike Parsons,[23] cimetidine (Tagamet)
being the first.

14.3.5 *H2 antagonists*

H2 receptor antagonists caught on rapidly, not only because they
fulfilled a previously unmet need but also because the new fashion of
endoscopy amongst gastroenterologists enabled visualisation of ulcers
and objective demonstration of healing. Even ailing pandas at London
Zoo suspected of having an ulcer were endoscoped, the cause confirmed and Tagamet given with instant cure! Cimetidine became the

world's first multi-billion dollar drug. H2 antagonists revolutionised clinical practice and gastroenterologists were suddenly in demand and invited to participate in 'Taga Tours' to foreign climes to debate, for example, whether these wonder pills should be taken before or after an evening meal.

14.3.6 *Bismuth*

However, just as endoscopy and renewed interest in ulcers helped to promote acid inhibition as treatment, so too they set the stage for it to be undermined. In 1981 a trial was published which showed that bismuth (previously recommended by Taylor and others throughout the 20th century) healed ulcers as fast as H2 antagonists and was apparently associated with a lower relapse rate.[24] At the time the scientific community was in thrall to concepts such as 'cytoprotection' and attributed the lower relapse rate on bismuth to an undefined higher quality of ulcer healing.

14.3.7 *Gastric bacteria*

Endoscopy ultimately undermined H2 antagonists as peptic ulcer treatments because the ability to take mucosal biopsy samples gave pathologists new insights and observations. One of these pathologists was Robin Warren who wrote:

> Then, in 1979, on my 42nd birthday, I noticed bacteria growing on the surface of a gastric biopsy. From then on, my spare time was largely centred on the study of these bacteria. Over the next two years, I collected numerous examples and showed that they were usually related to chronic gastritis, usually with the active change described by Richard Whitehead in 1972.[25]

Other pathologists also started to notice what appeared to be bacteria in the stomach and duodenum[15,16,26] (one, who shall remain nameless, claimed to me that the first duodenal biopsy in which he spotted bacteria also contained spermatozoa!), but did not take these observations as far as did Warren and Marshall.

14.4 The Research

14.4.1 *September–December 1981*

Following his introduction to Robin Warren, Barry Marshall collected biopsy samples and clinical information from 13 patients undergoing endoscopy between August and December 1981. Others had biopsied the ulcer itself but Robin Warren suggested that Barry Marshall take a sample of stomach away from any ulcer but within the area of gastritis in which the ulcer had developed. This was probably why they identified bacteria where others had previously failed.

14.4.2 *1982*

At the end of 1981, Marshall's training rotation took him to haematology but he was able to conduct an unfunded prospective study of 100 patients undergoing endoscopy. Even though he had to do the study while training in another discipline, Marshall completed the project in three to four months following ethical approval in early 1982. Today — and probably then — any funding body would likely have turned it down on a number of academic niceties. It was observational, it lacked a clear hypothesis and it had no power calculations: 100 patients were chosen so that, in the pre-computer era, calculations of percentages would be made easier. Barry Marshall himself says: 'I had no pre-conceived notion as to what diseases might be associated with the bacterium. Therefore the main goals of the study were to understand the histology and microbiology, rather than to discover the cause of peptic ulcer.'[27]

14.4.2.1 *First culture*

An obvious purpose of the study was to try to isolate and culture the bacteria. Samples were taken and set up for microaerophilic culture by the microbiologist John Pearman, using methods based upon work on the campylobacters which the spiral bacteria resembled. Nothing grew from the first 36 cultures, which were discarded routinely after 48 hours. Serendipity played a part in the first successful culture of *H. pylori*, which occurred on Easter Tuesday, 13 April 1982. At the time there was an outbreak of methicillin resistant *staphylococcus aureus* (MRSA) and most attention was focused on this. Consequently, the plates from the gastric biopsy samples taken from a duodenal ulcer patient (number 37) were not examined on Easter Saturday, but remained in the incubator untouched for a further three days. On return from the Easter holiday small transparent colonies were seen to be present on the plates and yielded almost pure cultures of *H. pylori*.[3, 4]

14.4.2.2 *Bacteria and ulcers*

In July 1982, one month after completing the study, Barry Marshall's training programme took him to Port Headland, a mining town 1,900 km north of Perth. In September he received tables of 'cross tabulations of bacteria versus everything else', and descriptive statistics from Rose Rendell, a student working in Norm Stenhouse's School of Medical Statistics. All 13 of the patients with duodenal ulcers had the bacteria on gastric histology, compared to about 50% of patients without ulcers. The quoted p value was 0.00044 for duodenal ulcer, 0.0086 for gastric ulcer (18 of 22 cases) and 0.00005 for all ulcers, even though there may not have been Bonferroni corrections for the other, 'cross tabs of bacteria versus everything else'! Remarkably, Barry noticed that the four patients with gastric ulcers but no *H. pylori* had no gastritis and were taking non-steroidal anti-inflammatory drugs (NSAIDs), the modern derivatives of Hoffman's aspirin.[3, 4]

14.4.2.3 *First reactions*

Marshall travelled back to Perth to present his preliminary findings to a sceptical group of physicians on 2 October. The Royal Perth Hospital was sufficiently unimpressed not to offer him a job, but Ian Hislop from Fremantle Hospital appointed him to an endoscopy training post so that he could continue his work, remarking, 'Barry, this is intriguing data. I think you are wrong but it is a curious finding and we need to look into it.'[27]

During the second half of 1982 the isolated bacteria were also characterised by John Armstrong and shown to have around five sheathed flagella, differentiating it from campylobacters which have an unsheathed flagellum.[2,3] It was found to be catalase and oxidase positive but on initial assessment no urease activity was detected. Given the enormous amounts of urease now known to be present in all *H. pylori* perhaps the bacterium was moribund or dead by the time the urease testing was done.

14.4.3 *1983*

14.4.3.1 *First publication*

Warren and Marshall wrote up their initial findings in two letters to the *Lancet*, published in June 1983.[1,2] One can speculate that they now realised they were on to something big and a little academic tension arose as to who should be first author, which they solved by writing two letters. Warren's letter, which described the distribution of the bacteria and their association with gastritis, was illustrated by a light microscopic section. The younger Marshall, in discussing what he referred to as 'Warren's bacteria', showed a predilection for electron microscopy. He suggested that the curved bacteria which had multiple flagellae did not fit any known species and concluded his letter by saying, 'If these bacteria are truly associated with antral gastritis, as described by Warren [sic] they may have a part to play in other poorly understood, gastritis-associated diseases [i.e. peptic ulcer and gastric cancer].'

He was right on both counts. Although the curved bacteria underwent serial reclassification to *Campylobacter*-like organisms then to *Campylobacter pyloridis* and to *Campylobacter pylori*, they were eventually declared to be a new microaerophilic species *H. pylori*, largely on the basis of the multiple flagella. Warren and Marshall were also soon to prove that the relationship with peptic ulcers was causative although it fell to others to do so for gastric cancer.[28,29] The letters stimulated no correspondence, though there was a passing mention in a *Lancet* editorial on 'Campylobacters'.[30] Later citations amounted to 2,045. However, Barry Marshall travelled to Europe and encountered interest from a number of investigators who were conducting their own studies.[31-33]

14.4.3.2 *Serology and a wild theory*

During 1983, Marshall and colleagues from Fremantle identified circulating antibodies to the bacterium in a substantial proportion of unselected individuals, a finding in line with their gastric biopsy study[34] and consistent with the notion that *H. pylori* colonisation was common. They asked: 'How do you acquire pyloric campylobacter and from whom? Without further comment we present the data in Table III.' Table III showed a high incidence amongst women attending a sexually transmitted diseases clinic. Given the paucity of information then it was an interesting idea to seek links between two spiral organisms but the implied association failed to take account of confounding variables.

14.4.3.3 *Bactericidal bismuth*

A further important finding was that bismuth was bactericidal.[35] Filter paper soaked in the proprietary preparation DeNol was used to show this *in vitro*, and for an *in vivo* demonstration Marshall persuaded his intern Vinod Ganju to take DeNol and undergo gastroscopy (Fig. 14.4). Taken with the confirmation that DeNol appeared to suppress ulcer relapse, a role for *H. pylori* in ulcer disease was starting to look very attractive. Robert Koch's first and second postulates had more or less been fulfilled, but the third and fourth had not.

14.4.4 *1984*

14.4.4.1 *Self-ingestion*

From January 1984, Marshall unsuccessfully tried to fulfil Koch's third and fourth postulates using pigs but he could not establish the infection over the next six months. Frustrated with this failure but, like Hoffman in the aspirin field before him, believing passionately in

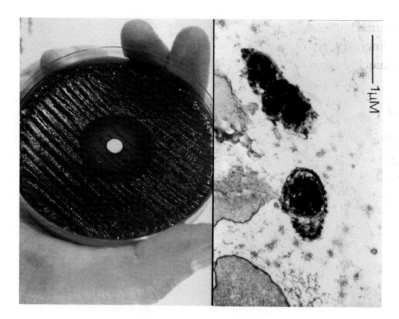

Fig. 14.4. Bismuth as an anti-*helicobacter* agent.

Left: Inhibition of *H. pylori* growth by bismuth citrate tablet.

Right: Electron micrograph of degenerating *H. pylori* in a mucosal biopsy taken 30 minutes after treatment with bismuth.

his discovery, Marshall also proceeded to conduct a secret experiment.[5] As with Hoffman, there was no proposal, no funding, no clear hypothesis and no statistics. On 14 July 1984, about a month after publishing (and perhaps flushed with the success of) their 100 patient study in the *Lancet,* he took cimetidine to lower acidity and assist bacterial survival. Two hours later he swallowed 50 ml of bacteria suspended in alkaline peptone water. It is still not clear whether he thought he was going to get an ulcer and if so, when. To begin with he felt well. Then, after five days, he became ill with dyspepsia, nausea, vomiting and halitosis. Barry noticed that the vomitus was not acidic. It was a simple critical insight into how *H. pylori* evades the sterilising influence of acid in the stomach.

After ten days he underwent endoscopy. Only two biopsy samples were taken. *H. pylori* was seen on histology (Fig. 14.2), together with gastritis, but it was not grown. Contrary to popular mythology, it did not require intensive treatment to eliminate it. The endoscopy was repeated on day 14. By now his symptoms had settled and there was no evidence of *H. pylori* in any of the eight samples. Tinidazole (an anti-microbial drug) was taken but only after the final endoscopy. Thus there were two salient findings, first that ingestion led to infection accompanied by gastritis, at least on histological evidence and, second, that persistent infection was difficult to achieve in an adult. Moreover, seroconversion did not occur. This was an early clue to understanding that *H. pylori* is an organism normally contracted in childhood. Barry was later to reflect that his actions were selfish but not as reckless as those of John Hunter, whose self-inoculation with *Treponema pallidum* ultimately led to his death from an aortic aneurism attributed to tertiary syphilis.[36]

For what it is worth, the self-ingestion experiment did not fulfil Koch's postulates. Barry Marshall did not get an ulcer, and since the bacterium was not recovered it could not be typed as being identical to the inoculating strain. But Koch's rather unwieldy and formulaic postulates are not worth that much. With the information already available, *H. pylori* would be accepted as the cause of ulcers if eradicating the organism eradicated the ulcer diathesis. In order to demonstrate this formally, Marshall designed a 2×2 clinical trial of cimetidine plus placebo, versus cimetidine plus tinidazole, versus bismuth plus placebo, versus bismuth plus tinidazole.[6] The Texan Pete Peterson, who had called Marshall a real cowboy for his self-ingestion experiment (a remark that Barry took to be complimentary), helped him to develop some 'rudimentary statistics' (which conveniently again required 100 patients to be studied!).

14.4.4.2 *Growing interest*

During the second half of 1984 Marshall's self-ingestion experiment fostered popular interest in his findings. Local doctors were impressed by the improvements seen in their patients and sent increasing numbers to be treated with antibiotics. Naturally there was also a great deal of scepticism from the medical establishment but equally a group of open-minded supporters soon developed, first in Europe and later in the US. These people were to broaden the investigative base[31-33] and would also form a new ulcer establishment.

14.4.4.3 *Urease testing*

One consequence was the finding that *H. pylori* had substantial urease activity, in contrast to the earlier failure to find it in Perth. Although the initial observation came from elsewhere,[37] it was Marshall who saw its diagnostic utility and developed and commercialised the world's first and most successful biopsy urease test, the CLO (*Campylobacter*-Like Organism) test, which is still widely used today. The principle is simple: a biopsy is put into a gel containing urea and a pH sensitive dye. A colour change indicates that *H. pylori* has converted urea to ammonia and thereby raised the pH (Fig. 14.5).

Simon Langton in the Biochemistry Department in Fremantle helped Barry to show that urea was often absent from the gastric juice of infected patients.[8] This suggested that the bacteria's urease activity was substantial and detectable *in vivo*. In fact, it put other urease-producing bacteria in the shade, making it the only tested bacteria with sufficient activity to produce enough ammonia to survive gastric acid. This realisation led to the development of a ^{14}C urea breath test,

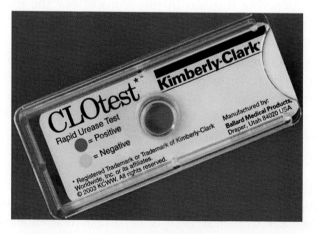

Fig. 14.5. A positive CLO (*Campylobacter*-Like Organism) test.

dependent on the principle that the CO_2 released by urease conversion would be absorbed and exhaled.[11] The dose of radiation was tiny and not hazardous but the ^{14}C breath test lost out to one based on the non-radioactive ^{13}C stable isotope test[38] developed by David Graham who, in a characteristically acerbic remark, claimed Barry Marshall had 'taken a good test and made it worse'!

14.4.5 1985

14.4.5.1 First randomised controlled trial of antibiotic treatments for ulcers

By his own account, Marshall met with considerable scepticism and hostility when he presented his proposal for an antibiotic trial to the Australian National Health and Medical Research Council. They doubted both his ability to use a serological test (despite it having already been developed) and to conduct a 100-patient study in the timescale of the grant. They awarded funding subject to a one-year review to assess recruitment.

They clearly did not take into account the earlier study which recruited 100 patients in 4 months, and the second 100-patient study was conducted as quickly as the earlier one (again at the Royal Perth Hospital) and far ahead of the schedule proposed by the Council. It is not clear whether this was in the protocol but the trial did not recruit all comers: by selectively including smokers Marshall was able to recruit 100 patients with ulcers from 300 screened. Treatment with antibiotics and successful eradication of *H. pylori* resulted in a marked reduction in ulcer recurrence,[6] thus establishing an entirely new approach to the treatment of gastroduodenal ulcers, which was confirmed in several other studies.[39–41] Marshall also noticed that smoking did not cause ulcer recurrence in the absence of *H. pylori*, a finding subsequently confirmed by Tom Borody.[42]

14.4.5.2 Teamwork

By now the key work had been done. Robin Warren subsequently published very little and Barry Marshall's output was limited to a further 60 or so papers. A remarkable four years of work and a handful of papers and letters had transformed understanding of peptic ulcer. I believe their success lay in their complementary characters: in early years both men showed themselves to be inquisitive. In Robin Warren this fed into a capacity for absorption that underlay his collection of 135 cases, which were central to the work. But he needed the more outgoing Barry Marshall, with his entrepreneurial eye for exploitation and development.

14.4.5.3 *Resistance*

The first description of *H. pylori* submitted to a scientific meeting was deemed to fall in the bottom 10% and their first full paper met with stiff criticism from referees.[43] Resistance came from various quarters: those experiencing cognitive dissonance as a result of the new paradigm; those whose Taga Tours travel plans seemed threatened; and from the academic establishment, suspicious of these upstarts. Academic correctness is an entity analogous to political correctness that can provide appropriate discipline for activity but can often be an uncreative systemisation of accumulated prejudices. One reason why there was such resistance to Warren and Marshall was that they were academically incorrect to an extent that seemed outrageous to some. With their research being done out of hours, ethical approval sometimes being omitted, clear prior hypotheses not always being evident, experiments evolving on the hoof and decisions about numbers of patients to study being taken in an unconventional way, they seemed like Australian cowboys — to make matters worse, one of them wore a bootlace tie! But it was the lack of conventional academic constraint that allowed what the *Lancet* called 'Marshall and Warren's inquisitive approach to unexplained phenomena'[44] to generate such a fast pace of discovery.

14.4.5.4 *Full circle*

By 1992 an NIH consensus conference placed *H. pylori* at the centre of ulcer management,[12] and in 1994 *H. pylori* was classified by the

World Health Organisation as a class 1 carcinogen.[13] Awards for the Australian pioneers started to flow and interest in the organism grew exponentially as others helped expand clinical understanding and application and scientific knowledge. My own role in this was limited. I was more interested in ulcers caused by non-steroidal anti-inflammatory drugs (NSAIDs), which damage the mucosa by inhibiting prostaglandin synthesis in gastric mucosa. Nick Hudson and I showed that this inhibition was entirely reversed by the mucosal inflammation present in *H. pylori*-infected individuals.[45] We speculated that *H. pylori* may not enhance NSAID ulcer risk and could even be protective under some circumstances. Facetiously we supplemented publication with a 'Save the *Helicobacter*' badge. I leave aside the question of whether we were right as argument still persists. What was interesting was the strength of feeling against our proposal, which echoed that which had greeted Warren and Marshall's initial proposal that bacteria might cause ulcers.[46] It was clear that the paradigm shift this caused had generated a new establishment, bound strongly together by a pioneering feeling and attached vigorously to the central belief in *H. pylori* as the cause of ulcers!

14.5 Impact on Medical Science

14.5.1 *Peptic ulceration*

The most obvious and immediate impact of the discovery of *H. pylori* was on the management of peptic ulcer. For the first time a condition previously thought to be life-long could be cured by a one week course of treatment. This was undoubtedly a major advance in the management of individual patients. However, at a population level the part played by medical strategies to detect and eradicate the organism has probably been relatively small compared to the decline that has been occurring as a result of reduced infection in childhood as sanitary conditions improved. Indeed, it is intriguing to speculate that had the natural decline in *H. pylori* preceded endoscopy by, say, another 25 years, the organism may never have been detected, at least in Western countries (in other populations, such as the Far East, *H. pylori* remains prevalent and ulcer disease problematic).

14.5.2 *Dyspepsia management*

Recognition that most serious gastric pathology is driven by *H. pylori* has led to a 'Test [for *H. pylori*] and Treat' strategy. Whether an ulcer happens to be present is irrelevant and the endoscopic detection of a gastric cancer seldom affects prognosis. Logical though it is, Test and Treat has not systematically been embraced and nor has endoscopy for dyspepsia been abandoned.

14.5.3 *NSAIDs and aspirin as a cause of ulcers and the development of selective cyclooxygenase (COX)-2 inhibitors*

Old habits die hard. I well remember participating in trials of prostaglandin analogues as peptic ulcer healing agents at a time when *H. pylori* was recognised as a cause of peptic ulcer. Not only was this, in retrospect, a vain venture since these drugs would be unlikely to compete with a curative therapy, but one of the main exclusion criteria was consumption of NSAIDs, as was traditional. It took some time and the identification of cyclooxygenase (COX)-2 for the paradigm shift associated with *H. pylori* to turn attitudes around so that NSAID-associated ulcers were focused on as a problem in their own right,[47] quite distinct from *H. pylori*-associated ulcers. I think the recognition of *H. pylori* as the cause of most ulcers helped not only to define more clearly the problem associated with NSAIDs but to draw attention in individual patients, who were neither infected nor taking NSAIDs, to the possibility that their ulcer was caused by Crohn's disease or Zollinger–Ellison syndrome.

14.5.4 *Reflux*

An indirect consequence of the discovery of the link between *H. pylori* and ulcers has been an increased focus on gastro-oesophageal disease as pharmaceutical firms with acid inhibitors looked for indications beyond peptic ulcer. Perhaps reflux would always have become the primary focus given its greatly increased prevalence in increasingly obese societies[48] but the demise of acid inhibition for non-NSAID ulcer therapy may have accelerated this process.

14.5.5 *Malignancies*

Warren and Marshall did not prove the link between *H. pylori* and gastric malignancy: that fell to others assessing seropositivity in serum banks.[28,29] Therapeutically the demonstration that eradication of *H. pylori* could cure MALT lymphoma was remarkable,[49] but no analogous advance has unequivocally emerged for gastric cancer. A great aspiration has been to reduce gastric cancer at a population level by mass eradication programmes in areas of high incidence. It is probably fair to say that firm evidence that this has been realised has not yet emerged.

14.5.6 *Genetic microbiology*

The most significant and successful work to follow Warren and Marshall relates to the identification of virulence factors, particularly toxins like Cag-A and Vac-A, which have been prototypic for a basic understanding of bacterial toxins beyond *H. pylori.*

14.5.7 *Evolution*

H. pylori was one of the first bacteria to be fully sequenced.[50] This revealed substantial genetic diversity, which has prompted interesting phylogenetic studies. These suggest that *H. pylori* accompanied the few thousand humans that migrated out of Africa 60,000 years ago and that they co-evolved as the human race populated the world.[51,52] A teleological advantage for *H. pylori* is easy to postulate: eliciting a controlled active chronic neutrophilic inflammatory response should release amino acids and other nutritional components for utilisation by the bacteria. One possible advantage to humans might be stimulation of increased acid production, reducing enteric infections in childhood but promoting death from gastric cancer after the reproductive phase of life.

14.5.8 *History of disease*

What we do not know is what pathology *H. pylori* engendered during the 60,000 year association. On the one hand dyspepsia and ulcers may be a modern phenomenon. For example, the annual number of patients admitted to Edinburgh Royal Infirmary for dyspepsia showed an extraordinary increase from none in 1730 to 900 per million population in 1760. It was only in the 19th century that gastric ulcer was frequently referred to in post-mortem examinations.[18] Duodenal ulcer followed in the 20th century. Subtle changes in the intragastric distribution of *H. pylori* and altered host responses related to age of ingestion could account for the evolution of different patterns of *H. pylori*-associated disease. On the other hand, ancient Greek writings undoubtedly describe patients with haematemesis and melaena.[15,16] Might it be that new toxic strains of *H. pylori* have developed in successive waves over the course of human history?

14.5.9 *Consequences of H. pylori loss*

The level of modern hygiene is unique in human history. This has aroused interest in the possibility that the human host is in some ways adapted to carrying *H. pylori*, with the suggestion that this results in hyperchlorhydria and worsening of acid-related oesophageal disease and development of Barrett's Oesophagus.[48] Reflux is also a consequence of obesity and here too the increased ghrelin and reduced gastric leptin that occur in the absence of *H. pylori* have been hypothesised to be contributory. A further possibility is that an absence of *H. pylori*, by driving the immune response away from a TH2 effect, may protect against atopic and allergic disorders.

14.5.10 *Save the Helicobacter!*

Barry Marshall now (sometimes) wears my 'Save the *Helicobacter*' badge. He has an institute that is working on *H. pylori* mutated to be harmless to humans, to be used as a vehicle for drugs and vaccines.[53, 54] The development of a vaccine to *H. pylori* in particular has been an unrealised aspiration, reflecting its dynamic ability to evade immune elimination. Time will tell whether there is yet a further twist in the *H. pylori* story — if so, it will once again come from Barry Marshall.

References

1. Warren RJ. Unidentified curved bacilli on gastric epithelium in active chronic gastritis. *Lancet* 1983; 321: 1273.
2. Marshall B. Unidentified curved bacilli on gastric epithelium in active chronic gastritis. *Lancet* 1983; 321: 1273–1275.
3. Warren RJ, Marshall B. Unidentified curved bacilli in the stomach of patients with gastritis and peptic ulceration. *Lancet* 1984; 323: 1311–1314.
4. Marshall BJ, McGechie DB, Rogers PA *et al.* Pyloric Campylobacter infection and gastroduodenal disease. *Med J Aust* 1985; 142: 439–444.
5. Marshall BJ, Armstrong JA, McGechie DB *et al.* Attempt to fulfil Koch's postulates for pyloric Campylobacter. *Med J Aust* 1985; 142: 436–439.
6. Marshall BJ, Goodwin CS, Warren JR *et al.* Prospective double-blind trial of duodenal ulcer relapse after eradication of Campylobacter pylori. *Lancet* 1988; 332: 1437–1442.
7. Marshall BJ, McGechie DB, Francis GJ *et al.* Pyloric campylobacter serology. *Lancet* 1984; 324: 281.
8. Marshall BJ. Langton SR. Urea hydrolysis in patients with Campylobacter pyloridis infection. *Lancet* 1986; 327: 965–966.
9. Marshall BJ, Barrett LJ, Prakash C *et al.* Urea protects Helicobacter (Campylobacter) pylori from the bactericidal effect of acid. *Gastroenterology* 1990; 99: 697–702.
10. Marshall BJ, Warren JR, Francis GJ *et al.* Rapid urease test in the management of Campylobacter pyloridis-associated gastritis. *Amer J Gastroenterol* 1987; 82: 200–210.
11. Marshall BJ, Surveyor I. Carbon-14 urea breath test for the diagnosis of Campylobacter pylori associated gastritis. *J Nucl Med* 1988; 29: 11–16.
12. NIH Consensus Development Panel on Helicobacter pylori in Peptic Ulcer Disease. NIH Consensus Conference. Helicobacter pylori in peptic ulcer disease. *JAMA* 1994; 272: 65–69.

13. International Agency for Research on Cancer. *IARC Monographs on the Evaluation of Carcinogenic Risks to Humans*. 1994; 61 Schistosomes, liver flukes and *Helicobacter pylori*.

14. Cruveilhier J. *Anatomie Pathologique du corps Humain*. Paris: Balliere; 1829–1842.

15. Unge P. *Helicobacter pylori* treatment in the past and in the 21st century. In: *Helicobacter Pioneers: Firsthand Accounts from the Scientists Who Discovered Helicobacters, 1892–1982*, Marshall B (ed.). Victoria, Australia: Blackwell Science Asia; 2002: 203–213.

16. Kidd M, Modlin IM. A century of *Helicobacter pylori*. *Digestion* 1988; 59: 1–15.

17. Taylor F. Ulcer of the Stomach. In: *The Practice of Medicine*, 11th ed., Taylor F (ed.). London: J & A Churchill; 1918: 688–694.

18. Baron JH, Watson F, Sonnenberg A. Three centuries of stomach symptoms in Scotland. *Aliment Pharmacol Ther* 2006; 24: 821–829.

19. Freedberg AS, Baron LE. The presence of spirochaetes in human gastric mucosa. *Am J Dig Dis* 1940; 7: 443–445.

20. Mann CC, Plummer ML. *The Aspirin Wars*. Boston: HBS Press; 1991.

21. Douthwaite AH, Lintott GAM. Gastroscopic observation of the effect of aspirin and certain other substances on the stomach. *Lancet* 1938; 232: 1222–1225.

22. Ito, S. Anatomic structure of the gastric mucosa. In: *Alimentary Canal*, Code CF (ed.). Washington: American Physiological Society; 1967: 705–741.

23. Black JW, Duncan WAM, Durant GJ *et al*. Definition and antagonism of histamine H2-receptors. *Nature* 1972; 236: 385–390.

24. Martin DF, May SJ, Tweedle DEF *et al*. Difference in relapse rates of duodenal ulcer after healing with cimetidine or tripotassium dicitrato bismuthate. *Lancet* 1981; 317: 7–10.

25. Warren, RJ. Autobiography. Nobelprize.org. Available at: http://nobelprize.org/nobel_prizes/medicine/laureates/2005/warren-auto-bio.html [Accessed 29 June 2011].

26. Steer HW, Colin-Jones DG. Mucosal changes in gastric ulceration and their response to carbenoxolone sodium. *Gut* 1975; 16: 590–597.

27. Marshall BJ. Heliobacter Connections, Nobel Lecture, December 8 2005. Available at: http://nobelprize.org/nobel_prizes/medicine/laureates/2005/marshall- lecture.pdf [Accessed 24 June 2011].

28. Parsonnet J, Friedman GD, Vandersteen DP *et al*. Helicobacter pylori infection and the risk of gastric carcinoma. *N Engl J Med* 1991; 325: 1127–1131.

29. Nomura A, Stemmermann GN, Chyou PH *et al*. Helicobacter pylori infection and gastric carcinoma among Japanese Americans in Hawaii. *N Engl J Med* 1991; 325: 1132–1136.

30. Editorial. New faces amongst the campylobacters. *Lancet* 1983; 322: 662.

31. McNulty CAM, Watson DM. Spiral bacteria of the gastric antrum. *Lancet* 1984; 323: 1068–1069.

32. Eldridge J, Lessells AM, Jones DM. Antibody to spiral organisms on gastric mucosa. *Lancet* 1984; 323: 1237.

33. O'Connor HJ, Axon ATR, Dixon MF. Campylobacter-like organisms unusual in type A (pernicious anaemia) gastritis. *Lancet* 1984; 324: 109–124.

34. Marshall, Mcgechie DB, Francis GJ *et al*. Pyloric campylobacter serology. *Lancet* 1984; 324: 281.

35. Marshall BJ, Armstrong JA, Francis GJ. Antibacterial action of bismuth in relation to Campylobacter pyloridis colonization and gastritis. *Digestion* 1987; 37 Suppl 2: 16–30.

36. Martinelli PT, Czelusta A, Peterson SR. Self-experimenters in medicine: heroes or fools? Part I. Pathogens. *Clinics in Dermatology* 2008; 26: 570–573.

37. Owen RJ, Martin SR, Borman P. Rapid urea hydrolysis by gastric campylobacters. *Lancet* 1985; 325: 111.

38. Graham DY. Klein PD. Evans Jr DJ *et al*. Campylobacter pylori detected noninvasively by the ^{13}C-urea breath test. *Lancet* 1987; 329: 1174–1177.

39. Rauws EAJ, Tytgat GNJ. Cure of duodenal ulcer associated with eradication of Helicobacter pylori. *Lancet* 1990; 335: 1233–1235.

40. Graham DY, Lew GM, Evans DG *et al*. Effect of triple therapy (antibiotics plus bismuth) on duodenal ulcer healing: a randomized controlled trial. *Ann Int Med* 1991; 115: 266–269.

41. Hentschel E, Brandstatter G, Dragosics B. Effect of ranitidine and amoxicillin plus metronidazole on the eradication of helicobacter pylori

and the recurrence of duodenal ulcer. *N Engl J Med* 1993; 328: 308–312.

42. Borody TJ. George LL. Brandl S *et al.* Smoking does not contribute to duodenal ulcer relapse after Helicobacter pylori eradication. *Am J Gastroenterol* 1992; 87: 1390–1393.

43. Marshall B. The discovery that *Helicobacter pylori*, a spiral bacterium, caused peptic ulcer disease. In: *Helicobacter Pioneers: Firsthand Accounts from the Scientists who Discovered Helicobacters, 1892–1982*, Marshall B (ed.). Oxford: Blackwell; 2002: 165–202.

44. Spirals and ulcers. *Lancet* 1984; 323: 1336–1337.

45. Hudson N, Balsitis M, Filipowicz B *et al.* Effect of Helicobacter pylori colonisation on gastric mucosal eicosanoid synthesis in patients taking non-steroidal anti-inflammatory drugs. *Gut* 1993; 34: 748–751.

46. Hawkey CJ. Personal review: *Helicobacter pylori*, NSAIDs and cognitive dissonance. *Aliment Pharmacol Therap* 1999; 13: 695–702.

47. Hawkey CJ.COX-2 Inhibitors. *Lancet* 1999; 353: 307–314.

48. Atherton, JC, Blaser MJ. Coadaptation of Helicobacter pylori and humans: ancient history, modern implications *J Clin Invest* 2009; 119: 2475–2587.

49. Wotherspoon AC. Doglioni C. Diss TC *et al.* Regression of primary low-grade B-cell gastric lymphoma of mucosa-associated lymphoid tissue type after eradication of Helicobacter pylori. *Lancet* 1993; 342: 575–577.

50. Tomb JF, White O, Kerlavage AR. The complete genome sequence of the gastric pathogen Helicobacter pylori. *Nature* 1997; 388: 539–547.

51. Linz B, Balloux F, Moodley Y *et al.* An African origin for the intimate association between humans and Helicobacter pylori. *Nature* 2007; 445: 915–918.

52. Moodley Y, Linz B, Yamaoka Y *et al.* The peopling of the Pacific from a bacterial perspective. *Science* 2009; 323: 527–530.

53. Marshall B, Schoep T. *Helicobacter pylori* as a vaccine delivery system. *Helicobacter* 2007; 12 Suppl. 2: 75–79.

54. Ondek Biologic Delivery Systems. Available at: http://www.ondek. com [Accessed 8 June 2011].

Chapter 15

THE DISCOVERY OF RNA INTERFERENCE — GENE SILENCING BY DOUBLE-STRANDED RNA

Richard P. Hull and Timothy J. Aitman

15.1 Introduction

The 2006 Nobel Prize in Physiology or Medicine was awarded to Professor Andrew Fire from Stanford University, California, and Professor Craig Mello from the University of Massachusetts Medical School, Worcester, for their discovery of the gene-silencing effect of double-stranded RNA (dsRNA) termed RNA interference (RNAi). Professor Göran K. Hansson, Chairman of the Nobel Committee for Physiology or Medicine summarised the impact of their discovery in his Nobel Prize presentation speech saying that it had 'unravelled a new principle for regulating the flow of genetic information', as well as adding a 'new dimension to our understanding of life and provided new tools for medicine.[1] Fire and Mello had identified a major regulatory step in their 'brilliant paper' where 'Double-stranded RNA activates an enzymatic mechanism that leads to gene silencing, with the genetic code in the RNA molecule determining which gene to silence'.[1] The significance of this discovery is highlighted by the fact that their Nobel Prize was awarded only eight years after the original publication of their findings.[2] Their description of RNAi has transformed our understanding of the mechanisms that underlie gene regulation in cells, as well as making RNAi an essential tool in biological research for manipulating gene expression and has great potential as a novel therapeutic modality for a wide spectrum of diseases.

In this chapter we will review the scientific backgrounds of both Nobel Laureates to understand how their scientific journeys led them to the discovery of RNAi, which has opened up new fields of research that are exploring the mechanisms controlling gene expression. We will conclude by examining the impact RNAi has had and will have in the future of biomedical research and clinical medicine.

15.2 Biographical and Scientific Background of the Laureates

15.2.1 *Andrew Fire*

Andrew Fire was born in 1959 and grew up in California. He attended the University of California at Berkeley, gaining a degree in mathematics, before studying for his PhD entitled '*In Vitro* Transcription Studies of Adenovirus', from 1978 to 1983 at the Massachusetts Institute of Technology under the mentorship of Nobel Laureate and geneticist Phillip Sharp. Following the completion of his PhD, Fire moved to the Medical Research Council Laboratory of Molecular Biology, Cambridge, UK as a Helen Hay Whitney Foundation Fellow, where he worked in the *Caenorhabditis elegans* group headed by the Nobel Laureate Sydney Brenner. Fire's research in Cambridge centred on microinjection technology and is where he first developed techniques for expressing foreign DNA in *C. elegans* worms. Fire returned to the US in 1986 as a researcher in the Department of Embryology at the Carnegie Institution of Washington in Baltimore, Maryland with his own independent research grant awarded by the National Institutes of Health to investigate gene regulation during the early development of *C. elegans*. He was appointed as a regular staff member at the Carnegie in 1989 and stayed there until 2003 when he moved back to California to Stanford University School of Medicine where he is currently Professor of Pathology and Genetics.

While at the Carnegie, Fire continued to work developing DNA transformation technology as a tool to investigate the function of cloned genes. A key tool that Fire wanted to apply to his work was the ability to disrupt the expression of specific genes. However, he was limited by the fact that his preferred method for mutating endogenous genes, using homologous recombination between injected DNA and the corresponding chromosomal locus, was not yet available in the *C. elegans* model. He began to explore an alternative approach that was first described by Jonathan Izant and Harold Weintraub in 1984 where antisense (nonsense) DNA strand transcription was used to inhibit gene activity.[3] Fire used a transgene, designed to generate antisense RNAs, to successfully inhibit gene expression in the body wall muscle of *C. elegans* and showed that the traits could be transmitted to subsequent generations.[4] As well as antisense constructs producing a targeted interference effect he found that sense constructs could also cause the effect. This finding was thought to be the result of unintended antisense RNA production from the DNA transgenes used to generate the sense strand. Fire concluded that the most likely mechanism of action was that the antisense RNA disrupted gene expression by hybridising to the sense transcript, which either blocked a late processing step, RNA transport, or translation. Interestingly he discounted a model where double-stranded RNAs (dsRNA) mediated degradation and inhibition of transcription because of the presence of sense RNA at normal levels, although he did not fully discount that dsRNA could have physiological effects on certain cells. Fire moved away from this avenue of interference research over the next few years, concentrating instead on trying to understand the role of gene regulation in specifying cell fate until he began his collaboration with Mello.

15.2.2 *Craig Mello*

Craig Mello was born in 1960 in New Haven, Connecticut, and attended Brown University where he majored in biochemistry and molecular biology, before moving to the University of Colorado in Boulder to begin his graduate studies. It was here that he first studied *C. elegans* as a member of David Hirsh's lab. Mello cites this 'fantastic' lab as key to his future training, which included his introduction to molecular biology by Dan Stinchcomb as well as to future collaborators such as Mike Krause, Jim Kramer and Ken Kemphues and Jim Priess with whom he carried out his postdoctoral work. Following David Hirsh's move to industry in his first year, Mello moved to Harvard University to continue working with Dan Stinchcomb, focusing mainly on identifying worm centromere activators using yeast as a model system. It was at this point that Fire and Mello first collaborated. Both men were working on developing techniques for DNA transformation in worms, building on the techniques described by Kimble *et al.*[5] and Stinchcomb *et al.*[6] Fire had made some early progress, developing a number of methods which Mello continued to refine, and this early collaboration between the two helped to make DNA transformation a routine method for the worm.[7] These methods were central to their later description of RNAi and highlight the advantages of the *C. elegans* model for studying the effects of DNA transformation. In their technique, fine sharp glass needles were inserted through the cuticle of the worm and positioned inside the large shared cytoplasm of a gonad which contains hundreds of germ-line nuclei. The experimental material could then be injected into the gonad with the procedure repeated for the other gonad and the worms then observed for the effects of the DNA transformation.

After successfully completing his doctoral studies at Harvard, Mello moved to the Fred Hutchinson Cancer Research Centre in Seattle, Washington, as a postdoctoral researcher in the lab of Jim Priess. Mello started his own lab in 1994 at the University of Massachusetts Medical School and subsequently became a Howard Hughes Medical Institute investigator in 2000. During this period, Mello worked on projects which focused on identifying genes that acted as regulators of early development in the worm and included another collaboration with Fire.[8] In 1995, the important discovery that direct injection of antisense RNA could be used to silence specific genes in *C. elegans* was made by Su Guo in Ken Kemphues' lab at Cornell University.[9] Mello was able to use this powerful tool to silence the genes he was studying and began to make progress in understanding the developmental mechanisms that determine cell fate in early embryos.[10] A key observation made by Guo and Kemphues, similar to that made by Fire in 1991, was that both sense and antisense RNA strands could cause gene silencing. The underlying mechanism behind this phenomenon was still not known but was thought to be a stochastic interaction where either strand could template the production of the other strand and build up silencing RNA levels. This mechanistic uncertainty led Mello in 1997 to term the silencing phenomenon RNA interference or RNAi.[10]

Mello's collaboration with Fire continued in 1997 with the publication of a paper exploring the mechanisms that underlie the repression of gene expression in the early embryonic development of *C. elegans*, though interestingly it did not involve the use of direct antisense RNA injections to silence target genes.[11] Both Fire in his Nobel Prize speech and Mary Montgomery, one of the *Nature* paper co-authors and a postdoctoral researcher in Fire's group, note that, as is so often the case within the scientific community, it was an informal discussion organised by Mello at a 1997 worm meeting in Madison, Wisconsin, that sparked the RNAi collaboration and laid the foundation for their RNAi discovery.[12, 13] The key hypothesis centred round the idea that dsRNA was the actual effector molecule, though Montgomery notes that the idea was greeted with a healthy scepticism during a lab meeting![12] This, however, did not stop their investigations continuing and the collaborative set of experiments that ensued, using the *C. elegans* model, led to the publication of their paper on RNAi in *Nature* in February 1998.[2]

15.3 The Discovery of Genetic Interference by Double-Stranded RNA

Fire and Mello's 1998 *Nature* paper entitled 'Potent and specific genetic interference by double-stranded RNA in *Caenorhabditis elegans*', described the key features of RNAi and gave insights to its underlying mechanisms.[2] Their central finding was that dsRNA was the effector molecule that caused RNAi and not highly purified sense or antisense RNA in isolation, as had previously been thought (Fig. 15.1). In earlier studies, interference had been demonstrated with either antisense or sense RNA, but these preparations were relatively impure

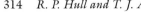

Fig. 15.1. RNA interference (RNAi) eliminates endogenous RNA transcripts and is mediated only by dsRNA. This figure, taken from Fire and Mello's 1998 *Nature* paper, has used *in situ* hybridization in *C. elegans* embryos following the injection into adult worms of antisense or dsRNA for the abundant transcript *mex-3* to demonstrate that RNAi is mediated by dsRNA and not antisense RNA and that it is able to eliminate endogenous RNA transcripts. a: Negative control showing lack of staining. b: Embryo from an uninjected parent worm demonstrating the normal abundance of *mex-3*. c: Embryo from a parent worm injected with antisense RNA to *mex-3* showing retention of *mex-3* transcripts though at a lower level than panel b. d: Embryo from a parent injected with dsRNA to *mex-3* demonstrating the complete elimination of endogenous *mex-3*. (Reprinted with permission from Macmillan Publishers Ltd: *Nature*, 391: 806–811, © 1998).

because the DNA transgene arrays or bacteriophage RNA polymerases used to generate the RNAs could also produce aberrant RNA products including, Fire and Mello believed, dsRNA molecules. The RNAi was highly specific, with only dsRNA sequences homologous to the target mRNA able to cause interference whilst dsRNA corresponding to introns or promoters did not. This finding suggested that RNAi was occurring at a post-transcriptional level; in addition, injection of dsRNA decreased or eliminated the endogenous mRNA transcripts suggesting they were degraded. RNAi could spread between tissues and be transmitted to progeny, suggesting the effect could be transmitted between cells as part of a potential RNA transport mechanism.

Fire and Mello rejected a simple antisense model to explain RNAi because they were able to achieve interference with only a few molecules of dsRNA per cell which was at least two orders of magnitude more effective than either sense or antisense RNA alone. They did not think that a simple antisense model could work because annealing between a few injected molecules of RNA and excess endogenous transcripts would not yield the observed phenotypes. Instead, they believed the findings were more in keeping with an active mechanism that involved a catalytic or amplification component. Another possibility was that the mechanism could be a non-specific response by cells to dsRNA and that the synergy they saw was due to potentiation of antisense effects by a 'panic mechanism'. However, Fire and Mello discounted this by showing that co-injection of unrelated dsRNA segments to the target gene did not potentiate the ability of single RNA strands to mediate inhibition. The actual mechanism underlying RNAi remained elusive at this time.

In their conclusions, Fire and Mello put their finding of RNAi into a wider context and accurately predicted the potential application of RNAi as a research tool. It was clear to them that RNAi had great potential as a genetic tool for studying gene function in *C. elegans* and could have an even wider application if the phenomenon was present in other nematodes, invertebrates and vertebrates. Fire and Mello believed that the mechanisms underlying RNAi must exist for some biological purpose and hypothesised that it could be used by organisms for physiological gene silencing. They also noted that their RNAi phenomenon may explain the other gene-silencing phenomena such as post-transcriptional gene silencing (PTGS) in plants.

15.4 Understanding the Mechanism Underlying RNAi

The discovery and description of RNAi opened up new avenues for research, and rapid progress was made in describing the mechanisms underlying RNAi and harnessing RNAi for biomedical research. Mello summed up this next period of exciting discovery aptly when he wrote that whilst 'some have likened this period to an RNA revolution...it is perhaps more apt to call it an RNA "revelation". RNA is not taking over the cell — it has been in control all along. We just didn't realize it until now.'[14]

Fire and Mello both followed up their *Nature* paper with further key insights into the phenomenon. Fire showed conclusively that the primary interference effects were post-transcriptional with no effect on initiation or elongation of transcription and, in addition, that RNAi reduced the accumulation of new transcripts in the nucleus, whilst almost eliminating all cytoplasmic accumulation of transcripts. These findings indicated that endogenous RNA was the target and the mechanism degraded target RNA prior to translation.[15] Mello observed that the RNAi effect was heritable and long-lived with potent interference lasting for several days after the initial injection of RNA in both the injected animal and its offspring.[16] Mello and Fire both found that the interfering RNA could be delivered by other methods such as feeding the worms *E. coli* engineered to express dsRNA or soaking them in a solution containing dsRNA. Whilst both were less potent than direct microinjection, the methods meant that larger scale genetic studies could be more easily performed.[17]

Fire believed that with these additional findings, the model could not be compatible with mechanisms that needed a stochiometric interaction between the injected RNA sequences and native transcripts. He discounted a replication-based mechanism where the dsRNA itself was amplified after its injection because they were unable to detect any replication of the injected dsRNA. Instead Fire proposed a three-step model to explain RNAi, which has marked similarities to the currently accepted mechanism of RNAi. Firstly, dsRNA would form part of a specialised ribonucleoprotein complex with partial unwinding of the duplex to allow homology-based target recognition. Following this there would be marking of the cellular RNA that had been recognised by cleavage or covalent modification, and then finally this target RNA would be degraded.[17] In his publications, Fire continued to comment on the similarities of RNAi with RNA-mediated silencing and co-suppression in plants, suggesting that dsRNA could act as a mediator in both phenomena. He proposed physiological roles for RNAi as a systemic defence against viruses and as a way for cells to modulate their gene expression and even suggested potential clinical applications for their discovery.[17, 18]

Mello also thought about RNAi in a wider context and was keen to understand how far evolution had gone in exploiting the phenomenon. He wondered whether there were RNA-based hormones that modulated gene expression in animals, whether cells fought infections by using RNAi to shut down viral genes and whether pathogens modified the host cell by capturing and overexpressing specific host gene segments. He suggested that RNAi indicated the existence of a powerful and specific avenue through which RNA from outside the cell can manipulate gene expression on the inside.[16]

Fire and Mello were not alone in investigating the RNAi phenomenon and their discovery prompted a flurry of follow-up publications. It soon became evident that RNAi was not unique to *C. elegans* and similar phenomena were reported in other organisms including *Drosophila*, *planaria* (flatworms), plants and *trypanosomes*. RNAi was found to share the same basic mechanisms as other silencing mechanisms such as post-transcriptional gene silencing and co-suppression, suggesting that they shared a common evolutionary origin. The next major breakthrough was made by Andrew Hamilton and David Baulcombe who had focused on the mechanisms underlying PTGS in plants. They identified that small RNAs, 25 nucleotides in length and homologous to the gene being suppressed, accumulated as part of the PTGS process and were likely to be the factor that determined its specificity.[19] These 21–25 nucleotide small RNAs were termed short interfering RNAs (siRNAs) and were shown to be the common factor that mediated interference in the RNA-silencing pathways of Drosophila[20] and *C. elegans*.[21] The enzyme Dicer, a member of the RNase III family of nucleases, was identified as the enzyme able to specifically cleave dsRNAs to produce these siRNAs and the enzyme was evolutionarily conserved in worms, flies, plants, fungi and mammals.[22] The RNA-induced silencing complex (RISC), an enzyme complex that degraded target mRNAs, had also been identified at this point during the investigations of the RNAi mechanism and was later shown to be an Argonaute protein.[23] The mechanisms behind RNAi were now becoming clearer and consisted of two major steps. The first step was the processing of a dsRNA by Dicer into a ~22 nucleotide-long siRNA. This guide siRNA was then incorporated into a nuclease complex, RISC, which could then target single-stranded mRNAs for degradation that were homologous to the guide siRNA (Fig. 15.2[24]).

The RNAi mechanisms were shown to have a physiological role in cells with the discovery that they were involved in the regulation of endogenous RNA species. As well as exogenous dsRNAs, Dicer can also process a class of native small RNAs, termed microRNAs (miRNAs).[25] microRNAs were identified first in *C. elegans* and linked with regulating their developmental timing and have also been identified in invertebrates and vertebrates.[26] A fellow RNase-III-type nuclease, Drosha, was also identified with a specific role for the processing of primary miRNAs into precursor miRNAs prior to their export into the cytoplasm for processing by Dicer.[27] The real potential of siRNA as a tool in research was also starting to be realised at this time. A significant advance was the demonstration that RNAi could be achieved with synthetic siRNAs.[20] This meant that the targeting step could be uncoupled from the dsRNA-processing step and showed that siRNA could be used as a tool for the specific regulation of gene expression in functional genomics and biomedical studies.[20] However, whilst these basic mechanisms underlying RNAi had been demonstrated in organisms such as *C. elegans* and *Drosophila*, it was still not clear whether RNAi functioned in mammalian cells, a major limitation for its wider application. The demonstration of RNAi in mouse embryos suggested that RNAi might exist in mammalian cells but it was still not certain whether this would be seen in somatic mammalian cells which had been shown to have non-specific defence responses to dsRNAs greater than 30 base pairs in length.[28] This significant breakthrough quickly came with the demonstration that RNAi could be achieved in cultured mammalian cells using 21-nucleotide siRNAs.[29] Both groups of authors noted that their findings opened the way for the use of siRNA as a tool for regulating gene expression and as a therapeutic modality in mammalian cells.[29]

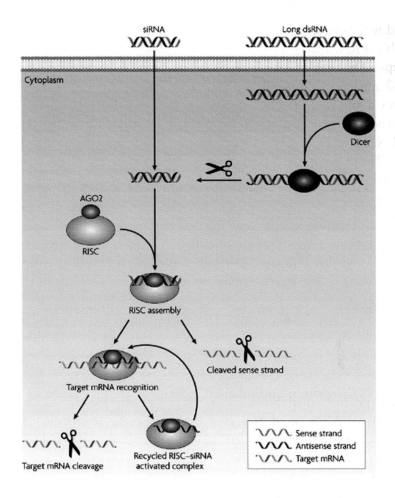

Fig. 15.2. The mechanism of RNA interference. Long double-stranded RNA (dsRNA) is introduced into the cytoplasm, where it is cleaved into small interfering RNA (siRNA) by the enzyme Dicer or, alternatively, siRNA can be introduced directly into the cell. The siRNA is then incorporated into the RNA-induced silencing complex (RISC) which results in the cleavage of the sense strand of RNA by argonaute 2 (AGO2). The activated RISC–siRNA complex seeks out, binds to and degrades complementary mRNA, which leads to the silencing of the target gene. The activated RISC–siRNA complex can then be recycled for the destruction of identical mRNA targets. (Figure and legend taken from Whitehead *et al.*, ref. 24. Reprinted with permission from Macmillan Publishers Ltd: *Nature Reviews Drug Discovery*, 391: 806–811, © 2009).

15.5 RNAi Functions in the Cell and Viral Infection

Over the last 12 years, an integral role for RNAi in regulating cellular functions has been demonstrated, as has been extensively reviewed elsewhere.[30] Its effects are, in the most part, inhibitory and its influence is widespread, affecting not only the post-transcriptional processing of transcripts but also chromatin structure, chromosome segregation, transcription, RNA processing, RNA stability and translation.[30] Advances are continuing to occur that are increasing our understanding of the many roles RNAi plays as well as the specific functions for the different small RNA species. miRNAs, for example, are key components of gene regulatory circuits, acting as adaptors for RISC to allow it to specifically recognise and silence particular mRNAs and are estimated to regulate as many as 50% of all mRNAs in vertebrates.[31] The RNAi machinery also plays a direct role in the formation and dynamic regulation of heterochromatin, a highly condensed form of chromatin. Heterochromatin acts as a base for the recruitment and spread of regulatory proteins that control numerous chromosomal processes including transcription, chromosome segregation and long range chromatin interactions in the yeast S. pombe, as well as C. elegans and mammals.[32] Indeed one view is that by its use of small RNAs as vectors to degrade transcripts and target heterochromatin to repetitive elements, the RNAi pathway has evolved over time to become an important defence mechanism for the genome.[30, 32]

RNAi is a major part of the antiviral response in plants and invertebrates and is thought to have first evolved as an innate immune response to viral infection.[33] In plants and invertebrates, RNAi is triggered by long dsRNAs which are key intermediates in the replication of RNA viruses except retroviruses. These long dsRNAs are cleaved by Dicer and the resulting siRNA is incorporated into the RISC and acts as a guide to target the complementary regions of the viral genomic or mRNA species. Viral RNAs are then cleaved by RISC leading to their degradation.[33] RNA viruses in turn have evolved gene products that inhibit RNAi in plants and invertebrates allowing them to survive and replicate. In contrast, in mammalian somatic cells these RNAi responses to viral infection are not seen and mammalian cells possess other innate responses to viral dsRNAs, including the interferon response.[33] This difference may have evolved to allow the RNAi machinery of mammalian cells to remain active during viral infection both to maintain normal cellular function but also to contribute to defence mechanisms. However, this absence of antiviral RNAi responses in mammalian cells does mean that viruses have the opportunity to harness the machinery and programme RISC with viral miRNAs. Such viral miRNAs have been shown to downregulate cellular or viral genes, to increase the sensitivity of virally infected cells to host innate or adaptive immune responses or stabilise viral latency as seen in herpes virus miRNAs, which downregulate the expression of viral immediate early proteins during an infection.[34]

15.6 The Impact of RNA Interference on Biomedical Research and Drug Discovery

RNAi has had a major impact on biomedical research primarily because it has enabled scientists to selectively knock down genes to understand their function in single gene studies, as well as allowing for larger genome-scale loss-of-function screens to identify candidate genes responsible for diseases or phenotypes.[35] RNAi was used to perform genome-scale screening in *C. elegans* within two years of its description by Fire and Mello.[36,37] The discovery that siRNAs could mediate RNAi in mammalian cells allowed for its even wider application.[29] RNAi-mediated knockdown has a number of advantages over classical genetic screens, particularly because the sequences of all identified genes are immediately known, lethal mutations are easier to identify and multiple genes with shared sequence can be knocked down, uncovering redundancy.[38] The scale of screens has rapidly increased with the production of arrayed libraries with chemically synthesised oligonucleotides covering thousands of genes. Such screening approaches have clear applications in drug discovery especially since the potential targets can range from oncogenes to growth factors to even single nucleotide polymorphisms.[39] It is therefore not surprising that it has become a method of choice for key steps in developing therapeutic agents, including target discovery, as well as for analysing the mechanisms of action of small molecules.[35]

15.7 The Potential for RNA Interference as a Novel Therapeutic Modality

The concept of RNA-based therapeutics comes directly from the work of Fire and Mello that described the phenomenon of RNA interference,[2] aided by the demonstration in mammalian cells by Sayda Elbashir et al.[29] that small interfering RNAs could trigger sequence specific gene inhibition. This means that a gene involved in human disease can be targeted specifically and be silenced by the exogenous introduction of siRNAs or constructs expressing short hairpin (sh)RNAs.[40] Such a specific gene-based approach means it has great potential for targeting disease-causing alleles within a tumour, for example, without targeting RNA from a wild type allele or by preventing the translation of a disease-causing protein.[40-42] RNAi may also have a role in treating infectious diseases through its targeting of pathogen-specific proteins, particularly those of viral origin, such as for respiratory syncytial virus infection and, more recently, as a post-exposure treatment for Ebola virus-induced haemorrhagic fever.[43, 44]

The translation of the RNAi discovery from its description as a novel mechanism underlying gene silencing in C. elegans to its emergence as a new therapeutic modality undergoing human clinical trials has been remarkably swift. As such, it is still in its early phases and the potential of RNAi to become a safe and effective therapeutic tool is only now starting to be realised, largely because a number of major challenges have had to be overcome. The key challenges have been to optimise the delivery of siRNA to the appropriate tissues and cells to achieve high potency with minimal off-target effects such as the triggering of unwanted immune responses.[40] The RNAi-based drugs that are currently in clinical trials are mostly synthetic siRNAs, which have the advantage of bypassing the Dicer cleavage step for entry into RISC, or expressed short hairpins.[40] miRNAs can also be targeted with complementary nucleotide sequences (anti-miRs) and these anti-miRs can block endogenous or exogenous (viral) miRNAs to neutralise their effects.

The delivery of the siRNA to the target tissue necessitates parenteral administration and continues to be a major hurdle for the successful application of RNAi as a therapeutic modality. A number of delivery vehicles are now being used, such as peptides recognised by cell-specific antibodies, as well as cationic lipids and cholesterol, all of which bring the exogenous siRNAs into the cell to allow their incorporation into endogenous RNAi machinery. Viral vectors can also be used to deliver the shRNA-based methods though shRNAs do have potential issues because virally delivered shRNAs can be expressed for long periods of time in the cell and can even saturate endogenous siRNA machinery, causing significant side effects.[40,45] Understanding and minimising off-target effects of the siRNA is an important part of the challenge to bring RNAi-based therapeutics to the clinic. For example, the promise from clinical trials that used direct injection of siRNA targeting vascular endothelial growth factor in macular degeneration was tempered by the finding that the effect was a siRNA class effect and not a specific interference effect. The siRNA did not actually enter the cells but acted by binding to extracellular Toll-like receptor 3 to activate immune pathways.[46] Whilst in this example the treatment was still safe, it does mean that unintended activation of the immune system could be a potential source of significant side effects, adding to the challenge of developing siRNA as a safe therapeutic modality.

The great potential of RNAi as a new therapeutic modality along with the results from preclinical trials for conditions such as macular degeneration and respiratory syncytial virus (RSV) infection[43] has resulted in early phase clinical trials (phase 1 and 2) using synthetic siRNAs for a wide range of diseases. These include age-related macular degeneration, RSV infection, asthma, hypercholesterolaemia, Pachyonycia congenita (also known as Jadassohn–Lewandowski Syndrome, an autosomal dominant dermatological condition due to mutations in genes encoding keratin proteins), solid tumours such as liver and lung cancer, metastatic melanoma, chronic myeloid leukaemia and acute kidney injury.[40, 47] shRNA is also being used to treat AIDS-related lymphoma and anti-miRNA is being used in a trial for hepatitis C.[24, 40] Although this rapid progress has been impressive it has not all been successful, with a number of development programmes being halted, such as one for wet age-related macular degeneration. By the end of 2010 there were still only two published trial reports, both of which were limited in that they enrolled only one patient each.[47] This is in contrast to the progress already achieved by antisense inhibition using oligonucleotides, where phase 3 studies in humans have been completed including the successful study in patients with homozygous familial hypercholesterolaemia of Mipomersen, an antisense oligonucleotide inhibitor of apoliprotein B synthesis.[48] Despite these challenges, the hope remains that RNAi can transform modern medicine and that an arsenal of effective and safe systemic RNAi therapies for a wide range of human diseases may be available within a few years.[49]

15.8 Conclusions

From the observation just 12 years ago that dsRNA mediated RNAi in *C. elegans*, we are now in a position where RNAi has redefined our understanding of how gene activity is regulated in our cells and has become an essential tool in biomedical research to manipulate gene expression. RNAi is helping to facilitate novel drug discovery and is

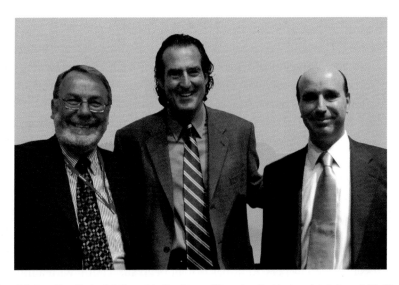

Fig. 15.3.   Dr Craig Mello with Professor Timothy J. Aitman (right) and Sir Peter Knight (left) following his lecture to Imperial College, London, on 21 April 2008 entitled, 'Return to the RNAi world: rethinking gene expression, evolution and medicine.'

even beginning to approach the clinic. It is the fundamental nature as well as the pace of scientific discovery and the far-reaching applications triggered by the Nobel Prize-winning discovery of RNAi by Fire and Mello that has made such an impact in changing medicine, and will continue to do so in the years to come.

It is the fate of Nobel Laureates to receive persistent requests for lectures to enlighten us on the route to their scientific discovery. Acceding to the request to lecture at Imperial College, London, in 2008 (Fig. 15.3), Craig Mello gave a comprehensive account of his perspective on the Nobel award for RNAi, including insightful comments about how the maturation of ideas, in this case between himself and his co-Laureate Andrew Fire, led to the key experiments permitting the leap in understanding that was judged worthy of a Nobel Prize.

Acknowledgements

We thank Matthias Merkenschlager, MRC Clinical Sciences Centre, for his helpful comments on this chapter.

References

1. The Nobel Prize in Physiology or Medicine 2006 — Presentation Speech. 2006; Available at: http://nobelprize.org/nobel_prizes/medicine/laureates/2006/presentation-speech.html. [Accessed 8 June 2011].

2. Fire A, Xu S, Montgomery MK *et al.* Potent and specific genetic interference by double-stranded RNA in Caenorhabditis elegans. *Nature* 1998; 391: 806–811.

3. Izant JG, Weintraub H. Inhibition of thymidine kinase gene expression by antisense RNA: a molecular approach to genetic analysis. *Cell* 1984; 36: 1007–1015.

4. Fire A, Albertson D, Harrison SW *et al.* Production of antisense RNA leads to effective and specific inhibition of gene expression in C. elegans muscle. *Development* 1991; 113: 503–514.

5. Kimble J, Hodgkin J, Smith T *et al.* Suppression of an amber mutation by microinjection of suppressor tRNA in C. elegans. *Nature* 1982; 299: 456–458.

6. Stinchcomb DT, Shaw JE, Carr SH *et al*. Extrachromosomal DNA transformation of Caenorhabditis elegans. *Mol Cell Biol* 1985; 5: 3484–3496.
7. Mello C, Fire A. DNA transformation. *Methods Cell Biol* 1995; 48: 451–482.
8. Mickey KM, Mello CC, Montgomery MK *et al*. An inductive interaction in 4-cell stage C. elegans embryos involves APX-1 expression in the signalling cell. *Development* 1996; 122: 1791–1798.
9. Guo S, Kemphues KJ. Par-1, a gene required for establishing polarity in C. elegans embryos, encodes a putative Ser/Thr kinase that is asymmetrically distributed. *Cell* 1995; 81: 611–620.
10. Rocheleau CE, Downs WD, Lin R *et al*. Wnt signaling and an APC-related gene specify endoderm in early C. elegans embryos. *Cell* 1997; 90: 707–716.
11. Seydoux G, Mello CC, Pettitt J *et al*. Repression of gene expression in the embryonic germ lineage of C. elegans. *Nature* 1996; 382: 713–716.
12. Montgomery MK. RNA interference: unraveling a mystery. *Nat Struct Mol Biol* 2006; 13: 1039–1041.
13. Fire A. *Les Prix Nobel. The Nobel Prizes 2006*. Stockholm: Nobel Foundation; 2007.
14. Mello CC, Conte D. Revealing the world of RNA interference. *Nature* 2004; 431: 338–342.
15. Montgomery MK, Fire A. Double-stranded RNA as a mediator in sequence-specific genetic silencing and co-suppression. *Trends Genet* 1998; 14: 255–258.
16. Tabara H, Grishok A, Mello CC. RNAi in C. elegans: soaking in the genome sequence. *Science* 1998; 282: 430–431.
17. Montgomery MK, Xu S, Fire A. RNA as a target of double-stranded RNA-mediated genetic interference in Caenorhabditis elegans. *Proc Natl Acad Sci USA* 1998; 95: 15502–15507.
18. Fire A. RNA-triggered gene silencing. *Trends Genet* 1999; 15: 358–363.
19. Hamilton AJ, Baulcombe DC. A species of small antisense RNA in post-transcriptional gene silencing in plants. *Science* 1999; 286: 950–952.

20. Elbashir SM, Lendeckel W, Tuschl T. RNA interference is mediated by 21- and 22-nucleotide RNAs. *Genes Dev* 2001; 15: 188–200.

21. Parrish S, Fire A. Distinct roles for RDE-1 and RDE-4 during RNA interference in Caenorhabditis elegans. *RNA* 2001; 7: 1397–1402.

22. Bernstein E, Caudy AA, Hammond SM *et al.* Role for a bidentate ribonuclease in the initiation step of RNA interference. *Nature* 2001; 409: 363–366.

23. Liu J, Carmell MA, Rivas FV *et al.* Argonaute2 is the catalytic engine of mammalian RNAi. *Science* 2004; 305: 1437–1441.

24. Whitehead KA, Langer R, Anderson DG. Knocking down barriers: advances in siRNA delivery. *Nat Rev Drug Discov* 2009; 8: 129–138.

25. Grishok A, Pasquinelli AE, Conte D *et al.* Genes and mechanisms related to RNA interference regulate expression of the small temporal RNAs that control C. elegans developmental timing. *Cell* 2001; 106: 23–34.

26. Lagos-Quintana M, Rauhut R, Lendeckel W *et al.* Identification of novel genes coding for small expressed RNAs. *Science* 2001; 294: 853–858.

27. Lee Y, Ahn C, Han J *et al.* The nuclear RNase III Drosha initiates microRNA processing. *Nature* 2003; 425: 415–419.

28. Wianny F, Zernicka-Goetz M. Specific interference with gene function by double-stranded RNA in early mouse development. *Nat Cell Biol* 2000; 2: 70–75.

29. Elbashir SM, Harborth J, Lendeckel W *et al.* Duplexes of 21-nucleotide RNAs mediate RNA interference in cultured mammalian cells. *Nature* 2001; 411: 494–498.

30. Carthew RW, Sontheimer EJ. Origins and mechanisms of miRNAs and siRNAs. *Cell* 2009; 136: 642–655.

31. Sharp PA. The Centrality of RNA. *Cell* 2009; 136: 577–580.

32. Grewal SIS, Jia S. Heterochromatin revisited. *Nat Rev Genet* 2007; 8: 35–46.

33. Cullen BR. Viral RNAs: lessons from the enemy. *Cell* 2009; 136: 592–597.

34. Gottwein E, Cullen BR. Viral and cellular microRNAs as determinants of viral pathogenesis and immunity. *Cell Host Microbe* 2008; 3: 375–387.

35. Echeverri CJ, Perrimon N. High-throughput RNAi screening in cultured cells: a user's guide. *Nat Rev Genet* 2006; 7: 373–384.

36. Fraser AG, Kamath RS, Zipperlen P *et al.* Functional genomic analysis of C. elegans chromosome I by systematic RNA interference. *Nature* 2000; 408: 325–330.
37. Gonczy P, Echeverri C, Oegema K *et al.* Functional genomic analysis of cell division in C. elegans using RNAi of genes on chromosome III. *Nature* 2000; 408: 331–336.
38. Boutros M, Ahringer J. The art and design of genetic screens: RNA interference. *Nat Rev Genet* 2008; 9: 554–566.
39. Hannon GJ, Rossi JJ. Unlocking the potential of the human genome with RNA interference. *Nature* 2004; 431: 371–378.
40. Tiemann K, Rossi JJ. RNAi-based therapeutics-current status, challenges and prospects. *EMBO Molecular Medicine* 2009; 1: 142–151.
41. Cooper TA, Wan L, Dreyfuss G. RNA and Disease. *Cell* 2009; 136: 777–793.
42. Stevenson M. Therapeutic potential of RNA interference. *N Engl J Med* 2004; 351: 1772–1777.
43. Bitko V, Musiyenko A, Shulyayeva O *et al.* Inhibition of respiratory viruses by nasally administered siRNA. *Nat Med* 2005; 11: 50–55.
44. Geisbert TW, Lee AC, Robbins M *et al.* Post-exposure protection of non-human primates against a lethal Ebola virus challenge with RNA interference: a proof-of-concept study. *Lancet* 2010; 375: 1896–1905.
45. Grimm D, Streetz KL, Jopling CL *et al.* Fatality in mice due to over-saturation of cellular microRNA/short hairpin RNA pathways. *Nature* 2006; 441: 537–541.
46. Kleinman ME, Yamada K, Takeda A *et al.* Sequence- and target-independent angiogenesis suppression by siRNA via TLR3. *Nature* 2008; 452: 591–597.
47. Vaishnaw A, Gollob J, Gamba-Vitalo C *et al.* A status report on RNAi therapeutics. *Silence* 2010; 1: 14.
48. Raal FJ, Santos RD, Blom DJ *et al.* Mipomersen, an apolipoprotein B synthesis inhibitor, for lowering of LDL cholesterol concentrations in patients with homozygous familial hypercholesterolaemia: a randomised, double-blind, placebo-controlled trial. *Lancet* 2010; 375: 998–1006.
49. Grimm D, Kay MA. Therapeutic application of RNAi: is mRNA targeting finally ready for prime time? *J Clin Invest* 2007; 117: 3633–3641.

APPENDIX: THE FIRST 100 NOBEL PRIZES IN PHYSIOLOGY OR MEDICINE

Year	Names	Topic	Nationalities
1901	von Behring	Diphtheria	Germany
1902	Ross	Malaria	UK
1903	Finsen	Lupus	Denmark
1904	Pavlov	Digestion	Russia
1905	Koch	TB	Germany
1906	Golgi, Cajal	CNS	Italy, Spain
1907	Laveran	Protozoa	France
1908	Mechnikov, Ehrlich	Immunity	Russia, Germany
1909	Kocher	Thyroid	Switzerland
1910	Kossel	Cell chemistry	Germany
1911	Gullstrand	Ocular function	Switzerland
1912	Carrel	Transplantation	USA
1913	Richet	Anaphylaxis	France
1914	Barany	Vestibular function	Austria
1919	Bordet	Immunity	Belgium
1920	Krogh	Capillary regulation	Denmark
1922	Hill, Meyerhof	Muscle metabolism	UK, Germany
1923	Banting, McLeod	Insulin	Canada, Canada
1924	Einthoven	ECG	Netherlands
1926	Fibiger	Carcinogenesis	Denmark
1927	Wagner-Jauregg	Malarial Rx for GPI	Austria
1928	Nicolle	Louse transmission of typhus	France
1929	Eijman, Hopkins	Vitamins	Netherlands, UK
1930	Landsteiner	Blood groups	Austria
1931	Warburg	Respiration	Germany
1932	Sherrington, Adrian	Neurones	UK, UK
1933	Morgan	Chromosomes	USA
1934	Whipple, Minot, Murphy	Vitamin B12	USA, USA, USA
1935	Spemann	Embryology	Germany
1936	Dale, Loewi	Nerve impulses	UK, Austria
1937	Szent-Gyorgyi	Vitamin C and muscle metabolism	Hungary

(*Continued*)

Year	Names	Topic	Nationalities
1938	Heymans	Chemoreceptors and Respiration	Belgium
1939	Domagk	Sulphonamides	Germany
1943	Dam, Doisy	Vitamin K	Denmark, USA
1944	Erlanger, Gasser	Nerve fibres	USA, USA
1945	Fleming, Chain, Florey	Penicillin	UK, UK, Australia
1946	Muller H	Mutagenesis	USA
1947	Cori, Cori, Houssay	Glucose metabolism	USA, USA, Argentina
1948	Muller P	DDT	Switzerland
1949	Hess, Moniz	CNS function, leucotomy	Switzerland, Portugal
1950	Kendall, Reichstein, Hench	Corticosteroids	USA, Switzerland, USA
1951	Theiler	Yellow fever vaccine	South Africa
1952	Waksman	Streptomycin	USA
1953	Krebs, Lipmann	Citric acid cycle, coenzyme A	UK, USA
1954	Enders, Weller, Robbins	Polio vaccine	USA, USA, USA
1955	Theorell	Oxidative enzymes, cytochrome C	Sweden
1956	Cournand, Forssmann, Richards	Cardiac catheterisation	USA, Germany, USA
1957	Bovet	Muscle relaxants	Italy
1958	Beadle, Tatum, Lederberg	Genes	USA, USA, USA
1959	Ochoa, Kornberg	RNA, DNA	USA, USA
1960	Burnet, Medawar	Immunity	Australia, UK
1961	von Bekesy	Cochlear function	USA
1962	Crick, Watson, Wilkins	Structure of DNA	UK, USA, UK/NZ
1963	Eccles, Hodgkin, Huxley	Neurology	Australia, UK, UK
1964	Bloch, Lynen	Cholesterol & FA metabolism	USA, Germany
1965	Jacob, Lwoff, Monod	Genes	France, France, France
1966	Rous, Huggins	Ca viruses, hormone Rx for Ca	USA, USA
1967	Granit, Hartline, Wald	Eyes	Switzerland, USA, USA
1968	Holley, Khorana, Nirenberg	Genetic code	USA, USA, USA
1969	Delbruck, Hershey, Luria	Viruses	USA, USA, USA
1970	Katz, von Euler, Axelrod	Neurotransmitters	UK, Switzerland, USA
1971	Sutherland	Hormone action, cyclic AMP	USA

(*Continued*)

Year	Names	Topic	Nationalities
1972	Edelman, Porter	Antibodies	USA, UK
1973	von Frisch, Lorenz, Tinbergen	Social behaviour	Germany, Austria, UK
1974	Claude, de Duve, Palade	Cell structure	Belgium, Belgium, USA
1975	Baltimore, Dulbecco, Temin	Viruses & genes	USA, USA, USA
1976	Blumberg, Gajdusek	Infectious disease	USA, USA
1977	Guillemin, Schally, Yalow	Neuropeptides	USA, USA, USA
1978	Arber, Nathans, Smith	Restriction enzymes, genes	Switzerland, USA, USA
1979	Cormack, Hounsfield	CAT scans	USA, UK
1980	Benacerraf, Dausset, Snell	Histocompatibility antigens	USA, France, USA
1981	Sperry, Hubel, Wiesel	Brain and ocular function	USA, USA, Sweden
1982	Bergstrom, Samuelsson, Vane	Prostaglandins	Sweden, Sweden, UK
1983	McClintock	Mobile genetic elements	USA
1984	Jerne, Kohler, Milstein	Monoclonal antibodies	Denmark, Germany, Argentina/UK
1985	Brown, Goldstein	Cholesterol metabolism	USA, USA
1986	Cohen, Levi-Montalcini	Growth factors	USA, Italy/USA
1987	Tonegawa	Genetic control of antibodies	Japan
1988	Black, Elion, Hitchings	Beta blockers, H2 antagonists	UK, USA, USA
1989	Bishop, Varmus	Retroviral oncogenes	USA, USA
1990	Murray, Thomas	Transplantation	USA, USA
1991	Neher, Sakmann	Ion channels	Germany, Germany
1992	Fischer, Krebs E	Phosphorylation	Switzerland/USA, USA
1993	Roberts, Sharp	Gene splicing	UK, USA
1994	Gilman, Rodbell	G-proteins	USA, USA
1995	Lewis, Nusslein-Volhard, Wieschaus	Embryology	USA, Germany, USA
1996	Doherty, Zinkernagel	Cell-mediated immune response	Australia, Switzerland
1997	Prusiner	Prions	USA
1998	Furchgott, Ignarro, Murad	Nitric oxide	USA, USA, USA
1999	Blobel	Cell signalling	USA
2000	Carlsson, Greengard, Kandel	CNS signalling	Sweden, USA, USA
2001	Hartwell, Hunt, Nurse	Control of cell cycling	USA, UK, UK

(Continued)

Year	Names	Topic	Nationalities
2002	Brenner, Horvitz, Sulston	Genetic regulation of organs/cells	UK, USA, UK
2003	Lauterbur, Mansfield	MRI	USA, UK
2004	Axel, Buck	Olfactory receptors	USA, USA
2005	Marshall, Warren	Helicobacter	Australia, Australia
2006	Fire, Mello	RNA interference	USA, USA
2007	Capecchi, Evans, Smithies	Gene targetting	USA, UK, UK
2008	zur Hausen, Barre-Sinoussi, Montagnier	HPV & HIV	Germany, France, France
2009	Blackburn, Greider, Szostak	Telomeres & telomerase	USA, USA, USA

Abbreviations used in Table

TB	Tuberculosis
CNS	Central Nervous System
ECG	Electrocardiograph
Rx	Treatment
GPI	General Paralysis of the Insane (tertiary syphilis)
DDT	Dichlorodiphenyltrichloroethane
RNA	Ribonucleic acid
DNA	Deoxyribonucleic acid
FA	Fatty acid
Ca	Cancer
AMP	Adenosine monophosphate
CAT	Computer-Assisted Tomography
G-proteins	Guanine nucleotide-binding proteins
MRI	Magnetic Resonance Imaging
HPV	Human Papillomavirus
HIV	Human Immunodeficiency Virus

Index